Studying a Study and Testing a Test

How to Read the Medical Evidence

Fifth Edition

Richard K. Riegelman, M.D., M.P.H., Ph.D.
*Professor of Epidemiology-Biostatistics, Medicine, and Health Policy
and Founding Dean
The George Washington University
School of Public Health and Health Services
Washington, D.C.*

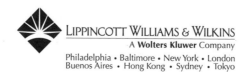

LIPPINCOTT WILLIAMS & WILKINS
A **Wolters Kluwer** Company

Philadelphia • Baltimore • New York • London
Buenos Aires • Hong Kong • Sydney • Tokyo

Acquisitions Editor: Danette Somers
Managing Editor: Michelle M. LaPlante
Project Manager: Bridgett Dougherty
Senior Manufacturing Manager: Ben Rivera
Marketing Manager: Kathy Neely
Cover Designer: MW Design
Design Coordinator: Holly Reid McLaughlin
Compositor: TechBooks
Printer: Edwards Brothers

© **2005 by Richard K. Riegelman**
Published by Lippincott Williams & Wilkins
530 Walnut Street
Philadelphia, PA 19106 USA
LWW.com

Printed in the USA

Library of Congress Cataloging-in-Publication Data
Riegelman, Richard K.
  Studying a study and testing a test : how to read the medical evidence /
Richard K. Riegelman.— 5th ed.
      p. ;   cm.
  Includes bibliographical references and index.
  ISBN-13: 978-0-7817-4576-5
  ISBN-10: 0-7817-4576-4
      1. Medical literature—Evaluation.   2. Medicine—Research—Evaluation.   I. Title.
    [DNLM: 1. Biometry.   2. Epidemiologic Methods.   3. Evidence-Based
Medicine—methods. WA 950 R554s 2005]
  R118.6.R54 2005
  610′.72—dc22
                                                                                2004020605

Contents

Section III. Rating a Rate

Section IV. Considering Costs and Evaluating Effectiveness

Section V. A Guide to the Guidelines

Section VI. Selecting a Statistic

Preface

Putting Progress Into Practice

The practice of medicine is changing at unprecedented speed. Today's reasonable assumption is outdated by tomorrow's evidence. A deluge of data faces us as we confront the onslaught of health research literature. How is the busy student, resident or practitioner to deal with this dilemma? Efficiently reading the research evidence is the key to successfully putting progress into practice.

The 5th edition of **Studying a Study and Testing a Test: How to Read the Medical Evidence** opens up the door to the practice of evidence-based medicine. For the first time, this new edition provides a unifying structure, the M.A.A.R.I.E. framework, for reading the full range of research articles encountered by students, residents and practitioners of medicine and public health. The M.A.A.R.I.E. framework is the key to the step-by-step questions-to-ask approach to efficiently reading the medical evidence.

The **Studying a Study Online** Web site is an integral part of the 5th edition. It can be found on the web at **www.StudyingaStudy.com**. This Web site provides practice using the M.A.A.R.I.E. framework, interactive flaw-catching exercises, the flowchart of statistics and examples of how to read real journal articles. The book and the Web site together are designed to be useful to the individual reader, residents' Journal Club, as well as students and faculty in a wide variety of clinical and public health disciplines.

Popular features from previous editions have been expanded in the 5th edition and updates added. A new section called A Guide to the Guidelines examines evidence-based recommendations for practitioners. New flaw-catching exercises appear throughout the book. The flowchart of statistics has been updated and more examples added.

The **Studying a Study and Testing a Test** approach to reading the health research literature aims to help students, residents, and practitioners practice evidence-based medicine built upon a strong foundation of research evidence. The aim is to help you efficiently review journal articles and feel confident in your ability to find the flaws that so often occur. It is important, however, to remember that every flaw is not fatal. The goal is to recognize the limitations of research and take them into account as you put the evidence into practice.

One final warning before you proceed. Reading the health research literature can be habit forming. You may even find it enjoyable.

Acknowledgements

The challenges associated with producing the 5th edition of Studying a Study and Testing a Test have been made easier by the support and encouragement I have received from students, colleagues, and of course the many readers of the previous editions from around the world.

This edition required writing a new section called A Guide to the Guidelines as well as extensively rewriting the Testing a Test and Rating a Rate sections. All of these benefited from feedback from students at the George Washington University School of Public Health and Health Services as well as the School of Medicine and Health Sciences.

The Studying a Study Online Web site is a joint project with my wife Linda. She has a unique ability to understand what technology can add to the learning process, an intuitive sense of how to make technology work, and the patience to explain it all to me. As the "content provider" I remain responsible for whatever goes wrong on the web but she deserves full credit for whatever goes right.

The staff of Lippincott Williams and Wilkins including their editors and web staff have been essential to moving this project to completion. The staff of TechBooks have made the editing of the 5th edition move very smoothly. I am especially grateful to Lyman Lyons, the copyeditor, who has helped ensure that every sentence makes sense and every word is carefully chosen.

Writing a 5th edition of a book is an especially enjoyable experience if it means that you get to build upon the past while looking to the future. This has been the case with the 5th edition of Studying a Study and Testing a Test. I hope you will enjoy reading it as much as I enjoyed writing it.

Richard Riegelman M.D., M.P.H., Ph.D.
Washington D.C. July 2004

1 Introduction and Flaw-Catching Exercise

The traditional course in reading the health literature consists of "Here's *The New England Journal of Medicine*. Read it!" This approach is analogous to learning to swim by the total immersion method. Some persons can learn to swim this way, of course, but a few drown, and many learn to fear the water.

In contrast to the method of total immersion, you are about to embark on a step-by-step, active-participation approach to reading the medical evidence. With the tools that you will learn, you will soon be able to read a journal article critically and efficiently. Considerable emphasis is placed on the errors that can occur in the various kinds of studies, but try to remember that not every flaw is fatal. The goal of literature reading is to recognize the limitations of a study and then put them into perspective. This is essential before putting the results into practice.

To make your job easier we use a common framework to organize our review of each of the types of investigations. Before developing and illustrating the components of the framework, however, let us begin with a flaw-catching exercise. A flaw-catching exercise is a simulated journal article containing an array of errors in each of the components of the framework. Read the following flaw-catching exercise and then try to answer the accompanying questions.

Cries Syndrome: Caused by Television or Just Bad Taste?

A medical condition known as Cries syndrome has been described as occurring among children 7 to 9 years old. The condition is characterized by episodes of uninterrupted crying lasting at least an hour per day for 3 consecutive days. The diagnosis also includes symptoms of sore throat, runny nose, and fever which precedes the onset of the crying and are severe enough to keep the child out of school.

Investigators identified 100 children with Cries syndrome. For each Cries syndrome child a classmate was chosen for comparison from among those who did not miss school. The study was conducted more than one month after the onset of symptoms. The investigators examined 20 variables, which included all the factors they could think of as being potentially associated with Cries syndrome. They collected data on all medication use, number of spankings, hours of television viewing, and number of hours at home, as well as 16 other variables.

Using pictures, they asked the children to identify the medications they had taken while they had Cries syndrome. Their classmates without Cries syndrome were also asked to use the pictures to identify medications taken during the same time period. The investigators then asked each child to classify each medication taken as a good-tasting or bad-tasting medication. The data on spankings were obtained from the primary caregiver. The investigators found the following data:

Percentage of children who reported taking bad-tasting medication
Cries syndrome: 90%
Controls: 10%

Average number of spankings per day
Cries syndrome: 1
Controls: 2

Average number of television viewing hours per day
Cries syndrome: 8 (range 5 to 12)
Controls: 2 (range 0 to 4)

Among the 20 variables, analyzed one at a time, the above were the only ones that were statistically significant using the usual statistical methods. The p values were 0.05 except for the hours of television, which had a P-value of 0.001. The investigators drew the following conclusions:

1. Bad-tasting medication is a contributory cause of Cries syndrome because it was strongly associated with Cries syndrome.
2. Spanking protects children from Cries syndrome because the controls had an increased frequency of being spanked.
3. Television viewing at least 4 hours per day is required for the development of Cries syndrome because all children with Cries syndrome and none of the controls watched television more than 4 hours per day during the period under investigation.
4. Because Cries syndrome patients were 9 times as likely to take bad-tasting medication, the investigators concluded that removing bad-tasting medication from the market would eliminate almost 90% of Cries syndrome cases among children like those in this investigation.
5. In addition, regular spanking of all children 7 to 9 years old should be widely used as a method of preventing Cries syndrome.

Now to get an idea of what you will be learning in the "Studying a Study" section, see if you can answer the following questions:

1. What type of investigation is this?
2. What is the study hypothesis?
3. Is the control group correctly assigned?
4. Are reporting and/or recall biases likely to be present in this study?
5. Does the method of data collection raise issues of precision and accuracy?
6. Is the estimate of the strength of the relationship performed correctly?
7. Is statistical significance testing performed correctly?
8. Is an adjustment procedure needed?
9. Is an association established between the use of bad-tasting medicine and Cries syndrome?
10. Is it established that the spankings occurred prior to the development of Cries syndrome?
11. Is it established that altering the frequency of spankings will alter the frequency of Cries syndrome?

12. Is it established that television viewing of at least 4 hours per day is a necessary cause of Cries syndrome?
13. Can the investigators conclude that removing bad-tasting medication from the market would reduce the frequency of Cries syndrome by almost 90% among children similar to those in the study?
14. Can the investigators conclude that regular spanking of all children 7 to 9 years old should be widely used as a method of preventing Cries syndrome?

To see how you have done, go to the *Studying a Study Online Web site at www.StudyingaStudy.com.*

This is a good time to locate and bookmark this Web site since it provides additional active participation exercises that will help you gain hands-on practice in using the skills that you will learn throughout this book.

Studying
a Study

I

2 Types of Studies and the M.A.A.R.I.E. Framework

Three basic types of investigations are found in the health research literature: *case-control studies, cohort studies,* and *randomized clinical trials.* Each type of investigation attempts to address a defined question or hypothesis by comparing one or more study groups with one or more control groups.[1]

An organizing framework can be used to evaluate each type of investigation. The framework is divided into six components:

- Method
- Assignment
- Assessment
- Results
- Interpretation
- Extrapolation

We call this the M.A.A.R.I.E. framework, an acronym using the first letter of each component: **M**ethod, **A**ssignment, **A**ssessment, **R**esults, **I**nterpretation, and **E**xtrapolation. Figure 2.1 outlines the application of the framework to a research study.

Method

Method issues are common to all types of health research. They require the investigators to clarify exactly what they are attempting to achieve by defining what they will investigate, who they will investigate, and how many they will investigate. Each of the six components in the M.A.A.R.I.E. framework can be divided into three specific issues. For method, the issues and key questions are as follows:

- **Study hypothesis:** What is the study question being investigated?
- **Study population:** What population is being investigated including the inclusion and exclusion criteria for the subjects in the investigation?
- **Sample size and statistical power:** How many individuals are included in the study and in the control groups? Are the numbers adequate to demonstrate statistical significance if the study hypothesis is true?

---

[1] The investigations discussed in this "Studying a Study" section are sometimes called *analytical studies.* Analytical studies compare study groups with control groups. However, investigations do not always have control groups. *Descriptive studies* obtain data on a group of individuals without comparing them to another group. Sometimes descriptive studies may use data external to the investigation to compare a group in the investigation with other groups or to the same group at an earlier period of time. These comparison groups are sometimes called *historical controls.* These types of investigations will be discussed in the "Rating a Rate" section later in this book. In special situations, descriptive studies may also be called *case-series, descriptive epidemiology studies,* or *natural history studies.* You will also encounter mixed types of studies such as *population-based case-control studies, nested case-control studies, and natural experiments.*

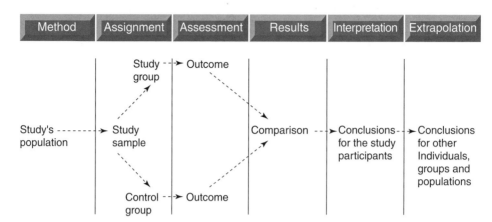

Figure 2.1. M.A.A.R.I.E. framework for studying a study.

Before investigators can decide which and how many individuals to include in an investigation, they need to define the study hypothesis. Then they can focus on the question of which individuals or population should be included in the investigation. Health research is not generally conducted by including everyone in the population of interest. Rather, health research is generally performed using only a subgroup, or *sample,* of all individuals who could in theory be included. For all types of health research, choosing whom to include and how many to include in an investigation are basic method issues. Thus, Method, the first component of the M.A.A.R.I.E. framework, defines the study question and sets the rules for obtaining the study and control samples. The M.A.A.R.I.E. framework continues with the following additional components:

Assignment: Selection of participants for study and control groups
Assessment: Measurement of outcomes or endpoint in the study and control groups
Results: Comparison of the outcome in the study and control groups
Interpretation: Meaning of the results for those included in the investigation
Extrapolation: Meaning for those not included in the investigation

To illustrate the application of the M.A.A.R.I.E. framework to case-control studies, cohort, and randomized clinical trials, let us outline the essential features of each type of study. We will then see how we can apply each type to the question of the potential risk of stroke with birth control pill use. The implications of the components of the M.A.A.R.I.E. framework differ slightly according to the type of investigation, as we discuss in this chapter.

We discuss each type of investigation by assuming that there is one study group and one control group. However, in all types of studies more than one study group and more than one control group can be included.

Applying the M.A.A.R.I.E. Framework

Case-Control Study

The unique feature of case-control studies of disease is that they begin by identifying individuals who have developed or failed to develop the disease being

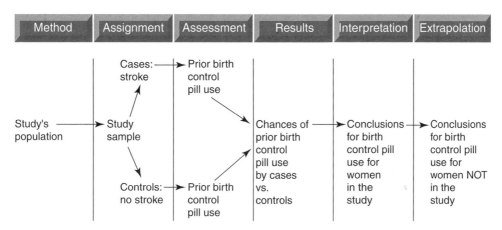

Figure 2.2. Application of the M.A.A.R.I.E. framework to a case-control study.

investigated. After identifying those with and without the disease, they look back in time to determine the characteristics of individuals before the onset of disease. In case-control studies, the *cases* are the individuals who have developed the disease, and the *controls* are the individuals who have not developed the disease. To use a case-control study to examine the relationship between birth control pill use and stroke, an investigator would proceed as follows:

Assignment: Select a study group of women who have had a stroke (cases) and a group of otherwise similar women who have not had a stroke (controls). Because the development of the disease has occurred without the investigator's intervention, this process is called *observed assignment*.

Assessment: Determine whether each woman in the case or study group and in the control group previously took birth control pills. The previous presence or absence of use of birth control pills is the outcome in a case-control study.

Results: Calculate the chances that the group of women with a stroke had used birth control pills versus the chances that the group of women without stroke had used birth control pills.

Interpretation: Draw conclusions about the meaning of birth control pill use for women included in the investigation

Extrapolation: Draw conclusions about the meaning of birth control pill use for categories of women not like those included in the investigation, such as women on newer low-dose birth control pills.

Figure 2.2 illustrates the application of the M.A.A.R.I.E. framework to this investigation.

Cohort Study

Cohort studies of disease differ from case-control studies in that they begin by identifying individuals for study and control groups before the investigator is aware of whether they have developed the disease. A *cohort* is a group of individuals who share a common experience. A cohort study begins by identifying a cohort that possesses the characteristics under study as well as a cohort that does not possess those characteristics. Then the frequency of developing the disease in each of the cohorts is obtained and compared. To use a cohort study to examine the relation-ship between birth control pill use and stroke, an investigator might proceed as follows:

Assignment: Select a study group of women who are using birth control pills and an otherwise similar control group of women who have never used birth control pills. Because the use of birth control pills is observed to occur without the investigator's intervention, this process is also called *observed assignment.*

Assessment: Determine who in the study group and the control group develops strokes. As opposed to a case-control study, the outcome for a cohort study is the subsequent presence or absence of a stroke.

Results: Calculate the chances of developing a stroke for women using birth control pills versus women not using birth control pills.

Interpretation: Draw conclusions about the meaning of birth control pill use for women included in the study.

Extrapolation: Draw conclusions about the meaning of birth control pill use for women not included in the study, such as women on newer low-dose birth control pills.

Figure 2.3 illustrates the application of the M.A.A.R.I.E. framework to a cohort study.

Randomized Clinical Trial

Randomized clinical trials are also called controlled clinical trials. As in cohort studies, individuals are assigned to study and control groups before determining who develops the disease. The unique feature of randomized clinical trials, how-ever, is the process for assigning individuals to study and control groups. In a randomized clinical trial, participants are randomized either to a study group or to a control group.

Randomization means that chance is used to assign a person to either the study or control group. This is done so that any one individual has a known, but not necessarily equal, probability of being assigned to the study group or the control

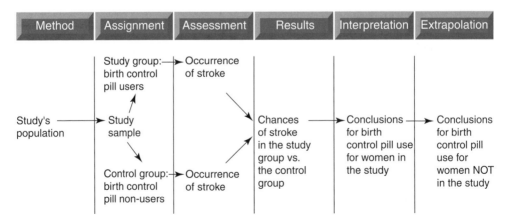

Figure 2.3. Application of the M.A.A.R.I.E. framework to a cohort study.

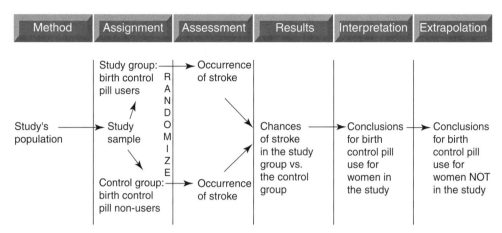

Figure 2.4. Application of the M.A.A.R.I.E. framework to a randomized clinical trial.

group. Ideally the study participants as well as the investigators are not aware of which participants are in which group. *Double-blind* assignment or masking means that neither the participant nor the investigators know whether the participant has been assigned to the study group or the control group.

To use a randomized clinical trial to examine the relationship between birth control pill use and stroke, an investigator might proceed as follows:

Assignment: Using randomization, women are assigned in a double-blind fashion to a study group that will be prescribed birth control pills or to a control group that will not be prescribed birth control pills.

Assessment: Observe these women to determine who subsequently develops stroke. As in a cohort study, in a randomized clinical trial the outcome is the presence or absence of stroke.

Results: Calculate the chances that women using birth control pills will develop a stroke versus women not using birth control pills.

Interpretation: Draw conclusions about the meaning of birth control pill use for women included in the study.

Extrapolation: Draw conclusions about the meaning of birth control pill use for women not included in the study, such as women on new low-dose birth control pills.

Figure 2.4 illustrates the application of the M.A.A.R.I.E. framework to a randomized trial.

Analysis of the Basic Study Types

The basic components and key questions we've outlined are common to the three basic types of investigations, the case-control, cohort, and randomized clinical trial. Each type, however, has its own strengths, weaknesses, and role to play in health research.

Case-control studies have the distinct advantage of being useful for studying rare conditions or diseases. If a condition is rare, case-control studies can detect differences between groups using far fewer individuals than other study designs. Often, much less time is needed to perform a case-control study because the disease has already developed. This method also allows investigators to simultaneously explore multiple characteristics or exposures that are potentially associated with a disease. One could examine, for instance, the many variables that are possibly associated with colon cancer, including diet, surgery, ulcerative colitis, polyps, alcohol, cigarettes, family history.

Case-control studies are often capable of showing that a potential "cause" and a disease or other outcome occur together more often than expected by chance alone. Thus case-control studies are useful as initial investigations designed to establish the existence of an association. Because case-control studies are able to examine rare diseases and rare outcomes, they can be used to investigate rare but serious side effects of treatment.

A special type of case-control study is called a *cross-sectional study*. A cross-sectional study, like a case-control study, starts with people with and without a condition. In a cross-sectional study the investigator determines whether each individual currently has the risk factor. That is, the condition and the risk factor are measured at the same point in time. Cross-sectional studies can be very useful to investigate conditions such as a genetic relationship, where we can be quite confident that a gene that is currently present was also present in the past.

The major objection to case-control studies is that they are prone to errors and biases that will be explained in the following chapters.

Cohort studies have the major advantage of demonstrating with greater assurance that a particular characteristic preceded a particular outcome being studied. As we will see, this is a critical distinction when assessing a cause-and-effect relationship. *Concurrent cohort studies or perspective cohort studies,* which follow patients forward over long periods of time, are expensive and time consuming. It is possible, however, to perform a cohort study without such a lengthy follow-up period. If reliable data on the presence or absence of the study characteristic are available from an earlier time, these data can be used to perform a *nonconcurrent cohort study,* often called a *retrospective cohort or database study*. In a nonconcurrent or retrospective cohort study, the assignment of individuals to groups is made on the basis of these past data. However, the groups are identified without the investigator being aware of the whether or not the participants developed the outcomes being assessed. After assignment has occurred, the investigator can then look at the data on disease occurrence.

For instance, if low-density lipoprotein (LDL) readings from a group of adults were available from 15 years before the current study began, those with and those without elevated LDL readings could be examined to assess the subsequent development of coronary artery disease, strokes, or other consequences of elevated LDL readings that might have occurred. The critical element, which characterizes all cohort studies, is the identification of individuals for study and control groups without knowledge of whether the disease or condition under investigation has developed.

Cohort studies can be used to delineate various consequences that may be produced by a single risk factor. For instance, researchers can simultaneously study the relationship between hypertension and stroke, myocardial infarction, heart failure, and renal disease. Cohort studies can produce more in-depth understanding of the effect of an etiologic factor on multiple outcomes.

Both case-control and cohort studies are *observational studies*; that is, they observe the assignment of individuals rather than impose the characteristics or interventions.

Randomized clinical trials are distinguished from observational studies by the randomization of individuals to study and control groups. Randomization helps to ensure that the study characteristic, and not some underlying predisposition, produces the study results. Randomized clinical trials are often used to study interventions that aim to prevent, cure, or palliate disease. They are capable of establishing whether an intervention has *efficacy,* that is whether it works under study conditions. When properly performed, randomized clinical trials are able to demonstrate all three definitive criteria for contributory cause or efficacy: association, prior association, and altering the cause alters the effect. The strengths and weaknesses of randomized clinical trials are explored in depth in chapter 9.

As we have seen, there are three key questions to ask pertaining to the method component of the M.A.A.R.I.E. framework. There are also three key questions to ask regarding each of the other components. These questions are briefly outlined in the following sections. These 15 questions along with the three questions from the method component make up the what we might call the Questions to Ask when Studying a Study. These questions form the basis for the M.A.A.R.I.E. framework and can serve as a checklist when reading journal articles. We will examine the questions in greater detail in the chapters that follow.

Assignment

The assignment component asks the following three questions about the characteristics of the study and control groups:

- **Process of Assignment:** What method is being used to identify and assign individuals to study and control groups, i.e., observed or randomization?
- **Confounding Variables:** Are there differences between the study and control groups, other than the characteristic under investigation, that may affect the outcome of the investigation?
- **Masking (or blinding):** Are the participants and/or the investigators aware of the participants' assignment to a particular study or control group?

Assessment

The process of assessment asks three basic questions about the quality of how the investigation's outcomes were measured:

- **Appropriate measurement:** Does the measurement of an outcome address the study question?
- **Accurate precise and measurement:** Is the measurement of an outcome an accurate and precise measure of the phenomenon that the investigation seeks to measure?
- **Complete and unaffected by observation:** Is the follow-up of participants nearly 100% complete and is it affected by the participants' or the investigators' knowledge of the study group or control group assignment?

Results

The results component quantitatively compares the measures of outcome obtained in the study group and in the control group. It requires us to ask the following three basic questions:

- **Estimation:** What is the magnitude or strength of the association or relationship observed in the investigation?
- **Inference:** What statistical techniques are used to perform statistical significance testing?
- **Adjustment:** What statistical techniques are used to take into account or control for differences between the study group and control group that may affect the results?

Interpretation

The interpretation component asks us to draw conclusions regarding the subjects in the investigation. Initially, it asks us to draw conclusions about cause-and-effect relationships, or what we will call *contributory cause* when we are talking about the etiology of a disease, or *efficacy* when we are asking whether an intervention works to improve outcome. We also ask whether the intervention produces harms and whether it works especially well or not well at all for *subgroups,* i.e., those with special characteristics. The three basic questions for interpretation are:

- **Contributory cause or efficacy:** Does the factor being investigated alter the probability that the disease will occur (contributing cause) or work to reduce the probability of an undesirable outcome (efficacy)?
- **Harms and interactions**: Are adverse effects or interactions that affect the meaning of the results identified?
- **Subgroups:** Are the outcomes observed in subgroups within the investigation different from the outcomes observed in the overall investigation?

Extrapolation

Extrapolation of health research studies asks how we can go beyond the data and the participants in a particular investigation to draw conclusions about individuals, groups, and populations that are not specifically included in the investigation. These groups may be your patients, your institution, or your community. These three key questions address extrapolation:

- **To similar individuals, groups, or populations:** Do the investigators extrapolate or extend the conclusions to individuals, groups, or populations that are similar to those who participated in the investigation?
- **Beyond the data:** Do the investigators extrapolate by extending the conditions beyond the dose, duration, or other characteristics of the investigation?
- **To other populations:** Do the investigators extrapolate to populations or settings that are quite different from those in the investigation?

The 6 components and 18 questions of the M.A.A.R.I.E. framework form the basis of the Studying a Study approach to reading the research literature. To see how this approach can be applied to reading actual journal articles please go to the *Studying a Study* Online Web site at www.StudyingaStudy.com.

Now let us take a more in-depth look at the M.A.A.R.I.E. framework by examining each of its 6 components and 18 questions.

3 Method

Investigations begin by identifying a study hypothesis as well as study and control samples to investigate a specific question in a defined population. Remember, the three key questions of method are:

- **Study hypothesis:** What is the study question being investigated?
- **Study population:** What population is being investigated and what are the inclusion and exclusion criteria for the subjects in the investigation?
- **Sample size and statistical power:** How many individuals are included in the study and in the control groups? Are the numbers adequate to demonstrate statistical significance if the study hypothesis is true?

Now let us examine these questions one at a time.

Study Hypothesis

The study's hypothesis, or study question, provides the starting point from which an investigation is organized. It defines the purpose of the investigation. Thus a study hypothesis is essential for all investigations that compare study and control groups. When reading the health research literature, therefore, the first question to ask is: What is the study hypothesis? Investigators should explicitly define a hypothesis. The hypothesis may be an association between a characteristic known as a *risk factor*[1] (e.g., birth control pills) and a disease (e.g., stroke), or between an intervention (e.g., reduction in blood pressure) and an improvement in outcome (e.g., reduced frequency of strokes).

It is often important to distinguish between what the investigators would ideally like to study and what they have in fact actually studied. Investigators may want to study the end-organ effects of hypertension, for example, but the inability to perform renal biopsies and cerebral angiograms may force them to carefully study retinal changes. Researchers may wish to investigate the long-term effects of a new drug to prevent osteoporosis, but time, money, and the desire to publish may limit their investigation to its short-term effects on bone metabolism and bone density.

To conduct an investigation, it is important to have a specific study hypothesis rather than a general relationship in mind. Consider the following example:

> An investigator wishes to study the relationship between hypertension and vascular damage. The investigator hypothesizes that the end-organ damage is associated with hypertension.

This hypothesis is not specific enough to study. A more specific one might be that an increased degree of narrowing of the retinal arteries, as measured on retinal

---

[1] The term "risk factor" will be used to imply only the existence of an association. A risk factor may also be referred to as a *risk marker*. At times the term risk factor is used in the literature to imply not only an association but a prior association—that is, the risk factor precedes the outcome in time. When this is the situation, the term *determinant* may be used.

photographs after 3 years of observation, will be associated with an increased level of diastolic blood pressure compared as measured by three blood pressure measurements at the beginning and at the end of the study. This provides a specific study question that can be addressed by an investigation.

Failure to clarify the hypothesis being tested makes it difficult for the researcher to choose the study design and the reader to assess its appropriateness. For instance, imagine the following situation:

> An investigator wishes to demonstrate that birth control pills are a contributory cause of strokes. The investigator conducts a case-control study using very careful methods. The results demonstrate a strong relationship between birth control pills and strokes. The investigator concludes that birth control pills are a contributory cause of stroke.

This investigator has failed to recognize that the use of a case-control study implies that the investigator is interested in demonstrating that birth control pills are associated with strokes rather than demonstrating that birth control pills are a contributory cause of strokes.

Study Population

The population being studied must be defined before beginning an investigation. This requires the investigators to define the characteristics of individuals who will be selected for the study group and control group. The study's populations may or may not represent the population of interest. The population of interest is called the *target population*. The target population is the large group of individuals to whom we wish to apply the results of the investigation. It is important to appreciate whether the study's population actually reflects the target population, as illustrated in the next example:

> A vaccine designed for high risk premature infants in intensive care units was investigated among healthy newborns. The healthy newborns were shown to have a strong antibody response to the vaccine and a high degree of clinical protection.

No matter how well designed this investigation, it's implications for high risk premature infants in the intensive care use will be limited. When the target population for an intervention, whether for prevention or cure, is known, it is important that the study's population reflect the target population.

In order to define the study population, investigators define what are called *inclusion criteria* and *exclusion criteria*. Inclusion criteria must be present for an individual to be eligible to participate in an investigation. Even if the inclusion criteria are met, presence of exclusion criteria means that the individual is not eligible for the investigation. Let us see why inclusion and exclusion criteria are needed by looking at the next example:

> An investigator wanted to study the effect of a new therapy for breast cancer. He selected all available breast cancer patients and found that the treatment, on average, resulted in no improvement in outcome. Later research revealed that the therapy provided a substantial improvement in outcome for women with Stage III breast cancer. The therapy, however, was shown to have no benefit if women with breast cancer had undergone previous radiation therapy.

If this investigation had been conducted by requiring Stage III breast cancer as inclusion criteria and previous radiation therapy as an exclusion criteria, the results would have been very different. Inclusion criteria serve to identify the types of individuals who should be included in the investigation. Exclusion criteria serve to remove individuals from eligibility because of special circumstances that may complicate their treatment or make interpretation more difficult.

Inclusion and exclusion criteria define the characteristics of those being studied. In addition, they narrow the group to which the results can be directly applied. For instance, if women diagnosed with Stage II breast cancer are not included in the study, it is not clear whether the results of the study apply to them.

Sample Size and Statistical Power

Having identified the study hypothesis and population, the reader of the health research literature should focus on the sample size of individuals selected for study and control groups. The question to ask is:

- Is there an adequate number of participants to demonstrate statistical significance if the study hypothesis is true?

The answer to this question is given by the *statistical power* of an investigation. Statistical power is the probability of demonstrating statistical significance if the study hypothesis is true. Research articles often identify the type II error rather than statistical power. *Type II error* is the complement of the statistical power. In other words, type II error is the probability of failing to demonstrate statistical significance if the study hypothesis is true.

Thus, if the type II error is 10%, the statistical power is 90%; if the type II error is 20%, the statistical power is 80%. Well-designed investigations should include enough individuals in the study and control groups to provide at least an 80% statistical power, or 80% probability of demonstrating statistical significance if the study hypothesis is true.

As we will see when we further discuss sample size in Chapter 9, statistical power depends on a series of assumptions. In addition, the number of individuals required to obtain the same statistical power is very different in case-control studies compared to cohort studies or randomized clinical trials. Failure to appreciate this distinction can lead to the following inconclusive cohort study:

> Investigators wished to study whether birth control pills are associated with the rare occurrence of strokes in young women. The researchers monitored 2,000 women on birth control pills and 2,000 women on other forms of birth control for 10 years. After spending millions of dollars in follow-up, they found two cases of stroke among the pill users and one case among the non–pill-users. The differences were not statistically significant.

In case-control studies of birth control pills and stroke, we are interested in determining whether the use of birth control pills is greater among those with stroke. Birth control pill use may be an overwhelmingly common characteristic of young women who have experienced a stroke. If so, the sample size required to conduct a case-control study may be quite small, perhaps 100 or less in each group.

On the other hand, when conducting a cohort study or randomized clinical trial, even if there is a very strong relationship between birth control pill use and stroke, it may be necessary to follow a large number of women who are taking and are not taking birth control pills to demonstrate a statistically significant relationship between birth control pills and strokes. When the occurrence of an outcome such as stroke is rare, say considerably less than 1%, many thousands of women may be required for the study and control groups in cohort and randomized clinical trials to provide an adequate statistical power to demonstrate statistical significance, even if the study hypothesis is true. In Chapter 9, we explore in more depth the implications of sample size.

Thus, the method component of the M.A.A.R.I.E. framework requires that we consider the study's hypothesis, the study's population being investigated, and the adequacy of the sample size. Equipped with an understanding of these key method questions, we are ready to turn our attention to the next component of our M.A.A.R.I.E. framework, assignment.

4 Assignment

The second component of the M.A.A.R.I.E. framework is assignment, the selection of participants for the study and control groups. Regardless of the type of investigation, there are three basic assignment issues:

- **Process:** What method is being used to assign participants to study and control groups?
- **Confounding variables:** Are there differences between the study and the control groups, other than the factor being investigated, that may affect the outcome of the investigation?
- **Masking:** Are the participants and/or the investigators aware of the participants' assignment to a particular study or control group?

Process

Case-control and cohort studies are both known as observational studies. In an observational study, no intervention is attempted, and thus no attempt is made to alter the course of a disease. The investigators observe the course of the disease among groups with and without the characteristics being studied.

In Chapter 2, we used the example of birth control pill use and strokes, and learned that the type of assignment performed in case-control and cohort studies is called observed assignment. This term implies that the researcher simply identifies individuals who meet the inclusion and exclusion criteria to become participants in an investigation.

The goal in creating study and control groups is to select participants for each of these groups who are as similar as possible, except for the presence or absence of the characteristic being investigated. Sometimes this goal is not achieved in a particular study because of a flawed method of observed assignment that creates what is called a *selection bias.*

Selection Bias

Few terms are less clearly understood or more loosely used than the word "bias." Bias is not the same as prejudice. It does not imply a prejudgment before the facts are known. Bias occurs when investigators unintentionally introduce factors into the investigation that influence the outcome of the study. Differences between the study and control groups result in a selection bias if these specific differences affect the outcome under investigation. The elements of selection bias are illustrated in the following hypothetical study:[1]

> A case-control study of premenopausal breast cancer compared the past use of birth control pills among 500 women who have breast cancer to the past use of the pill

---

[1] In reviewing this hypothetical case and others in this book, the reader should assume that all omitted portions of the study were properly performed.

among 500 age-matched women admitted to the hospital for hypertension or diabetes. Investigators found that 40% of the women with breast cancer had used birth control pills during the preceding five years, whereas only 5% of those with hypertension or diabetes in the control group had used the pill. The authors concluded that a strong association existed between the use of birth control pills and the development of premenopausal breast cancer.

To determine whether a selection bias may have existed when patients were assigned to the control group, we must first ask whether the women in the control group were similar to the women in the study group except that they did not have breast cancer. The answer is no. The women in the control group were quite different from the women in the study group because they had been admitted to the hospital for hypertension or diabetes. One must then ask whether this unique characteristic (hypertension or diabetes) was likely to have affected the results under investigation—that is, use of birth control pills.

The answer is yes. Because birth control pills are widely known to increase blood pressure and blood sugar, clinicians generally do not and should not prescribe birth control pills to women with hypertension or diabetes. Thus, the unique health characteristics of these women in the control group contributed to a lower use of birth control pills. This investigation's method of assignment, therefore, created a selection bias; the groups differed in a way that made a difference in outcome.

Selection bias can also occur in a cohort study, as illustrated in the following example:

> The effect of cigarette smoking on the development of myocardial infarctions was studied by selecting 10,000 middle-aged cigarette smokers and 10,000 middle-aged cigar smokers who have never smoked cigarettes. Both groups were observed for 10 years. The investigators found that the cigarette smokers had a rate of new myocardial infarction of 4 per 100 over 10 years, whereas the cigar smokers had a rate of new myocardial infarction of 7 per 100 over 10 years. The results were statistically significant. The investigators concluded that cigarette smokers have a lower risk of myocardial infarctions than cigar smokers.

Despite the statistical significance of this difference, the conclusion conflicts with the results of many other studies. Let us see if selection bias could have contributed to this.

The first question is whether the study and control groups differ. The answer is yes, because men constitute the vast majority of cigar smokers, whereas many more women smoke cigarettes than cigars. To establish the potential for a selection bias, we must also ask whether this difference could affect the outcome being measured. Again, the answer is yes. Middle-aged men have a higher risk of myocardial infarction. Thus, both elements of selection bias are present. The study and control groups differ with regard to a particular factor that could affect the outcome being measured.

Confounding Variables

Even when a study is properly designed so that selection bias is unlikely, *random error* due to chance alone may produce study and control groups that differ according to certain characteristics that might affect the results of the investigation. When these differences in characteristics affect outcome, we refer to them as *confounding variables*. Thus, a selection bias is a special type of confounding variable, which results from bias in the way the study group or control group subjects are selected. Remember, even in the absence of selection bias, differences in study group and control group characteristics can result by chance, i.e., random error. It is important to compare the study group and the control group subjects to determine whether they differ in ways that are likely to affect the outcome of the investigation even when there is no evidence of selection bias.

Most research articles include a table, usually the first table in the article, that identifies the characteristics that the investigators know about the study group and control group. This allows the researcher and the reader to compare the groups to determine whether large or important differences have been identified. These differences may be the result of bias or chance. In either situation, they need to be recognized and subsequently taken into account or adjusted for as part of the analysis of results.[2]

Matching and Pairing

One method for circumventing the problem of selection bias is to match individuals who are similar with respect to characteristics that might affect the study's results. For instance, if age is related to the probability of being a member of either the study group or the control group, and if age is also related to the outcome being measured, then the investigator may match for age. For instance, for every 65-year-old in the control group, investigators could choose one 65-year-old for the study group, and similarly with 30-year-olds, 40-year-olds, and so on. If properly performed, the process of matching guarantees that the distribution of ages in each group is the same.

Matching is not limited to making the groups uniform for age. It may be used for any characteristic related to the probability of experiencing the outcome under study. For example, if one were planning a cohort study addressing the relationship between birth control pills and breast cancer, family history of premenopausal breast cancer would be an important characteristic to consider for matching.

A disadvantage of matching groups is that the investigators cannot study the effect that the "matching characteristic" has on the outcome being measured. For instance, if they match for age and family history of premenopausal breast cancer, they lose the ability to study how age or family history affects the development of breast cancer. Furthermore, they lose the ability to study factors that are closely associated with the matched factor. This pitfall of matching is illustrated in the following example:

> One hundred patients with adult-onset diabetes were compared with 100 nondiabetic adults to study factors associated with adult-onset diabetes. The groups were matched to ensure a similar weight distribution in the two groups. The authors also found that the total calories consumed in each of the two groups was nearly identical, and concluded that the number of calories consumed was not related to the possibility of developing adult-onset diabetes.

[2] Note that the reader can evaluate only those characteristics the investigator identifies. Thus the reader should ask whether there are additional characteristics that would have been important to compare. The investigators can only adjust for difference that they identify. However, randomization, especially when the sample size is large, is capable of neutralizing differences the investigator does not recognize.

The authors of the study, having matched the patients by weight, then attempted to study the differences in calories consumed. Because there is a strong association between weight and calories consumed, it is not surprising that the authors found no difference in consumption of calories between the two groups matched for weight. This type of error is called *overmatching*.

The type of matching used in the diabetes example is called *group matching*. Group matching seeks an equal distribution of matched characteristics in each group. A second type of matching is known as *pairing* (a term used when one study group and one control group are included in an investigation). Pairing involves identifying one individual in the study group who can be compared with one individual in the control group. Pairing of individuals using one or a small number of characteristics can be a very effective way to avoid selection bias.

Pairing is a useful technique for preventing selection bias, but it needs to be used cautiously. While it may in theory be desirable to use a large number of characteristics, this may make identification of a control individual to pair with a study individual much more difficult, as illustrated in the next example:

> A case-control study was conducted of the relationship between lung cancer and exposure to a drug. The investigators attempted to pair the cases with controls matched for pack-year of cigarette smoking and exposure to environmental factors such as radon, age, and gender—all factors that were believed to be related to the chances of developing lung cancer. Unfortunately, the investigators were not able to complete the investigation because they could not identify controls that fulfilled these criteria.

Thus, for practical reasons it is important to limit matching to very important characteristics that will not prevent identification of subjects to use as controls.

This problem can sometimes be circumvented by using a study subject as his or her own control in what is called a *cross-over study*. In a cross-over study the same individuals are compared with themselves, for instance, while on and off medication. When properly performed, cross-over studies allow an investigator to use the same individuals in the study group and control group, and to then pair their results, thus keeping many factors constant.[3]

Cross-over studies must be used with great care, however, or they can produce misleading results, as the following hypothetical study illustrates:

> A study of the benefit of a new nonnarcotic medication for postoperative pain relief was performed by giving 100 patients the medication on postoperative day 1 and a placebo on day 2. For each patient, the degree of pain was measured using a well-established pain scale. The investigators found no difference between levels of pain on and off the medication.

When evaluating a cross-over study, one must recognize the potential for an effect of time and a carry-over effect of treatment. Pain is expected to decrease with time after surgery, so it is not accurate to compare the degree of pain on day 1 with the degree of pain on day 2.

Furthermore, one must be careful to assess whether there may be a carry-over effect in which the medication from day 1 continues to be active on day 2. Thus,

---

[3] All types of pairing allow the use of statistical significance tests, which increase the probability of demonstrating statistical significance for a particular size study group. Statistical significance tests used with pairing are called *matched tests*.

the absence of benefit in this cross-over trial should not imply that pain medication on day 1 after surgery is no more effective than a placebo on day 2.

Matching and pairing are two methods for preventing confounding variables that can be helpful techniques when properly used. It is important to recognize that they are not the only techniques available to address the issues of confounding variables. One can think of inclusion and exclusion criteria as another technique for ensuring that the study and control groups are similar. In addition, adjustment of data as part of the results component can be combined with matching or pairing to take into account the impact of confounding variables that are present.

Masking

Masking, or blinding, attempts to remove one source of bias by preventing each study participant and the investigators from knowing whether any one individual was assigned to a study group or to a control group.

The term *masking* is considered a more accurate reflection of the actual process and is currently considered the technically correct term, although the term *blinding* is still commonly used.

When masking is successful, we can be confident that knowledge of group assignment did not influence the outcomes that were measured. Masking of study subjects is a desirable technique that may be used in a randomized clinical trial. However, it is not usually feasible in either case-control or cohort investigations. In case-control studies, the patients have already experienced the outcome. In cohort investigations, the patients have already experienced the factors being investigated. Thus in both case-control and cohort investigations, it is important to consider whether the knowledge regarding the assignment influenced the measurement of the outcome. We will address this question of assessment in the next chapter.

5 Assessment

Assessment is the measurement of outcomes in the study group and in the control group. To understand the meaning of measuring outcomes, we need to remember that in case-control studies outcomes represent the presence or absence of previous characteristics or risk factors such as use of birth control pills or cigarette smoking. In cohort studies and randomized clinical trials, outcomes refer to the consequences of risk factors such as thrombophlebitis or lung cancer. Because the term "outcome" is sometimes thought of as meaning the consequences of risk factors, the term *endpoint* is also used to more clearly indicate the measurement being assessed in a case-control study as well as a cohort study or a randomized clinical trial. Thus the assessment process may be thought of as the process of measuring the outcome or endpoint in the study and control groups.

To assess the results of an investigation, researchers must define the outcome or endpoint they intend to measure. The measurement of the outcome or endpoint can be considered valid when it fulfills the following criteria:[1]

Appropriate: The measurement of the outcome addresses the study's question.
Accurate: On average, it has the same numerical value as the phenomenon being investigated. That is, it is free of systematic error or bias.
Precise: Produces nearly identical results when repeated under the same conditions. It has minimum variation as a result of the effects of chance. That is, there is minimum random error.

In addition, the implementation of the measurement should not introduce additional potential biases. The implementation should be as follows:

- **Complete:** The outcomes or endpoints of all participants have been measured.
- **Unaffected by the process:** Neither the participants' nor the investigators' knowledge of the study group or control group assignment affects the measurement of outcome. Also, the process of observation itself doesn't affect the outcome.

Let us look at the meaning and implications of each of these criteria

---

[1] The term "valid" unfortunately is used somewhat differently in different fields of investigation. The generic meaning of the term is that the measurement measures what it purports to measure. The concepts used here aims to incorporate the biological or social meaning of the term as well as the epidemiological and statistical concepts used in measurement. That is, "appropriate" implies that the measurement of outcomes measures a phenomenon that is closely correlated with the underlying biological or social phenomenon. "Accuracy and precision (or reproducibility)" correspond to the desired characteristics of statistical estimates and confidence intervals. "Complete and unaffected by the process of observation" indicates the absence of important systematic biases that may affect the accuracy and/or precision. Much of the confusion over the meaning of validity stems from different methods used to establish these criteria in different disciplines. Terms like internal, external, face, content, construct, and criterion validity may be thought of as reflecting different standards for judging whether these criteria are achieved.

Appropriate Measure of Outcome

To understand the importance of the appropriateness of a measure of outcome, let us first consider an example of how the use of an inappropriate measure of outcome can invalidate a study's conclusions.

> An investigator attempted to study whether users of brand A or brand B spermicide had a lower probability of developing tubal infections secondary to chlamydia. The investigator identified 100 women using each brand of spermicide, monitored these women, and performed annual cervical cultures for chlamydia for 5 years. The investigator found that women using brand A spermicide had $1^{1}/_{2}$ times as many positive cultures for chlamydia. The investigator concluded that brand B spermicide is associated with a lower rate of tubal infections.

Chlamydia cultures from the cervix do little to establish the presence or absence of tubal infection. The study may help to establish a higher frequency of chlamydia infection. However, if the intent is to study the relative frequency of tubal infection, the investigator has not chosen an appropriate outcome measurement. Investigators frequently are forced to measure an outcome that is not exactly the outcome they would like to measure. When this occurs, it is important to establish that the phenomenon being measured is appropriate to the question being investigated.

Increasingly, investigations seek to utilize outcomes that represent early evidence of the outcome of interest rather than wait until clear-cut or clinically important outcomes occur months or years later. For instance, when investigating coronary artery disease as an outcome, we'd rather detect the disease at the asymptomatic phase using testing rather than wait until there is clinical or ECG evidence of disease. Despite the desirability of using these early or *surrogate outcomes,* we need to be confident that these outcomes are closely related to the outcome of ultimate interest. As we will see in chapter 9 on randomized clinical trials, sometimes this is not so easy.

Accurate and Precise Measures of Outcome

Next, we look at what we mean by accurate and precise measures of outcome.[2] Precision is also referred to as *reliability* and as *reproducibility.* It is helpful to think of accuracy and precision as the two criteria for perfect performance. We can think of perfect performance as hitting the bull's-eye of a target on every shot. In order to be accurate on average, the bullet does not need to hit the bull's-eye every time. That is, it may be a little high one time and a little low the next time, but if these shots center around the bull's-eye, then the measurement is said to be accurate.

Precision, on the other hand, implies that the bullet always hits the same spot. Always in the same spot, however, may end up being on one side or other of the bull's-eye. Thus an ideal measurement is both accurate and precise. An accurate and precise measurement, by definition, hits the bull's-eye every time.

Measurement of outcome may lack either precision, accuracy, or both. When measurements lack precision and vary widely from measurement to measurement, we say they are not reproducible. Assuming this is due to chance, we call this

---

[2] Precision can also be viewed as narrow confidence intervals or the absence of substantial uncertainty.

random error. When a measurement is always off target in the same direction, we call this *systematic error* or *assessment bias.*

A large number of reasons for assessment bias have been identified. [3] It is helpful to think of these biases as the consequences of obtaining data from different types of sources of information. Thus, together they may be called *information biases.*

Information for measuring outcome may come from three basic sources:

1. The memory of study participants
2. The use of data from their previous records
3. Measurements by the study investigator

Information obtained from the memory of study individuals is subject to two special types of assessment bias—recall bias and reporting bias. *Recall bias* implies defects in memory, specifically defects in which one group is more likely to recall events than other groups. *Reporting bias* occurs when one group is more likely than the other to report what they remember. Consider the following example of how *recall bias* can occur:

> In a case-control study of the cause of spina bifida, 100 mothers of infants born with the disease and 100 mothers of infants born without the disease were studied. Among the mothers of spina bifida infants, 50% reported having had a sore throat during pregnancy versus 5% of the mothers whose infants did not develop spina bifida. The investigators concluded that they had shown an association between sore throats during pregnancy and spina bifida.

Before accepting the conclusions of the study, one must ask whether recall bias could explain its findings. One can argue that mothers who experienced the trauma of having an infant with spina bifida are likely to search their memory more intensively and to remember events not usually recalled by other women.

Thus, recall bias is more likely to occur when the subsequent events are traumatic, thereby causing subjectively remembered and frequently occuring events to be recalled that under normal circumstances would be forgotten. We cannot be certain that recall bias affected this case's outcome measurements, but the conditions are present in which recall bias occurs. Therefore, the result of this case-control study may be ascribed, at least in part, to recall bias. The presence of recall bias casts doubts on the alleged association between sore throats and the occurrence of spina bifida.

Reporting bias as well as recall bias may operate to impair the accuracy of the outcome measurement, as illustrated in the following example:

> A case-control study of the relationship between gonorrhea and multiple sexual partners was conducted. One hundred women who were newly diagnosed with gonorrhea were compared with 100 women in the same clinic who were found to be free of gonorrhea. The women who were diagnosed with gonorrhea were informed that the serious consequences of the disease could be prevented only by locating and treating their sexual partners. Both groups of women were asked about the number of sexual partners they had during the preceding 2 months. The group of women with gonorrhea reported an average of four times as many sexual partners as the group of

---

[3] The proliferation of names for biases that occur in specific setting can be avoided by using the structure of M.A.A.R.I.E. to divide bias into two types, bias in assignment and bias in assessment. Selection bias is the fundamental bias of assignment, and assessment bias is the fundamental bias in assessment. The specific types of bias discussed here, such as recall, reporting, and instrument, can be seen as specific types of assessment bias.

women without gonorrhea. The investigators concluded that on average women with gonorrhea have four times as many sexual partners as women without gonorrhea.

The women with gonorrhea in this study may have felt a greater obligation, hence less hesitation, to report their sexual partners than did the women without the disease. Reporting bias is more likely to occur when the information sought is personal or sensitive and one group is under greater pressure to report.

Thus, it is possible that women with gonorrhea may simply have been more thorough in reporting their sexual partners rather than actually having had more contacts. Reporting bias in addition to recall error may impair the accuracy of assessment in case-control studies because the participants in a case-control study are already aware of the occurrence or absence of the disease being studied.

When measurements are conducted or interpreted by the investigator, human factors can produce inaccuracies in measurement as a result of both assessment bias and chance. These errors can occur when two investigators perform the same measurements (*interobserver error*) or when the same individual performs the measurements more than once (*intraobserver error*).

Assessment bias may also occur as a result of inaccurate measurement by the testing instruments in all types of studies, as illustrated in the following example:

> The gastrointestinal side effects of two nonsteroidal antiinflammatory drugs for arthritis were assessed using an upper gastrointestinal (GI) X-ray. The investigator found no evidence that either drug was associated with gastritis.

The investigator did not recognize that an upper GI X-ray is a very poor instrument for measuring gastritis. Even if a drug caused gastritis, upper GI x-ray examination would not be adequate to identify its presence. Thus, any conclusion based on this measurement is likely to be inaccurate even if it reproducibly measures the wrong outcome.[4]

Whenever the measurement of outcome depends on subjective interpretation of data, the possibility of assessment bias exists. It is possible, however, to recognize and correct for this fundamental principle of human psychology. Human beings, including investigators, see what they want to see or expect to see. Correcting bias is accomplished by keeping the investigator, who makes the measurement of outcome, from knowing an individual's group assignment. Masked assessment can be used in case-control and cohort studies as well as in randomized clinical trials. Failure to use masked assessment can lead to the following type of bias:

> In a study of the use of nonsteroidal antiinflammatory drugs (NSAIDs), the investigators, who were the patients' attending physicians, questioned all patients to determine whether one of the NSAIDs was associated with more symptoms that could indicate gastritis. After questioning all patients about their symptoms, they determined that there was no difference in the occurrence of gastritis. They reported that the two drugs produced the same frequency of occurrence of gastritis symptoms.

In this study, the investigators making the assessment of outcome were aware of what the patients were receiving; thus, they were not masked. In addition, they were assessing the patients' subjective symptoms such as nausea, stomach pain, or indigestion in deciding whether gastritis was present. This is the setting in which masking is most critical. Even if the patients were unaware of which medication

---

[4] When gross instrument error occurs, as in this example, the measurement of outcome also can be considered inappropriate.

they were taking, the investigators' assessment may be biased. If the assessment conformed with their own hypothesis, their results are especially open to question. This does not imply fraud, only the natural tendency of human beings to see what they expect or want to see. The investigators' conclusions may be true, but their less-than-perfect techniques make it difficult or impossible to accept their conclusion.

Thus, masking in the process of assessment is important to eliminate this source of assessment bias.

Even in the absence of bias, chance can affect the outcome. Measurements of outcome may misclassify patients as having an outcome such as thrombophlebitis when they do not, or not having thrombophlebitis when they truly do. This type of misclassification when due to chance is known as *non-differential misclassification* or *classification error*. When a measurement is made which frequently misclassifies the outcomes, it is important to examine the consequences that occur, as illustrated in the next example:

> A cohort study tested for diabetes among those with and without a risk factor. The test used was known to have poor reproducibility. The investigators found that the association between the risk factor and the development of diabetes, while in the same direction as other investigations, was much weaker than expected.

The investigators may have diagnosed diabetes when it was not present or failed to diagnosis it when it was present. Assuming this applies to both the study group and the control group, we have an example of misclassification due to chance, or classification error. The consequences of classification error are to reduce the magnitude of the association below that which would be found in the absence of misclassification due to chance. Thus it is not surprising in this investigation that the association was in the same direction, but much weaker, than found in other studies.

Complete and Unaffected by the Process

Whenever follow-up of patients is incomplete, the possibility exists that those not included in the final assessment had a different frequency of the outcome than those included. The following example illustrates an error resulting from incomplete assessment:

> A cohort study of human immunodeficiency virus (HIV)-positive patients compared the natural history of the disease among asymptomatic patients with a CD4 count of 100 to 200 with a group of asymptomatic patients with a CD4 count of 200 to 400. The investigators were able to obtain follow-up with 50% of those with the lower CD4 counts and 60% of those with the higher CD4 counts. The investigators found no difference between the groups and concluded that the CD4 count is not a risk factor for developing acquired immunodeficiency syndrome (AIDS).

It can be argued that in this investigation, some of the patients who could not be followed-up were not available because they were dead. If this were the case, the results of the study might have been dramatically altered with complete follow-up. Incomplete follow-up can distort the conclusions of an investigation.

Follow-up does not necessarily mean that patients are actually examined or even that they have continued to be a part of an investigation. At times follow-up may be achieved by searching public records such as death certificates or by obtaining information from relatives or friends based on the participant's agreement to this type of follow-up when they entered the investigation. Using this meaning of follow-up, a high-quality investigation today should achieve nearly 100% follow-up.

Incomplete follow-up does not necessarily mean the patients were lost to follow-up as in the previous example. They may have been monitored with unequal intensity, as the next example illustrates:

> A cohort study of the side effects of birth control pills was conducted by comparing 1,000 young women taking the pill with 1,000 young women using other forms of birth control. Data were collected from the records of their private physicians over a 1-year period. Pill-users were scheduled for three follow-up visits during the year; non-pill-users were asked to return if they had problems. Among users of the pill, 75 women reported having headaches, 90 reported fatigue, and 60 reported depression. Among non-pill-users, 25 patients reported having headaches, 30 reported fatigue, and 20 reported depression. The average pill-user made three visits to her physician during the year versus one visit for the non-pill-user. The investigator concluded that use of the pill is associated with increased frequency of headaches, fatigue, and depression.

The problem of unequal intensity of observation of the two groups may have invalidated the results. The fact that pill-users, and not non-pill-users, were scheduled for visits to their physician may account for the more frequent recordings of headaches, fatigue, and depression. With more thorough observation, commonly occurring subjective symptoms are more likely to be recorded.

Even if a study's endpoint meets the difficult criteria of appropriate, accurate, precise, and complete assessment, one more area of concern exists. Investigators intend to measure events as they would have occurred had no one been watching. Unfortunately, the very process of conducting a study may involve the introduction of an observer into the events being measured. Thus, the reviewer must ask whether the process of observation altered the outcome, as illustrated in the following example:

> A cohort study was conducted of the relationship between obesity and menstrual regularity. One thousand obese women with menstrual irregularities who had joined a diet group were compared with 1,000 obese women with the same pattern of menstrual irregularities who were not enrolled in a diet group. The women were compared to evaluate the effects of weight loss on menstrual irregularities. Those in the diet group had exactly the same frequency of return to regular menstrual cycles as the nondiet group controls.

It is possible that the nondiet-group patients lost weight just like the diet-group patients because they were being observed as part of the study. Whenever it is possible for subjects to switch groups or alter their behavior, the effects of observation may affect an investigation. This is most likely to occur when the individuals in the control group are aware of the adverse consequences of their current behavior and feel pressured to change because they are being observed. This can occur only in a concurrent or prospective cohort study or in a randomized clinical trial, since these types of investigation are begun before any of the participants have developed the outcome.

We have now examined the criteria for a valid measurement of outcome—that is, the measurement should be appropriate, accurate, and precise, as well as complete and unaffected by the process of observation. We have examined the meaning of each of these criteria and have looked at problems that prevent a measurement from fulfilling these criteria. Now we are ready to use the fourth component of the M.A.A.R.I.E. framework, the results component, to compare the measurements obtained in the study group and in the control group.

6 Results

The fourth component of the M.A.A.R.I.E. framework is the results or analysis section. Like the previous components, results require us to address three key questions:

- **Estimation:** What is the magnitude or strength of the association or relationship observed in the investigation?
- **Inference:** What statistical techniques are used to perform statistical significance testing?
- **Adjustment:** What statistical techniques are used to take into account or control for difference between the study and control groups that may affect the results?

Estimation: Strength of Relationship

When measuring the strength of a relationship using data from samples, we are attempting to use that information to estimate the strength of the relationship within a larger group called a population. Thus, biostatisticians often refer to any measurement of the strength of a relationship as an *estimate* or *point estimate*. The data from the samples are said to estimate the population's *effect size,* which is the magnitude of the association or the difference in the larger population. First, we will look at the basic measure of the strength of an association that is most frequently used in cohort studies. Then we turn to the basic measure used in case-control studies. Let us assume that we are studying the association between birth control pills and thrombophlebitis. We want to measure the strength of the association to determine how the use of birth control pills affects the risk for thrombophlebitis. Therefore, we must first clarify the concept of *risk.*

When used quantitatively, risk implies the probability of developing a condition over a specified period of time. Risk equals the number of individuals who develop the condition divided by the total number of individuals who were possible candidates to develop the condition at the beginning of the period. In assessing the 10-year risk of developing thrombophlebitis, we would divide the number of women taking birth control pills who developed thrombophlebitis over a 10-year period by the total number of women in the study group who were taking birth control pills.

A further calculation is necessary to measure the relative degree of association between thrombophlebitis for women who are on birth control pills compared with women who are not on birth control pills. One such measure is known as *relative risk*. Relative risk is the probability of thrombophlebitis if birth control pills are used divided by the probability if birth control pills are not used. It is defined as follows:

$$\text{Relative risk} = \frac{\text{Probability of developing thrombophlebitis if birth control pills are used}}{\text{Probability of developing thrombophlebitis if birth control pills are not used}}$$

Generally,

$$\text{Relative risk} = \frac{\text{Probability of the outcome if the risk factor is present}}{\text{Probability of the outcome if the risk factor is absent}}$$

Let us illustrate how the risk and relative risk are calculated using a hypothetical example:

For 10 years, an investigator monitored 1,000 young women taking birth control pills and 1,000 young women who were nonusers. He found that 30 of the women on birth control pills developed thrombophlebitis over the 10-year period, whereas only 3 of the nonusers developed thrombophlebitis over the same time period. He presented his data using what is called a 2 × 2 table:

	Thrombophlebitis	No Thrombophlebitis	
Birth control pills	a = 30	b = 970	a + b = 1,000
No birth control pills	c = 3	d = 997	c + d = 1,000

The 10-year risk of developing thrombophlebitis on birth control pills equals the number of women on the pill who develop thrombophlebitis divided by the total number of women on the pill. Thus, the risk of developing thrombophlebitis for women on birth control pills is equal to:

$$\frac{a}{a+b} = \frac{30}{1,000} = 0.030$$

Likewise, the 10-year risk of developing thrombophlebitis for women not on the pill equals the number of women not on the pill who develop thrombophlebitis divided by the total number of women not on the pill. Thus, the risk of developing thrombophlebitis for women not on the pill is equal to:

$$\frac{c}{c+d} = \frac{3}{1,000} = 0.003$$

The relative risk equals the ratio of these two risks:

$$\text{Relative risk} = \frac{a/a+b}{c/c+d} = \frac{0.030}{0.003} = 10$$

A relative risk of 1 implies that the use of birth control pills does not increase the risk of thrombophlebitis. This relative risk of 10 implies that, on the average, women on the pill have a risk of thrombophlebitis 10 times that of women not on the pill.[1]

Now let us look at how we measure the strength of association for case-control studies by looking at a study of the association between birth control pills and thrombophlebitis.

An investigator selected 100 young women with thrombophlebitis and 100 young women without thrombophlebitis. She carefully obtained the history of prior use of birth control pills. She found that 90 of the 100 women with thrombophlebitis were

---

[1] Relative risks may also be presented with the group at lower risk in the numerator. These two forms of the relative risks are merely the reciprocal of each other. Thus, the risk of thrombophlebitis for those not taking birth control pills divided by the risk for those taking birth control pills would be 0.003/0.030 = 0.1 or 1/10.

using birth control pills compared with 45 of the women without thrombophlebitis. She presented her data using the following 2×2 table:

	Thrombophlebitis	No Thrombophlebitis
Birth control pills	a = 90	b = 45
No birth control pills	c = 10	d = 55
	a + c = 100	b + d = 100

Notice that in case-control studies the investigator can choose the total number of patients in each group (those with and without thrombophlebitis). She could have chosen to select 200 patients with thrombophlebitis and 100 patients without thrombophlebitis, or a number of other combinations.

Thus, the actual numbers in each vertical column, the cases and the controls, can be altered at will by the investigator. In other words, in a case-control study the number of individuals who have and do not have the disease does not necessarily reflect the actual frequency of those with and without the disease. Since the number of cases relative to the number of controls is determined by the investigator, it is improper to add the boxes in the case-control 2×2 table horizontally (as we did in the preceding cohort study) and calculate relative risk.

Thus we need to use a measurement that is not altered by the relative numbers in the study and control groups. This measurement is known as the *odds ratio.*

Odds ratios are often of similar magnitude as the relative risk. When this is the situation, it can be used as an approximation of relative risk. This is often the situation when the disease or condition under investigation occurs relatively infrequently.

To understand what we mean by an odds ratio, we first need to appreciate what we mean by odds, and how odds differs from risk. Risk is a probability in which the numerator contains the number of times the event, such as thrombophlebitis, occurs over a specified period of time. The denominator of a risk or probability contains the number of times the event could have occurred. Odds, like probability, contain the number of times the event occurred in the numerator. However, in the denominator odds contain only the number of times the event did not occur.

The difference between odds and probability may be appreciated by thinking of the chance of drawing an ace from a deck of 52 cards. The probability of drawing an ace is the number of times an ace can be drawn divided by the total number of cards, or 4 of 52, or 1 of 13. Odds, on the other hand, are the number of times an ace can be drawn divided by the number of times it cannot be drawn, or 4 to 48, or 1 to 12. Thus, the odds are slightly different from the probability, but when the event or the disease under study is rare, the odds are a good approximation of the probability.

The odds ratio is the odds of having the risk factor if the condition is present divided by the odds of having the risk factor if the condition is not present. The odds of being on the pill if thrombophlebitis is present are equal to:

$$\frac{a}{c} = \frac{90}{10} = 9$$

Likewise, the odds of being on the pill for women who do not develop thrombophlebitis are measured by dividing the number of women who do not have thrombophlebitis and are using the pill by the number of women who do not have thrombophlebitis and are not on the pill. Thus, the odds of being on the pill if thrombophlebitis is not present are equal to:

$$\frac{b}{d} = \frac{45}{55} = 0.82$$

Like the calculation of relative risk, one can develop a measure of the relative odds of being on the pill if thrombophlebitis is present versus being on the pill if thrombophlebitis is not present. This measure of the strength of association is the odds ratio. Thus,

$$\text{Odds ratio} = \frac{\text{Odds of being on the pill if thrombophlebitis is present}}{\text{Odds of being on the pill if thrombophlebitis is not present}}$$

$$= \frac{a/c}{b/d} = \frac{9}{0.82} = 11$$

An odds ratio of 1, parallel with our interpretation of relative risk, implies the odds are the same for being on the pill if thrombophlebitis is present and for being on the pill if thrombophlebitis is absent. Our odds ratio of 11 means that the odds of being on birth control pills are increased 11-fold for women with thrombophlebitis.

The odds ratio is the basic measure of the degree of association for case-control studies. It is a useful measurement of the strength of the association. In addition, as long as the disease (thrombophlebitis) is rare, the odds ratio is approximately equal to the relative risk.

It is possible to look at the odds ratio in reverse, as one would do in a cohort study, and come up with the same result. For instance,

$$\text{Odds ratio} = \frac{\text{Odds of developing thrombophlebitis if pill is used}}{\text{Odds of developing thrombophlebitis if pill is not used}}$$

The odds ratio then equals:

$$\frac{a/b}{c/d} = 11$$

Notice that this is actually the same formula for the odds ratio as the one shown previously, i.e., both can be expressed as ad divided by bc. This convenient property allows one to calculate an odds ratio from a cohort or randomized clinical trial instead of calculating the relative risk. This makes it easier to compare the results of a case-control study with those of a cohort study or randomized clinical trial.

Thus, relative risk and odds ratio are the fundamental measures we use to quantitate the strength of an association between a risk factor and a disease. A special type of odds ratio (or relative risk) is calculated when pairing is used to conduct an investigation. Remember, there are two basic approaches to dealing with potential confounding variables. Investigators can match as part of the assignment process, and they can adjust as part of the analysis. When the type of matching known as pairing is used to ensure identical distribution of potential confounding variables between study and control groups, a special type of odds ratio should be used to estimate the strength of the association.

As an example, let us suppose in a case-control study that each pair includes one case with thrombophlebitis and one control without thrombophlebitis. The odds ratio then compares the odds of using and not using birth control pills by comparing the half of the pair with thrombophlebitis to the half without thrombophlebitis.

Assume that a case-control study of birth control pills and thrombophlebitis was conducted using 100 pairs of patients with thrombophlebitis and controls without thrombophlebitis. The cases and controls were paired so that each member of the pair was the same age and parity (number of children). The results of a paired case-control study are presented using the following 2×2 table:[2]

	Controls using birth control pills	Controls not using birth control pills
Cases using birth control pills	30	50
Cases not using birth control pills	5	15

The odds ratio in a paired case-control study uses only the pairs in which the exposure (e.g., the use of birth control pills) is different between the case and control members of a pair. The pairs in which the cases with thrombophlebitis and the controls without thrombophlebitis differ in their use of birth control pills are known as *discordant pairs*.

The odds ratio is calculated using discordant pairs as follows:

$$\frac{\text{Number of pairs with cases using birth control pills and controls not using birth control pills}}{\text{Number of pairs with controls using birth control pills and cases not using birth control pills}} = \frac{50}{5} = 10$$

This odds ratio is interpreted the same way as an odds ratio calculated from unpaired studies.[3] Pairing can also be used in cohort studies and randomized clinical trials.

Inference: Statistical Significance Testing or Hypothesis Testing

Most investigations are conducted on only a sample of a larger group of individuals who could have been included in the study. Researchers, therefore, are frequently confronted with the question of whether they would achieve similar results if the entire population was included in the study, or whether chance selection may have produced unusual results in their particular sample.

---

[2] The table for a paired case-control study tells us about what happens to a pair instead of what happens to each person. Thus, the frequencies in this paired 2×2 table add up to 100 (the number of pairs) instead of 200 (the number of persons in the study).

[3] Pairing, however, has an advantage of greater statistical power. Everything else being equal, statistical significance can be established using smaller numbers of study and control group patients. Also note that there is a special type of case-control study called a *population-based case-control study* in which the ratio of cases to controls reflects the ratio found in a larger population. In that special situation it is possible to calculate a relative risk from a case-control study.

Unfortunately, there is no direct method for answering this question. Instead, investigators are forced to test their study hypothesis using a circuitous method of proof by elimination. This method is known as *statistical significance testing* or *hypothesis testing.*

Statistical significance testing, in its most common form, quantitates the probability of obtaining the observed data (or a more extreme result supporting the study hypothesis) if no differences between groups exist in the larger population. Statistical significance testing assumes that individuals used in an investigation are representative or randomly selected from a larger group or population. This use of the term *random* is confusing because statistical significance testing is used in studies in which the individuals are not randomly selected. This apparent contradiction can be reconciled if one assumes that the larger population consists of all individuals with the same characteristics as those required for entry into the investigation. Thus, statistical significance tests actually address questions about larger populations made up of individuals just like those used in the investigation. Statistical significance testing aims to draw conclusions or inferences about a population by studying samples of that population. Therefore, biostatisticians often refer to statistical significance testing as *inference.*

Statistical Significance Testing Procedures

Statistical significance testing, which is also called hypothesis testing, assumes that only two types of relationships exist. Either differences between groups within the study population exist or they do not exist. When we conduct statistical significance tests on study data, we assume at the beginning that no such differences exist in the population. The role of statistical significance testing is to evaluate the results obtained from the samples to determine whether these results would be so unusual—if no difference exists in the larger population—that we can conclude that a difference does exist in the large population. Notice that the issue is whether or not a difference or association exists. Statistical significance testing itself says little or nothing about the size or importance of the potential difference or association.

Statistical significance testing begins with a *study hypothesis* stating that a difference exists in the larger population. In performing statistical significance tests, it is assumed initially that the study hypothesis is false, and a *null hypothesis* is formulated stating that no difference exists in the larger population. Statistical methods are then used to calculate the probability of obtaining the observed results in the study sample, or more extreme results, if no difference actually exists in the larger population.

When only a small probability exists that the observed results would occur in samples if the null hypothesis were true, then investigators can reject the null hypothesis. In rejecting the null hypothesis, the investigators accept, by elimination, the existence of their only other alternative—the existence of a difference between groups in the larger population. Biostatisticians often refer to the study hypothesis as the *alternative hypothesis* because it is the alternative to the null hypothesis.

The specific steps in statistical significance testing are as follows:

1. State study hypothesis
2. Formulate null hypothesis

3. Decide statistical significance cutoff level
4. Collect data
5. Apply statistical significance test
6. Reject or fail to reject the null hypothesis

STATE STUDY HYPOTHESIS

Before collecting the data, the investigators state in a study hypothesis that a difference exists between the study group and the control group in the larger population.

FORMULATE NULL HYPOTHESIS

The investigators then assume that no true difference exists between the study group and the control group in the larger population.

DECIDE STATISTICAL SIGNIFICANCE CUTOFF LEVEL

The investigators determine what level of probability will be considered small enough to reject the null hypothesis. In the vast majority of health research studies, a 5% chance or less of occurrence is considered unlikely enough to allow the investigators to reject the null hypothesis. However, we are generally left with some possibility that chance alone has produced an unusual set of data. Thus, a null hypothesis which is in fact true will be rejected in favor of the study hypothesis as much as 5% of the time.[4]

COLLECT DATA

The data may be collected using a study design such as case-control, cohort, or randomized clinical trial.

APPLY STATISTICAL SIGNIFICANCE TEST

If differences between the study and control groups exist, the investigators determine the probability that these differences would occur if no true difference exists in the larger population from which both the study and control group individuals in the samples have been selected. This probability is known as the *P*-value.

In other words, they calculate the probability that the observed data or more extreme data would occur if the null hypothesis of no difference were true. To do so, the investigators must choose from a variety of statistical significance tests. Because each type of test is appropriate to a specific type of data, investigators must take care to choose the proper test, as we discuss in Section VI, Selecting a Statistic.

To understand how a statistical significance test uses *P*-values, let's consider an example that uses small numbers to allow easy calculation.

---

[4] Investigators also need to decide whether to use a one-tailed or two-tailed statistical significance test. A *two-tailed* test implies that the investigator is willing to accept data that deviate in either direction from the null hypothesis. A *one-tailed* test implies that the investigator is only willing to accept data that deviate in the direction of the study hypothesis. We will assume a two-tailed test unless otherwise indicated.

Assume that an investigator wants to study the question: "Are there an equal number of males and females born in the United States?" The investigator first hypothesizes that more males than females are born in the United States; a null hypothesis that an equal number of males and females are born in the United States is then formulated. Then, the investigator decides the statistical significance cutoff level, which is usually set at 5%, or $P = 0.05$. Next, the investigator samples four birth certificates and finds that there are four males and zero females in the sample of births.

Let us now calculate the probability of obtaining four males and zero females if the null hypothesis of equal numbers of males and females is true:

Probability of one male	0.50 or 50%
Probability of two males in a row	0.25 or 25%
Probability of three males in a row	0.125 or 12.5%
Probability of four males in a row	0.0625 or 6.25%

Thus, there is a 6.25% chance of obtaining four males in a row even if an equal number of males and females are born in the United States.[5] Thus, the P-value equals 0.0625. All P-values tell us the same basic information. They tell us the probability of producing the observed data, assuming that the null hypothesis is true. Technically they are said to measure the probability of obtaining the observed data, or more extreme data, if no true difference between groups actually exist in the larger population.

REJECT OR FAIL TO REJECT THE NULL HYPOTHESIS

Having obtained a P-value, the investigators proceed to reject or fail to reject the null hypothesis. If the P-value is 0.05 or less, i.e., the probability of the results occurring by chance is less than or equal to 0.05, then the investigators can reject the null hypothesis.

In this situation the probability is small that chance alone could produce the differences in outcome if the null hypothesis is true. By elimination, the investigators can then accept the study hypothesis that a true difference exists in the outcome between study and control groups in the larger population.

What if the probability of occurrence by chance is greater than 0.05—that is, the P-value is greater than 0.05 as in the preceding example? The investigators then are unable to reject the null hypothesis. This does not mean that the null hypothesis, that no true difference exists in the larger population, is true. It merely indicates that the probability of obtaining the observed results is too great to reject the null hypothesis and thereby accept by elimination the study hypothesis. When the P-value is greater than 0.05, we say that the investigation has failed to reject the null hypothesis. The burden of proof, therefore, is on the investigators to show that the data obtained in the samples are very unlikely before rejecting the null hypothesis in favor of the study hypothesis. The following example shows how the significance testing procedure operates in practice.

[5] A one-tailed statistical significance test has been used. The births have been assumed to be independent of each other in calculating probabilities. To simplify the calculations, an example has been chosen in which no more extreme possibility exists.

An investigator wanted to test the hypothesis that there is a difference in the frequency of mouth cancer among those who chew tobacco and those who do not chew tobacco. She formulated a null hypothesis stating that mouth cancer occurs with no greater frequency among those who chew tobacco than among those who do not chew tobacco. She then decided that she would reject the null hypothesis if she obtained data that would occur only 5% or less of the time if the null hypothesis was true. She next collected data from a sample of the general population of those who chew tobacco and those who do not chew tobacco. Using the proper statistical significance test, she found that if no difference existed between those who chew tobacco and those who do not chew tobacco in the general population, then data as extreme or more extreme than her data would be observed by chance only 3% of the time—i.e., a P-value of 0.03. She concluded that because her data were quite unlikely to occur if there were no difference between the study group and the control group, she would reject the null hypothesis. The investigator thus accepted by elimination the study hypothesis that a difference in the frequency of mouth cancer exists between those who chew tobacco and those who do not chew tobacco.

When a statistically significant difference between groups is obtained, we say there is an *association* between the study group and the characteristic being studied. That is, there is an association between chewing tobacco and mouth cancer. By association we mean that the two occur together more frequently than is expected by chance alone. Remember that we have defined small as a 5% chance or less that the observed results would have occurred if no true difference exists in the larger population.

The 5% figure may be too large if important decisions depend on the results. The 5% figure is based on some convenient statistical properties; however, it is not a magic number. It is possible to define small as 1%, 0.1%, or any other probability. Remember, however, that no matter what level is chosen, there will always be some probability of rejecting the null hypothesis when no true difference exists in the larger population. Statistical significance tests can measure this probability, but they cannot eliminate it.

Table 6.1 reviews and summarizes the steps for performing a statistical significance test.

Table 6.1. *How a statistical significance test works*

State study hypothesis	Develop the study question: A difference exists between groups in a population.
Formulate null hypothesis	Reverse the hypothesis: No difference exists between groups in the population.
Decide statistical significance cutoff level	Equal to or less than 5% unless otherwise indicated and justified
Collect data	Collect data from samples of the larger population.
Apply statistical significance test	Determine the probability of obtaining the observed data or more extreme data if the null hypothesis were true (i.e., choose and apply the correct statistical significance test).
Reject or fail to reject the null hypothesis	Reject the null hypothesis and accept by elimination the study hypothesis if the statistical significance cutoff level is reached (P-value equal to or less than 0.05); fail to reject the null hypothesis if the observed data have more than a 5% probability of occurring by chance if there is no difference between groups in the larger population (P-value greater than 0.05).

Errors in Statistical Significance Testing

Several types of errors commonly occur in using statistical significance tests:

- Failure to state one hypothesis before conducting the study—the multiple comparison problem
- Failure to draw correct conclusions from the results of statistical significance tests by not considering the potential for a *Type I error*
- Failure to draw correct conclusions from the results of statistical significance tests by not considering the potential for a *Type II error*

Multiple Comparison Problem

The multiple comparison problem occurs when an investigator attempts to investigate multiple hypotheses in the same investigation or attempts to analyze the data without first creating a hypothesis.

The following example illustrates the consequences of failing to state the hypothesis before conducting the study:

> An investigator carefully selected 100 individuals known to have long-standing hypertension and 100 individuals of the same age known to be free of hypertension. He compared them using a list of 100 characteristics to determine how the two groups differed. Of the 100 characteristics studied, two were found to be statistically significant at the 0.05 level using standard statistical methods: (1) Hypertensives generally have more letters in their last name than nonhypertensives, and (2) hypertensives generally are born during the first 3 1/2 days of the week, whereas nonhypertensives are usually born during the last 3 1/2 days of the week. The author concluded that although these differences had not been foreseen, longer names and birth during the first half of the week are different between groups with and without hypertension.

This example illustrates the importance of stating the hypothesis beforehand. Whenever a large number of characteristics are used to make a large number of comparisons, it is likely by chance alone that some of them will be statistically significant. It can be misleading to apply the usual levels of statistical significance unless the hypothesis has been stated before collecting and analyzing the data. If differences are looked for without formulating one study hypothesis or only after collecting and analyzing the data, much stricter criteria should be applied than the usual 5% probability.

The multiple comparison problem can also occur when investigators analyze the data two or more times. When multiple hypotheses are being examined or the data is being analyzed multiple times, a suggested rule of thumb for the reader of the health literature is to divide the observed P-value by the number of hypotheses being tested for statistical significance or the number of times the data is analyzed. The resulting P-value can then be used to reject or fail to reject the null hypothesis. For instance, imagine that an investigation examined five hypotheses at the same time. To reach a P-value that would have the same meaning as $P = 0.05$ for one hypothesis, the P-value must be equal to 0.01. That is:

$$\frac{0.05}{\text{Number of comparison}} = \frac{0.05}{5} = 0.01$$

This *P*-value of 0.01 should be interpreted just like a *P*-value of 0.05 if one study hypothesis was stated before beginning the study.[6,7]

Type I Errors

Some errors are inherent in the method of statistical significance testing. A fundamental concept of statistical significance testing is the possibility that a null hypothesis will be falsely rejected and a study hypothesis will be falsely accepted by elimination. This is known as a Type I error.

In traditional statistical significance testing, there is as much as a 5% chance of incorrectly accepting by elimination a study hypothesis even when no true difference exists in the larger population from which the study samples were obtained. The level of Type I error that is built into the design of an investigation before it is conducted is known as the *alpha level*. Statistical significance testing does not eliminate uncertainty; it aims to measure the uncertainty that exists. Careful readers of studies are, therefore, able to appreciate the degree of doubt that exists and can decide for themselves whether they are willing to tolerate that degree of uncertainty.

Let us see how failure to appreciate the possibility of a Type I error can lead to misinterpreted study results.

> The author of a review article evaluated 20 well-conducted studies that examined the relationship between breastfeeding and breast cancer. Nineteen of the studies found no difference in the frequency of breast cancer between breastfeeding and formula-feeding. One study found a difference in which the breastfeeding group had an increase in breast cancer. The results of this one investigation were statistically significant at the 0.05 level. The author of the review article concluded that because the study suggested that breastfeeding is associated with an increased risk of breast cancer, breastfeeding should be discouraged.

When 20 well-conducted studies are performed to test a study hypothesis that is not true for the larger population, a substantial possibility exists that one of the studies may show an association at the 0.05 level simply by chance. Remember the meaning of statistical significance with a *P*-value of 0.05: It implies that the

---

[6] This method, called *Bonferroni's correction,* is a useful approximation for small numbers of variables. As the number of comparisons increases much above 5, the required *P*-value tends to be too small before statistical significance can be declared. This approach reduces the statistical power of a study to demonstrate statistical significance for any one variable. Thus, many biostatisticians argue it is better to use the multivariable method, which will be discussed in Section VI, Selecting a Statistic. Also note that when a hypothesis is indicated prior to collecting the data, most, if not all, of the variables used in the investigation are collected for purposes of adjustment for potential confounding variables. Thus when analyzing data in this situation, one is not dealing with multiple comparisons. Other methods are used to correct for multiple analyses of the data. The correction needed for multiple analyses is not as large as the correction needed for multiple hypotheses.

[7] Remember that statistical significance testing or hypothesis testing is a method of drawing inferences in a world in which we must decide between the study hypothesis and the null hypothesis based only on the data within the study. It is possible, however, to look at inference as a process that incorporates some probability that the hypothesis is true. In this process, the investigator must estimate this probability before the study begins. This might be done on the basis of the results of previous studies or other medical knowledge. When this prior probability is obtained, statistical methods are available to estimate the probability that the hypothesis is true after the results of the study are obtained. This *Bayesian process* is parallel to the use of diagnostic testing, which we discuss in Section II, Testing a Test. An advantage of the Bayesian approach is that *P*-values need not be adjusted to account for the number of variables.

results have a 5% probability, or a chance of 1 in 20, of occurring by chance alone when no difference exists in the larger population.

Thus, 1 study in 20 that shows a difference should not be regarded as evidence for a difference in the larger population. It is important to keep in mind the possibility that no difference may exist even when statistically significant results have been demonstrated. If the only study showing a relationship had been accepted without further questioning, breastfeeding might have been discouraged without considering its many benefits.

Type II Errors

A *Type II* error says that failure to reject the null hypothesis does not necessarily mean that no true difference exists in the larger population. Remember that statistical significance testing directly addresses only the null hypothesis. The process of statistical significance testing allows one to reject or fail to reject that null hypothesis. It does not allow one to prove a null hypothesis. Failure to reject a null hypothesis merely implies that the evidence is not strong enough to reject the assumption that no difference exists in the larger population.

A Type II error occurs when we are prevented from demonstrating a statistically significant difference even when a difference actually exists in the larger population. This happens when chance produces an unusual set of data that fails to show a difference, even though one actually exists in the larger population. Efforts to perform statistical significance testing always carry with them the possibility of error.

Investigators may make the problem far worse by using samples that are smaller than recommended based on careful study design. Thus, the chance of making a Type II error increases as the sample's size decreases.

Statistical techniques are available for estimating the probability that a study of a particular size could demonstrate a statistically significant difference if a difference of a specified size actually exists in the larger population. These techniques measure the *statistical power* of the study. The statistical power of a study is its probability of demonstrating statistical significance. Thus, statistical power equals one minus the Type II error. In many studies the probability is quite large that one will fail to show a statistically significant difference when a true difference actually exists. No arbitrary number indicates how great a Type II error one should tolerate. However, well-designed studies often aim for a Type II error between 10% and 20%. A Type II error of 10% is often the goal, with a 20% Type II error being the maximum tolerated consistent with good study design. Without actually stating it, investigators who use relatively small samples may be accepting a 30%, 40%, or even greater probability that they will fail to demonstrate a statistically significant difference when a true difference exists in the larger population. The size of the Type II error tolerated in the design of an investigation is known as the *beta level*. Table 6.2 summarizes and compares Type I and II errors.

The following example shows the effect of sample size on the ability to demonstrate statistically significant differences between groups:

> A study of the adverse effects of cigarettes on health was undertaken by monitoring 100 cigarette smokers and 100 similar nonsmokers for 20 years. During the 20 years, 5 smokers developed lung cancer, whereas none of the nonsmokers were afflicted. During the same time period, 10 smokers and 9 nonsmokers developed myocardial

Table 6.2. *Inherent errors of statistical significance testing*

	Type I Error	Type II Error
Definition	Rejection of null hypothesis when no true difference exists in the larger population	Failure to reject the null hypothesis when a true difference exists in the larger population
Source	Random error	Random error and/or sample size that is too small to allow adequate statistical power
Frequency of occurrence	Alpha level prior to conducting the investigation indicates the probability of a Type 1 error that will be tolerated. After results are obtained, the *P*-value indicates the probability of a Type I error.	Beta level prior to conducting the investigation indicates the probability of a Type II error that will be tolerated. If the sample size is small, the probability of a Type II error can be very large, i.e., 50% or greater.

infarction. The results for lung cancer were statistically significant, but the results for myocardial infarction were not. The authors concluded that a difference in lung cancer frequency between smokers and nonsmokers had been demonstrated, and a difference between smokers and nonsmokers for myocardial infarction had been refuted.

When true differences between groups are very large, as they are between smokers and nonsmokers in relation to lung cancer, only a relatively small sample may be required to demonstrate statistical significance. When there are true but smaller differences, it requires greater numbers to demonstrate a statistically significant difference.

This study would not refute a difference in the probabilities of myocardial infarction in cigarette smokers and nonsmokers. It is very likely that the number of individuals included were too few to give the study enough statistical power to demonstrate the statistical significance of a difference. A study with limited statistical power to demonstrate a difference also has limited power to refute a difference.

When the size of an investigation is very large, just the opposite issue may arise. It may be possible to demonstrate statistical significance even if the size or magnitude of the association is very small. Image the following results.

> Investigators monitored 100,000 middle-age men for 10 years to determine which factors were associated with coronary artery disease. They hypothesized beforehand that uric acid might be a factor in predicting the disease. The investigators found that men who developed coronary artery disease had a uric acid measure of 7.8 mg/dL, whereas men who did not develop the disease had an average uric acid measure of 7.7 mg/dL. The difference was statistically significant with a *P*-value of 0.05. The authors concluded that because a statistically significant difference had been found, the results would be clinically useful.

Because the difference in this investigation is statistically significant, it is most likely real in the larger population. However, it is so small that it probably is not clinically important. The large number of men being observed allowed investigators to obtain a statistically significant result for a very small difference between groups.

However, the small size of the difference makes it unlikely that uric acid measurements could be clinically useful in predicting who will develop coronary artery disease. The small difference does not help the clinician to differentiate those who will develop coronary artery disease from those who will not. In fact, when the test is performed in the clinical laboratory, this small difference is probably less than the size of the laboratory error in measuring uric acid.

In earlier chapters, we learned that statistical significance testing tells us very little about the size of a difference or the strength of an association; that is the role of estimation. Thus, it is important to ask not only whether a difference or association is statistically significant, but whether it is large or substantial enough to be clinically useful. The world is full of myriad differences between individuals and between groups. Many of these, however, are not great enough to allow us to usefully separate individuals into groups for purposes of disease prevention, diagnosis, and therapy.[8]

Confidence Intervals

Statistical significance testing does not directly provide us with information about the strength of an observed association. It is attractive to use a method that provides a summary measure (often called a *point estimate*) of the strength of an association and that also permits us to take chance into account using a statistical significance test.

The calculation of *confidence intervals* is such a method. Confidence intervals combine information from samples about the strength of an observed association with information about the effects of chance on the likelihood of obtaining the observed results. It is possible to calculate the confidence interval for any percentage confidence. However, the 95% confidence interval is the most commonly used. It allows us to be 95% confident that the larger population's difference or association lies within the confidence interval.

Confidence intervals are often calculated for odds ratios and relative risks. The calculation of these intervals can be complex. The reader of the literature, however, may see an expression for relative risk such as "10 (95% confidence interval, 8,12)" or sometime just "10 (8,12)," which expresses the observed relative risk (lower confidence limit, upper confidence limit) The term *confidence limit* is used to indicate the upper or lower extent of a confidence interval.

Imagine a study in which the relative risk for birth control pills and thrombophlebitis was 10 (8,12). How would you interpret this confidence interval? The 10 indicates the relative risk observed in the sample. The confidence interval around this relative risk allows us to say with 95% confidence that the relative risk in the larger population is between 8 and 12. Because the lower confidence limit is 8, far greater than 1, this allows us to be quite confident that a substantial relative risk is present not only in our sample, but in the larger population from which our sample was obtained.

These expressions of confidence limits, in addition to providing additional information on the size of the estimates of relative risks or odds ratios, have another advantage for the health literature reader: They allow us to rapidly draw conclusions

---

[8] It is sometimes necessary to distinguish between statistically significant, substantial, and clinically important differences. At times, statistically significant and large or substantial differences between groups are not useful for decision making. For example, we may decide medically or socially to treat individuals the same regardless of large differences in factors such as intelligence, height, or age.

about the statistical significance of the observed data. When using 95% confidence intervals, we can quickly conclude whether or not the observed data are statistically significant with a *P*-value less than or equal to 0.05.

This calculation is particularly straightforward for relative risk and odds ratio. For these, 1 represents the point at which the probabilities or odds of disease are the same, whether or not the risk factor or intervention is present. Thus, a relative risk or odds ratio of 1 is actually an expression of the null hypothesis, which says the probability or odds of disease are the same whether the risk factor is present or absent.

Thus, if the 95% confidence interval around the observed relative risk does not extend below 1, we can conclude that the relative risk is statistically significant with a *P*-value less than or equal to 0.05. The same principles are true for odds ratios. Let us look at a series of relative risks and 95% confidence intervals for studies on birth control pill and thrombophletitis:

A. 4 (0.9, 7.1)
B. 4 (2, 6)
C. 8 (1, 15)
D. 8 (6, 10)

The number to the left of the parenthesis is the relative risk, which is obtained from the data in the investigation. The numbers within the parentheses are the lower and upper limits of the 95% confidence interval. The 95% confidence limits on relative risk in B and D do not include 1. In C they include 1 but do not extend below 1.

Thus, B, C, and D are statistically significant with a *P*-value less than or equal to 0.05. Example A is not statistically significant because its lower confidence limit extends below 1.

When the observed relative risk (or odds ratio) is greater than 1 (e.g., 4 or 8), we need to look at the lower confidence limit to see whether it extends below 1.[9,10]

In example A, the 95% confidence interval for the relative risk extends below 1. This implies that it is possible that birth control pills actually reduce the risk and thus leaves us with enough uncertainty regarding birth control pills and thrombophlebitis that we cannot declare statistical significance. In examples B, C, and D, we can have 95% or more confidence that birth-control pills are associated with an increase in the probability of thrombophlebitis, and thus we can declare statistical significance.

As a reader of the literature, you will increasingly find the observed value and the confidence limits included in the results section. This is helpful because it

---

[9] For odds ratios, the formula for the confidence interval is the observed value plus or minus 1.96 times the square root of $(1/a+1/b+1/c+1/d)$, where a,b,c,d are the values in the 2×2 table.

[10] When the observed odds ratio is less than 1 (e.g., 0.8), we need to look at the upper 95% confidence limit to see whether it extends above 1. When the 95% confidence interval extends beyond 1 from either direction, the results are not statistically significant. By tradition, when the 95% confidence interval reaches, but does not extend beyond 1, the results are considered statistically significant. Thus, a *P*-value of .05 is considered statistically significant. Note that to avoid confusion, all the confidence intervals illustrated have been symmetrical around the observed value. Often confidence intervals are not symmetrical.

allows you to gain a "gestalt," or a feel, for the data. It allows you to draw your own conclusion about the importance of the size or strength of the point estimate. Finally, if you want to convert to the traditional statistical significance testing format for hypothesis testing, you can often make an approximate calculation to determine whether the results are statistically significant with a *P*-value of 0.05 or less.[11]

Thus confidence intervals can help us answer the first two questions of statistics: the estimation of the magnitude of the effect and inference or statistical significance.

Adjustment: Addressing the Effect of Confounding Variables

As we discussed in chapter 4, confounding variables can result from either random error or bias. Chance may produce random error. Unlike bias, the effect of chance is unpredictable. It may either favor or oppose the study hypothesis in a way that cannot be predicted beforehand.

Bias, on the other hand, implies a systematic effect on the data in one particular direction that predictably favors or opposes the study hypothesis. Bias results from the way the patients were assigned or assessed.

Bias and chance may each produce differences between study and control groups, resulting in study and control groups that differ in ways that can affect the outcome of the study.

In Chapter 4, we also noted that the investigator is obligated to compare the characteristics of individuals in the study group with those in the control group to determine whether they differ in known ways. If the groups differ, even without being statistically significant, the investigator must consider whether these differences could have affected the results. Characteristics that differ between groups and that may affect the results of the study are potential confounding variables. These potential confounding variables may result either from selection bias or from differences between the study and control groups produced by random error. If a potential confounding variable is detected, the investigator is obligated to consider this in the analysis of results using a process we call *adjustment of data.*[12]

In the most straightforward form of adjustment, known as *stratification,* the investigator may separate into groups those who possessed specific levels of the confounding variable. Members of the study group and the control group with the same level of confounding variable are then compared to see whether an association between exposure and disease exists. For instance, if gender is a potential confounding variable, the investigator might subdivide the study group and the control group into men and women, and then compare study group versus control

---

[11] Confidence intervals around differences can also be calculated. When comparing the confidence intervals between two groups, however, it is important to recognize that statistical significance is addressed by asking whether the confidence intervals of each group overlap the value in the other group. A common misconception holds that the confidence intervals themselves cannot overlap.

[12] Many biostatisticians encourage the use of adjustment, even when the differences are small or the importance of differences is not apparent. This has become common if not routine with the availability of sophisticated computer software. Also note that multiple variable methods allow for use of data that can include large numbers of potential categories rather than being restricted to data like gender or race that has two or a limited number of potential categories.

group men and study group versus control group women to determine whether differences exist when the groups of the same gender are compared. Statistical techniques known as *multivariable methods* are available for adjusting one or more variables at a time, as we discuss in Section VI, "Selecting a Statistic." Failure to recognize and adjust for a confounding variable can result in serious errors, as illustrated in the following example:

> An investigator studied the relationship between coffee consumption and lung cancer by monitoring 500 heavy coffee drinkers and 500 coffee abstainers for 10 years. In this cohort study, the risk for lung cancer in heavy coffee drinkers was 2 times that of coffee abstainers. The author concluded that coffee, along with cigarettes, was established as a risk factor in the development of lung cancer.

Coffee consumption may look like it is related to lung cancer but this apparent association is most likely the result of the fact that coffee drinking is associated with cigarette smoking. Assume that smoking cigarettes is not only a contributing cause of lung cancer but is associated with coffee consumption. Thus when we try to investigate the relationship between coffee consumption and lung cancer, cigarette smoking is a confounding variable. That is, cigarette smoking must be taken into account through the process known as adjustment.

Figure 6.1 depicts the relationship between coffee drinking, cigarette smoking, and lung cancer. In adjusting for cigarette smoking, the investigator could divide coffee drinkers into cigarette smokers and nonsmokers and do the same with the coffee abstainers. The investigator would then compare nonsmoking coffee drinkers with nonsmoking coffee abstainers to determine whether the relationship between coffee drinking and lung cancer still holds true. Only after determining that eliminating the impact of cigarette smoking does not eliminate the relationship between coffee drinking and lung cancer can the author conclude that coffee drinking is associated with the development of lung cancer.

The process of adjustment may be combined with the use of matching or pairing in an effort to prevent and take into account confounding variables. Much of the more sophisticated uses of statistical methods relates to effort to take into account confounding variables, as we will see in Section VI, "Selecting a Statistic." For

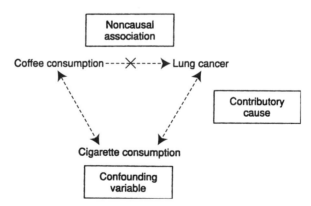

Figure 6.1. Relationship among contributory cause, confounding variable, and noncausal association.

now, we have learned that the key issues of analysis of results relate to estimating the magnitude of the effect, performing statistical significance testing, and taking into account confounding variables through the process known as adjustment. Now we are ready to use what we have learned in the results component of the M.A.A.R.I.E. framework to interpret the meaning of the results for those who participated in the investigation.

7 Interpretation

Interpretation asks us to address questions about the meaning of the investigation's results for those who have participated in the investigation. There are three types of questions that can be addressed by interpretation.

- Contributory cause or efficacy: Does the factor(s) being investigated alter the probability that the disease will occur (contributory cause) or work to reduce the probability of an undesirable outcome (efficacy)?
- Harms and Interactions: Are adverse effects or interaction that affect the meaning of the results identified?
- Subgroups: Are the outcomes observed in subgroups within the investigation different from those observed in the overall investigation?

Questions of contributory cause or efficacy are the first questions that are addressed by interpretation, and at times may be the only questions. Questions of adverse outcomes and questions about subgroups may only be important when there is evidence for contributory cause or efficacy. Therefore we will take a close look at the issues of contributory cause and efficacy and then outline key concepts for understanding adverse outcomes and subgroups.

Contributary Cause or Efficacy

In chapter 2, we introduced a definition of cause and effect termed *contributory cause*. This same definition is used to establish efficacy. To definitively establish the existence of a contributory cause or efficacy, all three of the following criteria must be fulfilled:

1. **Association:** Does the investigation establish a statistically significant association which provides convincing evidence that those with the "cause" also have an increased probability of experiencing the "effect"?
2. **Prior association:** Does the investigation establish that the "cause" precedes the "effect"?
3. **Altering the cause alters the effect:** Does the investigation establish that altering or modifying the frequency or severity of the "cause" alters the frequency or severity of the disease or other "effect"?

Association

Establishing the first criterion of contributory cause, association, requires that we examine the magnitude and the statistical significance of the relationship established in the analysis of results. To establish the existence of an association, we expect a statistically significant relationship.

Remember, statistical significance testing is designed to help us assess the role of chance when we observe a difference or an association in any of the forms of investigation that we have examined. Thus, the evidence provided in the results section is the basis for determining that an association exists between those with the factor and those with the outcome under investigation. This is what we mean by an association, or what is sometimes called an *association at the individual level*.[1]

Prior Association and Cause-Effect Link

To establish the second and third criteria, we must rely on more than statistical analysis. It may appear simple to establish that a cause precedes a disease, but let us look at two hypothetical studies in which the authors may have been fooled into believing that they had established cause preceding effect.

> Two investigators conducted a case-control study to determine whether antacids were taken by patients with myocardial infarction (MI) the week preceding an MI. They were looking for causes of the condition. MI patients were compared with patients admitted for elective surgery. The authors found that the MI patients were 10 times more likely to have taken antacids as the controls were during the week preceding admission. The authors concluded that taking antacids is associated with subsequent MIs.

The authors believed that they established not only the first criterion of causation (an association at the individual level) but also the second criterion (that the cause precedes the effect).

But did they? If individuals have angina before MIs, they may misinterpret the pain and try to alleviate it by self-medicating with antacids. Therefore, the medication is taken to treat the disease and does not truly precede the disease. This study failed to establish that the cause precedes the effect because it did not clarify whether the disease led the patients to take the medication or whether the medication precipitated the disease. This example illustrates what is called *reverse causality*. It illustrated the potential difficulty encountered in separating cause and effect in case-control studies. Case-control studies, however, may be capable of providing convincing evidence that the cause precedes the effect. This occurs when there is good documentation of previous characteristics that are not affected by knowledge of occurrence of the disease.

Cohort studies often have an advantage in establishing that the possible cause occurs before the effect. The following example, however, illustrates that even in cohort studies we may encounter reverse causality.

> A group of 1,000 patients who had stopped smoking cigarettes within the last year were compared with 1,000 current cigarette smokers matched for total pack-years of smoking. The two groups were monitored for 6 months to determine with what frequency they developed lung cancer. The study showed that 5% of the study group who had stopped smoking cigarettes were diagnosed with lung cancer as opposed to only 0.1% of the currently smoking controls. The authors concluded that stopping cigarette smoking was associated with the subsequent development of lung cancer. Therefore, they advised current smokers to continue smoking.

[1] Note that in the context of contributory cause and efficacy, association implies individual association. That is, those with the factor or risk factor under investigation are those with the increased or decreased probability of experiencing the outcome. As will be discussed in the Rating a Rate section, associations may exist at the group or population level that do not necessarily exist at the individual level.

The cessation of cigarette smoking appears to occur before the development of lung cancer, but what if smokers stop smoking because of symptoms produced by lung cancer? If this was true, then lung cancer stops smoking, and not vice versa. Thus, one must be careful in accepting that the hypothesized cause precedes the effect. The ability of cohort studies to establish that the cause precedes the effect is enhanced when the time lapse between cause and effect relative to the natural history of the disease is longer than in this example. Short time intervals still leave open the possibility that the presumed cause has been influenced by the presumed effect instead of the reverse.

Altering the Cause Alters the Effect

Even if one has firmly established that the possible cause precedes the effect, to completely fulfill the criteria for contributory cause, it is necessary to establish that altering the cause alters the probability of the effect.[2] This criterion can be established by performing an intervention study in which the investigator alters the cause and determines whether this subsequently contributes to altering the probability of the effect. Ideally, this criterion is fulfilled by performing a randomized clinical trial. Randomized clinical trials may not be ethical or practical thus we need to examine other ways to establish cause and effect.

When contributory cause cannot be definitively established using a randomized clinical trial, we may need to make our best judgments about the existence of a cause-and-effect relationship. For this situation a series of *ancillary, adjunct,* or *supportive criteria* for contributory cause have been developed. These include the following:

1. **Strength of association.** A strong association between the risk factor and the disease as measured, for example, by a large relative risk.
2. **Consistency of association.** Consistency is present when investigations performed in different settings on different types of patients produce similar results.
3. **Biological plausibility.** Biological plausibility implies that a known biological mechanism is capable of explaining the relationship between the cause and the effect. The biological plausibility of the relationship is evaluated on the basis of clinical or basic science principles and knowledge. For instance, hypertension is a biologically plausible contributory cause of strokes, coronary artery disease, and renal disease because the mechanism for damage is known and the type of damage is consistent with that mechanism. On the other hand, data

---

[2] It is important to recognize that contributory cause is an empirical definition. It does not require an understanding of the intermediate mechanism by which the contributory cause triggers the effect. Historically, numerous instances have occurred in which actions based on a demonstration of contributory cause reduced disease despite the absence of a scientific understanding of how the result actually occurred. Puerperal fever was controlled through hand washing before the bacterial agents were recognized. Malaria was controlled by swamp clearance before its mosquito transmission was recognized. Scurvy was prevented by citrus fruit before the British ever heard of vitamin C. Once we understand more about the direct mechanisms that produce disease, we are able to distinguish between indirect and direct contributory causes. What we call a direct cause of disease depends on the current state of knowledge and understanding of disease mechanism. Thus, over time, many direct causes may come to be regarded as indirect causes. In addition, it is important to distinguish these terms from the legal concept of proximal cause. *Proximal cause* refers to actions that could prevent a particular outcome and should not be confused with the definition of causation used here.

suggesting a relationship between hypertension and cancer would not be biologically plausible, at least on the basis of current knowledge.

Biological plausibility also implies that the timing and magnitude of the cause are compatible with the occurrence of the effect. For instance, we assume that severe, long-standing hypertension is more likely to be a contributory cause of congestive heart failure or renal disease than mild hypertension of short duration.

4. **A dose-response relationship.** A dose-response relationship implies that changes in levels of exposure to the risk factor are associated with changes in the frequency of disease in a consistent direction.

Data that support each of these four criteria help bolster the argument that a factor is actually a contributory cause. When these criteria are fulfilled, it reduces the likelihood that the observed association is due to chance or bias. The criteria, however, do not definitively establish the existence of a contributory cause.

None of these four criteria for contributory cause are essential. A risk factor with a modest but real association may in fact be one of a series of contributory causes for a disease. Consistency is not essential because it is possible for a risk factor to operate in one community but not in another. This may occur because of the existence in one community of other prerequisite conditions. Biological plausibility assumes that we understand the relevant biological processes. Finally, a dose-response relationship, although frequent in biological relationships, is not required for a cause-and-effect relationship. Even when it is present, it usually only exists over a limited range of values. For cigarettes and lung cancer, one or two cigarettes per day may not measurably increase the probability of lung cancer, and the difference between three and four packs per day may not be detectable. Dose response relationships may be confusing, as illustrated in the next example:

> An investigator conducted a cohort study of the association between radiation and thyroid cancer. He found that low-dose radiation had a relative risk of 5 of being associated with thyroid cancer. He found that at moderate levels of radiation, the relative risk was 10, but at high levels, the relative risk was 1. The investigator concluded that radiation could not cause thyroid cancer because no dose-response relationship of more cancer with more radiation was demonstrated.

The relative risk of 10 is an impressive association between radiation and thyroid cancer. This should not be dismissed merely because the relative risk is diminished at higher doses. It is possible that low-dose and moderate-dose radiation contributes to thyroid cancer, whereas large doses of radiation actually kill cells and thus do not contribute to thyroid cancer.

For many biological relationships, a little exposure may have little measurable effect. At higher doses, the effect may increase rapidly with increases in dose. At still higher doses, there may be little increase in effect. Thus, the presence of a dose-response relationship may depend on which part of the curve is being studied. When a relationship suggests that one specific agent produced one and only one specific outcome, the evidence for causation is also strengthened.

These ancillary, adjunct, or supportive criteria for judging contributory cause are just that: They do not in and of themselves settle the issue. If present, they may help support the argument for contributory cause. These criteria helps in understanding issues raised in a controversy and the limitations of the data.

Other Concepts of Causation

The concept of contributory cause has been very useful in studying disease causation. Contributory cause, however, is not the only concept of causation that has been used in clinical medicine. In the nineteenth century, Robert Koch developed a series of conditions that must be met before a microorganism can be considered the cause of a disease. The conditions, known as *Koch's postulates,*[3] include a requirement that the organism is always found with the disease. This condition is often called *necessary cause.*

Necessary cause goes beyond the requirements we have outlined for establishing contributory cause. Historically, this was very useful in the study of infectious disease when a single agent was responsible for a single disease. However, if the concept of necessary cause is applied to the study of chronic diseases, it is nearly impossible to prove a causal relationship. For instance, even though cigarettes have been well established as a contributory cause of lung cancer, cigarette smoking is not a necessary condition for developing lung cancer; not everyone with lung cancer has smoked cigarettes.

Under the rules of strict logic, causation also requires a second condition known as *sufficient cause.* This condition says that if the cause is present, the disease will also be present. In our cigarette and lung cancer example, sufficient cause would imply that if cigarette smoking is present, lung cancer will always follow.

Even in the area of infectious disease, cause and effect may not be straightforward; for instance, mononucleosis is a well-established clinical illness for which the Epstein-Barr virus has been shown to be a contributory cause. However, other viruses such as cytomegalovirus also have been shown to cause mononucleosis. In addition, evidence may show that Epstein-Barr has been present in a patient without ever causing mononucleosis, or it may manifest itself by being a contributory cause of other diseases, such as Burkitt's lymphoma. Thus, despite the fact that the Epstein-Barr virus has been established as a contributory cause of mononucleosis, it is neither a necessary nor a sufficient cause of this syndrome. If we require necessary and sufficient cause before concluding that a cause-and-effect relationship exists, we will be able to document very few, if any, cause-and-effect relationships in clinical medicine or public health. The next example illustrates the consequences of strictly applying necessary cause to health studies:

> In a study of the risk factors for coronary artery disease, investigators identified 100 individuals from a population of 10,000 MI patients who experienced MIs despite normal blood pressure, normal LDL and HDL cholesterol, regular exercise, no smoking, and no family history of coronary artery disease. The authors concluded that they had demonstrated hypertension, high LDH and low HDL cholesterol, lack of exercise, smoking, and family history were not the causes of coronary artery disease because not every MI patient possessed a risk factor.

The authors of this study were using the concept of necessary cause as a concept of causation. Instead of necessary cause, however, let us assume that all these factors

---

[3] Koch's postulates have been too strict for use in infectious disease causation as well. A modified version referred to by the National Institutes of Health as Modern Koch's Postulates require: (a) Epidemiological association: The suspected cause must be strongly associated with the disease; (b) Isolation: The suspected pathogen can be isolated and propagated outside the host; and (c) Transmission pathogenesis: Transfer of the suspected pathogen to an uninfected host, man or animal, produces the disease in that host. See www:niaid.nih.gov/factsheets/evidhiv.htm (May 20, 2004).

had been shown to fulfill the criteria for contributory cause of coronary artery disease. Contributory cause, unlike necessary cause, does not require that everyone who is free of the cause will be free of the effect. The failure of known contributory causes to be present in all cases of disease emphasizes the limitations of our current knowledge about all the contributory causes of coronary artery disease and encourages further investigations into additional risk factors. It illustrates the limitations of our current state of knowledge, since if all the contributory causes were known, then everyone with disease would possess at least one such factor.

Thus, even when a contributory cause has been established, it will not necessarily be present in each and every case.

In summary, contributory cause is a useful definition of causation. It requires a demonstration that: The cause and the effect occur together in an individual more often than expected by chance alone; the presumed cause precedes the effect; and altering the cause alters the effect in some individuals. It does not require that all people who are free of the contributory cause will be free of the effect. It does not require that all people who possess the contributory cause will develop the effect. In other words, a contributory cause may be neither necessary nor sufficient, but it must be contributory. Its presence must increase the probability of the occurrence of disease and its reduction must reduce the probability of the disease.[4]

Harms and Interactions

Complete interpretation of the results requires us to look beyond contributory cause or efficacy to examine not only the benefits of an intervention but also its potential harms. The approach used for judging the importance of potential harms is different from the approach used for potential benefits or efficacy. As we have seen, investigations are often specifically designed with the aim of demonstrating statistically significant results for the primary endpoint. Unless safety is itself the primary endpoint, most investigations will not be capable of demonstrating the statistical significance of adverse effect observed in an investigation. The importance of understanding this principle is illustrated in the next example.

> An investigation found that a new treatment for thrombophlebitis had efficacy in more rapidly resolving clots than conventional treatment. Pulmonary emboli occurred in a slightly greater percentage of those receiving the new treatment. The investigators concluded that this side effect was not important since the results were not statistically significant.

Despite the small numbers and absence of statistical significance, this finding may be very important. We cannot ignore increases in side effect merely because they are not statistically significant, since most investigations do not have the statistical power to allow us to use statistical significance testing for adverse effects.

---

[4] The concept of contributory cause is very useful because it is directly linked to the demonstration that interventions may alter the outcome. It should not be concluded that a contributory cause that has been demonstrated is the only contributory cause, or that the intervention that has been investigated is necessarily the best possible or even the best available intervention. Multiple factors may be demonstrated to be contributory causes and multiple interventions may alter the cause and thereby alter the effect. The demonstration of specific contributory causes may camouflage the larger social determinants of cause-and-effect relationships, such as poverty, pollution, or climate change. These have been called the *causes of causes*.

In addition to interpretations of benefits and harms of interventions, we may be able to learn about the interactions between factors that produce outcome. Interactions between treatments such as drugs is an important part of the evaluation of harms in clinical practice. Let us extend our previous example to illustrate this point.

> The data on patients receiving the new treatment and experiencing pulmonary emboli were examined. It was found that these patients had especially rapid dissolution of their clots. The authors concluded that there may be an interaction between the speed of clot breakdown and the probability of pulmonary emboli. They argued that this relationship makes biological sense, and stress the potential harm of this new treatment.

The authors correctly focused on the potential interaction. They relate this interaction to what is known about the biology and wisely are cautious about the use of this new treatment.[5]

Despite the importance of interactions, statistical methods for identifying and integrating interactions into data analysis are limited. Formal statistical methods usually require statistical significance before labeling the relationship between two factor as interaction. Because of the low statistical power for identifying interaction, the absence of statistical interaction should not be equated with the absence of biological interaction.[6]

At times the impact of interactions are so great that they can be demonstrated to be statistically significant. In these situations they are added as an additional factor or variable along with the confounding variables. When interactions are found to be statistically significant, it is important to focus on their interpretation, as illustrated in the next example.

> Cigarette smoking is found on average to have a relative risk of 10 for lung cancer. Exposure to environmental factors including asbestos, uranium, and radon are found on average to have a relative risk of 3 for lung cancer. When cigarette exposure and environmental exposure were both present, the average relative risk was found to be 30.

This is a type of interaction known as *multiplicative interaction*. Mulitiplicative interaction implies that the risks multiply rather than add together. If the risks added together, we would expect an average relative risk of 13 when both cigarette exposure and environmental exposure is present. This is an important finding, since it suggests that addressing either of the factors will have a much greater than expected impact on the chances of developing lung cancer.

---

[5] At times the distinction is made between statistical and biological interaction. This is an example of biological interaction. Despite the biological interaction discussed here, it is unlikely that statistical interaction would be demonstrated. Statistical interaction, even when present, may depend on the scale of measurement used—that is, it may exist for ratios such as relative risk and not exist for differences.

[6] It has been argued that use of a P-value of 0.05 is not appropriate for statistical significance tests of interaction because of the low power of the tests. In addition, an argument exists that interaction should not be subject to statistical significance testing at all. Note that we do not subject confounding variables to statistical significance tests. However, interactions are very common, and if we introduce a large number of interaction terms into a regression analysis, its statistical power to demonstrate statistical significance for the primary relationship is reduced. Perhaps this is the reason that there is great resistance to raising the acceptable P-value for defining interaction or for eliminating the use of statistical significance testing for interaction.

Subgroups

In addition to examining the contributory cause or efficacy and the side effects and interactions, investigators often examine the meaning of the investigation for subgroups of individuals with special characteristics.

Examination of subgroups, or subgroup analysis, is an important and error-prone component of interpretation. Ideally we would like to examine subgroups especially when an intervention has been shown to have efficacy. For instance, we'd like to know whether a treatment with efficacy works best for mild vs. severe disease, young vs. old, males vs. females, etc. Knowing the results for each of these subgroups and many others would assist us in applying the results in practice.

Despite the potential usefulness of subgroup analysis, it must be done carefully because there are so many potential subgroups. If all of the potential subgroups are analyzed, we are faced with what we have called the multiple comparison problem—look at enough groups and some of them will inevitably be statistically significant if we use the standard statistical methods.

A number of methods exist for circumventing this problem. One approach argues that subgroup analysis should not be done unless the results obtained using the entire study have demonstrated statistical significance. In this approach multiple subgroups may be examined, but we need to take into account the number of subgroups examined.

Another approach argues that before the investigation begins a limited number of potentially important subgroups can be identified for later subgroup analysis. These might include those with more severe disease or those receiving more intensive treatment. The investigator then would examine these subgroups regardless of the results for the overall investigation. Both of these approaches can be used with caution. However, it is important not to examine subgroups to try to give meaning to an investigation when no overall statistically significant results are found, as illustrated in the following example.

> An investigation of a new treatment for lung cancer found no statistically significant difference between the new treatment and the conventional treatment. However, after examining a large number of subgroups, the investigators found that those who had left-side primary lesions had a statistically significant improvement in longevity.

As with multiple comparisons in general, when we look at multiple subgroups we will often eventually find one or more that is statistically significant. Without an overall finding of statistical significance and without an initial hypothesis that left-side primary lesions will respond better, we need to be very cautious in interpreting the results.

Now we have examined the meaning of the results for those in the investigation. However, our job in not quite done. When reading research, we are interested not only in the meaning for those in the investigation but for those we will encounter in practice. These may be individual patients, at-risk groups, or populations in communities. Thus the last component of the M.A.A.R.I.E. asks us to draw conclusion about those who are not included in the investigation.

That is the role of extrapolation, as we will see in the next chapter.

8 Extrapolation

In the preceding chapters, we illustrated the errors that can be made in the first five component of the M.A.A.R.I.E. framework: method, assignment to study and control groups, assessment of outcome, analysis of results, interpretation of study results. Having completed this process, the investigator next asks what this all means for individuals not included in the study and for situations not directly addressed by the study. In conducting extrapolation, the reader must ask how the investigators applied the results to:

- Individuals, groups, or populations who are similar to the average participant in the investigation
- Situations that go beyond the range of the study's data
- Populations or settings that differ from those in the investigation

This is not the investigators' job alone. In fact, they are not in the best position to perform extrapolation. The investigators often want their study's conclusions to have the broadest possible implications. But they cannot know the characteristics of the individuals, institutions, or communities to whom the reader wishes to apply the study's conclusions. Thus, the reader needs to be the expert on extrapolation.

Let us start by seeing how we can use the outcome data of a study to extrapolate to similar individuals, similar groups at risk, and similar populations or communities. We will then explore extrapolation beyond the data and to different populations and settings.

Extrapolation to Similar Individuals, Groups, or Populations

The most cautious form of extrapolation asks the investigator to extend the conclusions to individuals, at-risk groups, and populations that are similar to those included in the investigation. This process can usually proceed using a quantitative approach without the need for subjective judgments on the part of the investigator.

In this form of extrapolation, one way we may be interested in extrapolating study results is to assess their overall meaning for an individual who is similar to the average individual included in the investigation. In doing this, we assume that the study's findings are as applicable to other very similar individuals who possess the risk factor being studied as it was for the individuals who were actually included in the investigation.

Many case-control and cohort studies estimate the odds ratio or relative risk associated with the development of the disease if a risk factor is present compared with when it is not present. The odds ratio and relative risk tell us the strength of the relationship between the risk factor and the disease. If a cause-and-effect relationship is present and the effect of the risk factor is completely reversible, the relative risks tell us important information regarding the individual patient. On average, a relative risk of 10 means the individual patient has a 10 times higher risk of developing the disease over a specified period of time if the risk factor is present than he or she does if the risk factor is not present.[1]

Relative risk does not, however, tell us the absolute magnitude of the risk of developing the disease if the risk factor is present compared with when it is not present. A relative risk of 10 may indicate an increase in risk from 1 per 1,000,000 for those without the risk factor to 1 per 100,000 for those with the risk factor. Alternatively, a relative risk of 10 may indicate an increase in risk from 1 per 100 for those without the risk factor to 1 per 10 among those with the risk factor. Thus, despite the same relative risk, what is called the *absolute risk* for individuals can be very different.

Failure to understand the concept of absolute risk can lead to the following type of extrapolation error:

> A patient has read that the relative risk of death from leukemia is increased four times with use of a new chemotherapy for Stage III breast cancer; the relative risk of dying from Stage III breast cancer without chemotherapy is 3. She therefore argues that the chemotherapy is not worth the risk.

The absolute risk of dying from Stage III breast cancer, however, is far greater than the risk of death from future leukemia. The infrequent and later occurrence of leukemia means that even in the presence of a risk factor that increases the risk fourfold, the absolute risk of dying from leukemia is still very small compared with the very high risk of dying from breast cancer.

Thus, the absolute risk strongly favors the benefits of treatment despite the small probability of harm. The patient in this example has failed to understand the important difference between relative risk and absolute risk. Thus, it is desirable to have information on both the relative risk and absolute risk when extrapolating the results of a study to a particular individual or when comparing one risk to another.

When extrapolating to individuals, it is essential to appreciate that the data from an investigation address issues of averages. Imagine that an intervention is found to have efficacy in an investigation that includes participants with diastolic blood pressure ranging from 90 to 120 mm Hg with an average of 100 mm Hg. The extrapolation to similar individuals should initially address the implications for those similar to the average person in the study, i.e., those with a diastolic blood pressure of 100 mm Hg. Those between 90 and 100 mm Hg might be regarded as a subgroup. There are most likely only a small number of participants in the study with a diastolic blood pressure of 90 mm Hg. Extrapolating results to individuals with a diastolic blood pressure of 90 mm Hg can dramatically increase the number of individuals to whom the results apply, even if there is no evidence that the benefit results from treating individuals with a diastolic blood pressure of 90 mm Hg. Failure to focus on the average can lead to the following extrapolation error:

> An investigation was conducted on a new medication that lowers serum homocysteine levels. Approximately half the population have a level of serum homocysteine of 10 μmol/L or greater. Patients whose only risk factor for coronary artery disease was

---

[1] How well estimates of relative risk apply to an individual is actually determined by how similar the individuals included in the study are to the individual to whom we wish to apply the results. Application of results to an individual assumes that the study sample is composed entirely of persons exactly like that individual. It is not enough that only some persons like that individual are included in the study sample. Thus prediction for one individual based on group investigations is even more difficult than prediction for the average person.

a high serum homocysteine level ranging from 10 to 30 μmol/L, with an average of 15 μmol/L, were included in the investigation. Five hundred individuals were included in the study group and in the control group, including ten individuals with a homocysteine level between 10 and 11 μmol/L. The investigation demonstrated a clinically important and statistically significant reduction in coronary artery disease among the study group compared to the control group. The investigators concluded that all adults in the United States with a serum homocysteine level of 10 μmol/L or greater should be considered candidates for the new medication.

The investigators imply that approximately half of all American adults should be considered for this new medication. They drew this conclusion because they focused on the full range of values (10 to 30 μmol/L) included in the investigation rather than the average of 15 μmol/L. This was especially dangerous since there were so few individuals included with a serum homocysteine level near the lower end of the range. Thus, unless there is convincing data from those with a homocysteine level of 10 μmol/L, extrapolation should address the average individual in the investigation.

Extrapolation to At-Risk Groups

Relative risk and absolute risk are often used to make estimates about individual patients. Sometimes, however, we are more interested in the average impact that a risk factor may have on groups of individuals with the risk factor or on a community of individuals with and without the risk factor.

When assessing the impact of a risk factor on a group of individuals, we use a concept known as *attributable risk percentage*.[2] Calculation of attributable risk percentage does not require the existence of a cause-and-effect relationship. However, when a contributory cause exists, attributable risk percentage tells us the percentage of a disease that may potentially be eliminated from individuals who have the risk factor if the effects of that risk factor can be completely removed.[3]

Attributable risk percentage is defined as follows:

$$\frac{\text{Probability of disease if risk factor present} - \text{Probability of disease if risk factor absent}}{\text{Probability of disease if risk factor present}} \times 100\%$$

Attributable risk percentage can be easily calculated from relative risk using the following formula when the relative risk is greater than 1:

$$\text{Attributable risk percentage} = \frac{\text{Relative Risk} - 1}{\text{Relative Risk}} \times 100\%$$

The following table uses this formula to convert relative risk to attributable risk percentage:

---

[2] Attributable risk percentage has also been called attributable fraction (exposed), etiologic fraction (exposed), attributable proportion (exposed), percentage risk reduction, and protective efficacy rate.

[3] This interpretation of attributable risk percentage requires that the effects of the risk factor can be immediately and completely removed.

Relative risk	Attributable risk percentage
1	0
2	50%
4	75%
10	90%
20	95%

Notice that even a relative risk of 2 may produce as much as a 50% reduction in the disease among those with the risk factor.[4]

Failure to understand this concept may lead to the following extrapolation error:

> A large, well-designed cohort study was conducted on men who exercised regularly versus men, matched for risk factors for coronary artery disease, who did not exercise regularly. The study found that those who did not exercise regularly had a relative risk of 1.5 of developing coronary artery disease. The investigators concluded that even if this was true, the relative risk was too small to be of any practical importance.

Despite the fact that the relative risk is only 1.5, notice that it converts into a substantial attributable risk percentage:

$$\text{Attributable risk percentage} = \frac{1.5 - 1}{1.5} \times 100\% = 33\%$$

This means that among men who do not exercise regularly, one-third of their risk of coronary artery disease could potentially be eliminated if the effect of their lack of exercise could be eliminated. This may affect a large number of individuals because coronary artery disease is a frequently occurring disease and lack of regular exercise is a frequently occurring risk factor.

An alternative way of expressing this information, which is applicable to cohort studies and controlled clinical trials, is known as the *number needed to treat*. The number needed to treat indicates how many patients similar to the average study participant must be treated, as the average study group patient was, to obtain one less bad outcome or one more good outcome.[4] It is calculated as follows:

$$\text{Number needed to treat} = \cfrac{1}{\begin{array}{c}\text{Probability of the}\\\text{adverse outcome in}\\\text{the control group}\end{array} - \begin{array}{c}\text{Probability of the}\\\text{adverse outcome in}\\\text{the study group}\end{array}}$$

Imagine that an investigation demonstrated a reduction of coronary artery disease over 5 years from 20 per 1,000 in a control group to 10 per 1,000 in the study group. The number needed to treat for 5 years to produce one less case of coronary artery disease would be calculated as follows:

$$\text{Number needed to treat} = \frac{1}{20/1{,}000 - 10/1{,}000} = \frac{1}{10/1{,}000} = 100$$

---

[4] A relative risk less than 1 can be converted and expressed as a relative risk greater than 1 by using the reciprocal—i.e., a relative risk of 0.5 can also be expressed as a relative risk of 2. However, using the reciprocal of a relative risk less than 1 alters the meaning since the factor in the numerator is now the factor that increases the risk. It is confusing to compare relative risks greater than 1 with relative risks less than 1 since relative risks greater than 1 do not have an upper limit while relative risks less than 1 cannot be less than 0. Thus there are advantages of expressing all relative risks as greater than 1.

The number needed to treat of 100 indicates that 100 individuals like the average participant in the study needs to be treated for 5 years to produce one less case of coronary artery disease.[5]

Extrapolation to Populations or Communities

When extrapolating the results of a study to a community or population of individuals with and without a risk factor, we need to use another measure of risk known as the *population attributable risk percentage (PAR).*[6]

If a cause-and-effect relationship is present, the population attributable risk percentage tells us the percentage of the risk in a population that can potentially be eliminated.[7] To calculate the PAR percentage, we must know more than the relative risk (expressed as greater than 1). It requires that we know or be able to estimate the proportion of individuals in the population who possess the risk factor (b from 0 to 1). If we know the relative risk and the proportion of individuals in the population with the risk factor (b), we can calculate PAR percentage using the following formula:[8]

Population attributable risk percentage (PAR%)

$$= \frac{b \, (\text{Relative risk} - 1)}{b \, (\text{Relative risk} - 1) + 1} \times 100\%$$

This formula allows us to relate relative risk, proportion of the population with the risk factor (b), and PAR percentage as follows:

Relative risk	b	PAR% (Approximate)
2	0.01	1%
4	0.01	3%
10	0.01	8%
20	0.01	16%
2	0.10	9%
4	0.10	23%
10	0.10	46%
20	0.10	65%
2	0.50	33%
4	0.50	60%
10	0.50	82%
20	0.50	90%
2	1.00	50%
4	1.00	75%
10	1.00	90%
20	1.00	95%

Notice that if the risk factor is uncommon in the population (e.g., 1% or b = 0.01), the relative risk must be substantial before the PAR percentage becomes impressive. On the other hand, if the risk factor is common (e.g., 50% or b = 0.50), even a small

[5] The number needed to treat may be less than 0. Negative numbers indicate that the control group patients, on average, had a better outcome. Thus, a negative number needed to treat indicates how many patients must be treated to produce an additional bad outcome.

[6] Population attributable risk percentage has also been called attributable fraction (population), attributable proportion (population), and etiologic fraction (population).

[7] This interpretation of PAR percentage like attributable risk percentage requires that a cause-and-effect relationship is present and that the consequences of the cause are immediately and completely reversible. PARs from two or more causes may add to more than 100%. This is also the situation for PAR%.

[8] When the odds ratio is a good approximation of relative risk, it may be used to calculate population attributable risk.

relative risk means the potential community impact may be substantial. When the prevalence of the risk factor is 1, or 100% (i.e., when everyone has the risk factor), notice that the PAR percentage equals the attributable risk percentage. This is expected because attributable risk percentage uses a study group of individuals who all have the risk factor.

Failure to understand the concept of population attributable risk percentage can lead to the following extrapolation error:

> Investigators report that a hereditary form of high cholesterol occurs in 1 per 100,000 Americans. They also report that those with this form of hyperlipidemia have a relative risk of 20 for developing coronary artery disease. The authors concluded that a cure for this form of hyperlipidemia would have a substantial impact on the national problem of coronary artery disease.

Using the data and our formula for population attributable risk percentage, we find that elimination of coronary artery disease secondary to this form of hyperlipidemia produces a population attributable risk percentage of about one fiftieth of 1%. Thus, the fact that this type of hyperlipidemia is so rare a risk factor for a common disease means that eliminating its impact cannot be expected to have a substantial impact on the overall occurrence of coronary artery disease.

When calculating the population attributable risk percentage, we often need to bring in data on the prevalence of the risk factor in the population from other studies. At times, however, an investigation may itself reflect the prevalence of a risk factor. This type of investigation is said to be *population based*. A population-based investigation allows us to calculate all of our measures using data produced by the investigation itself without relying on outside data.[9]

Extrapolation beyond the Range of the Data

Extrapolation to new situations or different types of individuals is even more difficult and is often the most challenging step when reading research. It is difficult because the investigator and the reviewers are usually not able to adequately address the issues of interest to a particular reader. It is up to you, the reader. The investigator does not know your community or your patients. Despite the difficulty with extrapolating research data, it is impossible to be a health practitioner without extrapolation from the research. Often, we must go beyond the data on the basis of reasonable assumptions. If one is unwilling to do any extrapolation, then one is limited to applying research results to individuals who are nearly identical to the average participant in an investigation.

Despite the necessity of extrapolating research data, it is important to recognize the types of errors that can occur if the extrapolation is not carefully performed. When extrapolating to different groups or different situations, two basic types of errors can occur—those due to extrapolations beyond the data, and those that occur as a result of the difference between the study population and the target population, which is the group to whom we wish to apply the results.

In research studies, individuals are usually exposed to the factors thought to be associated with the outcome for only a limited amount of time at a limited range of exposure. The investigators may be studying a factor such as hypertension that

---

[9] When the investigation is population based, it is possible to calculate all the key measures directly from the 2×2 table. This includes incidence with and without the risk factor, relative risk, attributable risk percentage, number needed to treat, prevalence of the risk factor, and population attributable risk percentage.

results in a stroke, or a therapeutic agent such as an antibiotic that has efficacy for treating an infection. In either case, the interpretation must be limited to the range and duration of hypertension experienced by the subjects or the dosage and duration of the antibiotic used in the study. When the investigators draw conclusions that extrapolate beyond the dose or duration of exposure experienced by the study subjects, they frequently are making unwarranted assumptions. They may assume that longer exposure continues to produce the same effect experienced by the study subjects. The following example illustrates a potential error resulting from extrapolating beyond the range of the data:

> A new antihypertensive agent was tested on 100 patients with hard-to-control hypertension. In all 100 patients with hard-to-control hypertension, the agent lowered diastolic blood pressure from 120 to 110 mm Hg at dosages of 1 mg/kg, and from 110 to 100 mm Hg at dosages of 2 mg/kg. The authors concluded that this agent would be able to lower diastolic blood pressure from 100 to 90 mm Hg at doses of 3 mg/kg.

It is possible that clinical evidence would document the new agent's efficacy at 3 mg/kg. Such documentation, however, awaits empirical evidence. Many antihypertensive agents have been shown to reach maximum effectiveness at a certain dosage and do not increase their effectiveness at higher dosages. To conclude that higher dosages produce greater effects without experimental evidence is to make a linear extrapolation beyond the range of the data.

Another type of error associated with extrapolation beyond the range of the data concerns potential side effects experienced at increased duration, as illustrated by the following hypothetical example:

> A 1-year study of the effects of administering daily estrogen to 100 menopausal women found that the drug relieved hot flashes and reduced the rate of osteoporosis as opposed to age-matched women given placebos who experienced no symptom relief. The authors found no adverse effects from the estrogens and concluded that estrogens are safe and effective. Therefore, they recommended that estrogens be administered long term to women, beginning at the onset of menopause.

The authors have extrapolated the data on using estrogens from a 1-year period of follow-up to long-term administration. No evidence is presented to show that if 1 year of administration is safe, so is long-term, continuous administration of estrogen. It is not likely that any long-term adverse effects would show up in a 1-year study. Thus, the authors have made potentially dangerous extrapolations by going beyond the range of their data.

Linear extrapolation may sometimes be necessary in clinical and public health practice, but we must recognize that linear extrapolation has taken place so we can be on the lookout for new data that may undermine the assumptions and thus challenge the conclusion obtained by linear extrapolation.[10]

[10] Extrapolation beyond the data also includes prediction of future events. Prognosis is a special form of prediction in that one is trying to predict the future events for a single individual. Prediction of average outcome is really a special case of extrapolation beyond the data when the data is extended beyond the time period of the investigation. The types of assumptions, however, that need to be made for prediction of future events are often very strenuous. We usually need to assume that current trends will continue, which is an assumption that is rarely fulfilled. Prognosis for specific individuals is especially difficult when based on group data, since there is far more variation among individuals than for the average outcome. However, when making predictions about the future of one particular individual, an extremely valuable source of data may be available. An individual's past response, be it to surgery, grief, or opportunity, is often the best available predictor of their future response, often far better than can be obtained using data from groups of individuals.

Extrapolation to Different Populations or Settings

When extrapolating to a target population, it is important to consider how that group differs from the study's population sampled in the investigation. The following scenario illustrates how differences between countries, for instance, can complicate extrapolation from one country to another:

> In a study involving Japan and the United States, 20% of the Japanese participants were found to have hypertension and 60% smoked cigarettes, both known contributory causes of coronary artery disease in the United States. Among U.S. participants, 10% had hypertension and 30% smoked cigarettes. Studies in Japan did not demonstrate an association between hypertension or cigarettes and coronary artery disease, whereas similar studies in the United States demonstrated a statistically significant association. The authors concluded that hypertension and cigarette smoking must protect the Japanese from myocardial infarctions.

The authors have extrapolated from one culture to a very different culture. Other explanations for the observed data are possible. If U.S. participants frequently possess another risk factor, such as high LDL cholesterol, which until recently has been rare in Japan, this factor may override cigarette smoking and hypertension and help to produce the high rate of myocardial infarctions in the U.S. population.

Extrapolation within countries can also be difficult when differences exist between the group that was investigated and the target population to which one wants to apply the findings, as illustrated in the next example:

> A study of the preventive effect of treating borderline tuberculosis (TB) skin tests (6–10 mm) with a year of isoniazid was conducted among Alaskan Native Americans. The population had a frequency of borderline skin tests of 2 per 1,000. The study was conducted by giving isoniazid to 200 Alaskan Native Americans with borderline skin tests and placebos to 200 others with the same borderline condition. Twenty cases of active TB occurred among the placebo patients and only one among the patients given isoniazid. The results were statistically significant at the 0.01 level. A health official from the state of Virginia, where borderline skin tests occur in 300 per 1,000 skin tests, was impressed with these results. He advocated that all patients in Virginia who had borderline skin tests be treated with isoniazid for 1 year.

In extrapolating to the population of Virginia, the health official assumed that borderline skin tests mean the same thing for Alaskan Native Americans as for Virginians. Other data suggest, however, that many borderline skin tests in Virginia are not due to TB exposure. They are frequently caused by an atypical mycobacteria that carries a much more benign prognosis and does not reliably respond to isoniazid. By not appreciating this factor in the residents of Virginia, the health official may be submitting many individuals to useless and potentially harmful therapy.

Extrapolation of study results is always a difficult but extremely important part of reading the health research literature. Extrapolation involves first asking what the results mean for people like the average individual included in the investigation. Thus, one must begin by looking closely at the types of patients and settings in which the investigation was conducted. This enables the reader to consider what the results mean for similar at-risk groups and finally communities or populations of individuals with and without the characteristics under study.

Often, the reader wants to go one step further and extend the extrapolation to individuals and situations that are different from those in the study. This extrapolation beyond the data must take into account the differences between the types of individuals included in the investigation and the target group. Recognizing the assumptions we make in extrapolation forces us to keep our eyes open for new information that challenges these assumptions and potentially invalidates our conclusions.

We have now examined how to apply the M.A.A.R.I.E. framework to the three basic study designs: case-control, cohort, and randomized clinical trial. Now we turn our attention to applying this framework to the special characteristics of randomized clinical trials and then to nonconcurrent or retrospective cohort studies. Finally, we will use the M.A.A.R.I.E. framework to examine efforts to combine data from studies, which is known as *meta-analysis*.

9 Randomized Clinical Trials

Randomized clinical trials are now widely considered the gold standard by which we judge the efficacy of therapy. The U.S. Food and Drug Administration (FDA) requires them for drug approval;[1] the National Institutes of Health (NIH) rewards them with funding; the journals encourage them by publication; and increasingly, practitioners read them and apply their results. When feasible and ethical, randomized clinical trials are a standard part of health research. Thus, it is critically important to appreciate what these trials can tell us, what can go wrong, and what questions they cannot address.

Randomized clinical trials today are usually conducted using an elaborate set of rules and procedures. The details for conducting the study also need to be defined in what is called the study's *protocol*. Prior to beginning a randomized clinical trial, the investigation must be reviewed by an Investigational Review Board (IRB) to evaluate the quality of the study design, the ethics of conducting the study, and the safeguards provided for patients, including a review of the informed consent statement that potential participants will be asked to sign. The IRB is asking whether it is reasonable for a potential participant to be asked to participate. Once approved by the IRB, those who are asked to participate in the study must be informed and provide their informed consent.[2] The reporting of randomized clinical trials has become relatively uniform over the last few years largely due to the publication of the CONSORT statement (*Con*solidated *S*tandards *o*f *R*eporting *T*rials).[3]

CONSORT states that randomized clinical trials are to be published using a template showing the flow of participants. Figure 9.1 is the recommended template for reporting the data from randomized clinical trials. The terms used are parallel to the first four components of the M.A.A.R.I.E. framework.

- Enrollment = Method
- Allocation = Assignment
- Follow-up = Assessment
- Analysis = Results

Let us use the M.A.A.R.I.E. framework to examine the unique features of randomized clinical trials.

---

[1] The United States Food and Drug Administration generally requires convincing results from two independently conducted, well-designed randomized clinical trials for approval of a new drug. These investigations may be conducted in the United States or abroad.

[2] An additional review under the Health Insurance Portability and Accountability Act (HIPAA) regulations is also now required to ensure the confidentiality of study data.

[3] For the complete CONSORT statement and its revisions and detailed explanations, see www.consort-statement.org (May 20, 2004).

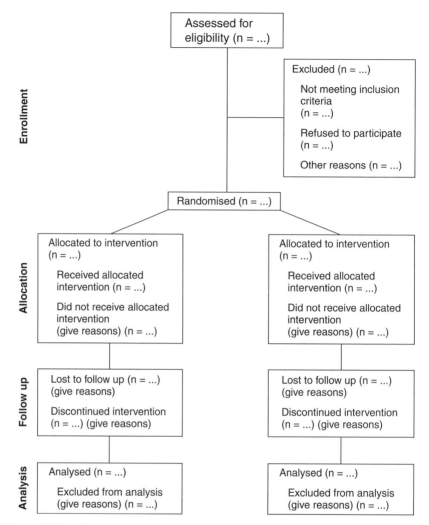

Figure 9.1. Revised template of the CONSORT diagram showing the flow of participants through each stage of a randomized trial. (Adapted from Consort Statement www.consort-statement.org (May 20, 2004)).

Method

Randomized clinical trials generally are used to establish the efficacy of treatment. Thus their study hypothesis usually indicates that on average those in the study group will have a better outcome than those in the control group.

Randomized clinical trials are capable of demonstrating all three criteria of contributory cause. When applied to a treatment, the term *efficacy* is used instead of *contributory cause*. *Efficacy* means that in the study group being investigated, the therapy increased the probability of a desirable outcome. Efficacy, however, needs to be distinguished from effectiveness. *Effectiveness* implies that the therapy works under usual conditions of practice as opposed to the conditions of an investigation.

Randomized clinical trials usually have a very specific study hypothesis since they seek to determine whether the therapy works when given according to a defined dosage schedule, by a defined route of administration, and to a defined type of patient.[4]

Thus randomized clinical trials are expected to have a detailed protocol, including specific inclusion and exclusion criteria. All participants are expected to fulfill these criteria. All those who are assessed for eligibility usually do not end up being participants in the investigation. They may not meet the inclusion criteria, they may refuse to participate, or there may be other reasons. Thus the CONSORT statement's template begins by identifying the number assessed for eligibility and then indicates the number who were excluded and the reasons for their exclusion.

Randomized clinical trials are not suitable for the initial investigation of a new treatment. When used as part of the drug approval process, randomized clinical trials are traditionally referred to as *phase III trials*. As defined by the FDA, *phase I trials* refer to the initial efforts to administer the treatment to human beings. They aim to establish a dosage regimen and to evaluate potential toxicities. They provide only a preliminary look at the potential efficacy of the therapy. Phase I trials aim to establish the indications and regimen for administering the new therapy and to determine whether the new therapy warrants further study. *Phase II trials* are usually small-scale controlled or uncontrolled trials that aim to establish whether full-scale randomized clinical trials should be conducted.

The FDA has traditionally required two independently conducted randomized clinical trials before reviewing a drug for approval for one particular indication. Once on the market, clinicians may use the drug for other indications which is called *off-label* prescribing. Ideally, a randomized clinical, or phase III, trial should be performed before the drug is widely used for new indications.[5] For new drugs that do not have market approval, this is relatively easy. However, for many procedures and drugs that have been previously marketed and used for other indications, the treatment may have been widely used before randomized clinical trials could be implemented. This is a problem, because once the treatment has been widely used, physicians and often patients have developed firm ideas about the value of the therapy. In that case, they may not believe it is ethical to enter into a randomized clinical trial or to continue participation if they discover that the patient has been assigned to the control group.

Once the time is considered right for a randomized clinical trial, the next question is whether it is feasible to perform one. To answer this, the investigator must define the question being asked in a randomized clinical trial.

Most randomized clinical trials aim to determine whether the new or experimental therapy results in a better outcome than a placebo or standard therapy. To determine whether a trial is feasible, investigators need to estimate the necessary sample size. They must estimate how many patients are required to have a reasonable chance of demonstrating a statistically significant difference between the new

---

[4] It is possible to perform a randomized clinical trial to assess the effectiveness of therapy by using a representative sample of the types of patients to be treated with the therapy and the usual methods that are being used clinically.

[5] Also note that the FDA's procedures are undergoing change, with a goal of selectively introducing new treatments into practice earlier.

therapy and the placebo or standard therapy. The required sample size depends on the following factors:[6]

1. **Size of the Type I error that the investigators will tolerate.** This is the probability of demonstrating a statistically significant difference in samples when no true difference exists between treatments in the larger population. The alpha level for the Type I error is usually set at 5%.
2. **Size of the Type II error that the investigators will tolerate.** This is the probability of failing to demonstrate a statistically significant difference in study samples when a true difference of a selected magnitude actually exists between treatments. As we discussed previously, investigators should aim for Type II error (or beta level) of 10% and accept no more than 20%. A Type II error of 20% indicates an 80% statistical power, since the statistical power plus the Type II error add up to 100%. The 80% statistical power implies 80% probability of being able to demonstrate a statistically significant difference between the samples if a true difference of the estimated size actually exists in the larger populations.
3. **Percentage of individuals in the control group who are expected to experience the adverse outcome (death or other undesired outcomes) under study.** Often this can be estimated from previous studies.
4. **Improvement in outcome within the study group that the investigators seek to demonstrate as statistically significant.** Despite the desire to demonstrate statistical significance for even small real changes, the investigators need to decide the minimum size of a difference that would be considered clinically important. The smaller this difference between study group and control group therapy that one expects, the larger the sample size required.[7]

Let us take a look at the way these factors affect the required sample size. Table 9.1 provides general guidelines for sample size for different levels of these factors.

Table 9.1 assumes one study group and one control group of equal size. It also assumes that the investigators are interested in the study results whether the results are in the direction of the study treatment or in the opposite direction. Statisticians refer to statistical significance tests that consider data favoring deviations from the null hypothesis in either direction as *two-tailed tests*. Table 9.1 assumes a Type I error of 5%.

Let us take a look at the meaning of these numbers for different types of studies:

Imagine that an investigator wishes to conduct a randomized clinical trial on a treatment designed to reduce the 1-year risk of death from adenocarcinoma of the ovary.

---

[6] This is all the information that is required for an either/or variable. When calculating sample size for variables with multiple possible outcomes, one must also estimate the standard deviation of the variable.

[7] The frequency of the outcome under investigation may be estimated from past studies, especially for the control group. It is often more difficult to estimate the expected frequency in the study group. Overly optimistic estimates of the results of the new therapy will result in sample size estimates that are too small to demonstrate statistical significance. The treatment used in the control group may influence the estimated frequency of the outcome in the control group. Use of a placebo may have advantages from the perspective of sample size since it may result in a lower rate of desired outcomes in the control group and thus reduce the number of participants needed. Today the standards for an ethical study require that a placebo not be used if other treatements are available that have greater efficacy than a placebo. One of the consequences of this policy is to increase the sample size needed for randomized clinical trials.

Assume that the 1-year risk of death using standard therapy is 40%. The investigator expected to be able to reduce the 1-year risk of death to 20% using a new treatment. He believes, however, that the treatment could possibly increase rather than reduce the risk of death. If he is willing to tolerate a 20% probability of failing to obtain statistically significant results, even if a true difference of this magnitude exists in the larger populations, how many patients are required in the study group and control group?

To answer this question, we can use Table 9.1 as follows:

Locate the 20% probability of an adverse outcome (death) in the study group on the horizontal axis.

Next, locate the 40% probability of an adverse outcome in the control group on the vertical axis. These intersect at 117, 90, and 49. The correct number is the one that lines up with the 20% Type II error. The answer is at least 90.

Thus, 90 women with advanced adenocarcinoma in the study group and 90 in the control group are needed to have a 20% probability of failing to demonstrate statistical significance if the true 1-year risk of death is actually 40% using the standard treatment and 20% using the new therapy. Notice that the sample size required for a Type II error of 10% is 117. Thus, a compromise sample size of about 100 in each group would be reasonable for this study.

Also notice that the table includes the numbers required for a 50% Type II error, an error that should not be tolerated. Here 49, i.e., about 50 participants, in each group would produce a 50% Type II error.

Thus a sample size of 100 is an approximate estimate of the number of individuals needed in each group when the probability of an adverse outcome is substantial and the investigators hope to be able to reduce it in half with the new treatment while keeping the size of the Type II error less than 20%.

Table 9.1. *Sample size requirement for controlled clinical trials*[a]

Adverse outcome in the control group	Type II error	Probability of adverse outcome in the study group			
		1%	5%	10%	20%
2%	10%	3,696	851	207	72
	20%	2,511	652	161	56
	50%	1,327	351	90	38
10%	10%	154	619	—	285
	20%	120	473	—	218
	50%	69	251	—	117
20%	10%	62	112	285	—
	20%	49	87	218	—
	50%	29	49	117	—
40%	10%	25	33	48	117
	20%	20	26	37	90
	50%	12	16	22	49
60%	10%	13	16	20	34
	20%	11	13	16	27
	50%		78	10	16

[a]All sample sizes obtained from this table assume a 5% Type I error.

Now let us contrast this situation with one in which the probability of an adverse outcome is much lower even without intervention:

> An investigator wishes to study the effect of a new treatment on the probability of neonatal sepsis secondary to delayed presentation of premature rupture of the membranes. We assume that the probability of neonatal sepsis using standard treatment is 10%, and the study group therapy aims to reduce the probability of neonatal sepsis to 5%, although it is possible that the new therapy will increase the risk of death.

Using the chart as before, we located 619, 473, and 251. Thus, we see that 619 individuals are needed for the study group and 619 individuals are needed for the control group to limit to 10% the probability of making a Type II error as is the aim for well designed studies. If we were willing to tolerate a 20% Type II error, 473 individuals would be required in each group. Thus approximately 500 individuals each in the study and the control groups is required to be able to demonstrate statistical significance when the true difference between adverse outcomes in the larger population is 10% versus 5%.

The neonatal sepsis example is typical of the problems we study in clinical practice. It demonstrates why large sample sizes are required in most randomized clinical trials before they are likely to demonstrate statistical significance. Thus, it is not usually feasible to investigate small improvements in therapy using a randomized clinical trial.

Let us go one step further and see what happens to the required sample size when a randomized clinical trial is performed on a preventive intervention in which the adverse outcome is uncommon even in the absence of prevention:

> Imagine that a new drug for preventing adverse outcomes of pregnancy in women with hypertension before pregnancy is expected to reduce the probability of adverse pregnancy outcomes from 2% to 1%, although the new therapy could possibly increase the risk of adverse outcomes.

From Table 9.1, we can see that at least 2,511 individuals are required in each group even if the investigator is willing to tolerate a 20% Type II error. These enormous numbers point out the difficulty in performing randomized clinical trials when one wishes to apply preventive therapy, especially when the risk of adverse outcomes is already quite low.[8]

Even when a randomized clinical trial is feasible, it may not be ethical to perform one. These trials are not considered ethical if they require individuals to submit to substantial risks without a realistic expectation of a substantial benefit. In general, investigations that use a placebo when standard therapy has been shown to have efficacy are not considered ethical. A randomized clinical trial may be conducted using standard therapy in the control group, but this may require an increase in the sample size. Thus, despite the advantages of randomized trials in defining the efficacy of a therapy, they are not always feasible or ethical.

---

[8] These sample sizes are designed for the *primary endpoint,* which should be an endpoint expected to occur relatively frequently and to be biologically important. However, it may not be the most important endpoint of interest. For instance, in a study of coronary artery disease, a myocardial infarction may be a primary endpoint. Other endpoints that have even more clinical importance but occur less frequently, such as disability or death, are often measured as *secondary endpoints.* In general, primary but not secondary endpoints are used for calculating sample size.

In summary, the method component of randomized clinical trial usually hypothesizes the efficacy of an intervention; it has very specific inclusion and exclusion criteria; and its sample size is calculated to provide at least 80% statistical power to demonstrate statistical significance.

Assignment

Participants in a randomized clinical trial are not usually selected at random from a larger population. Usually, they are volunteers who meet a series of inclusion and exclusion criteria defined by the investigators.

To become a participant, an eligible individual must provide what we have called informed consent. Informed consent is more than a signed legal document. It requires that potential participants be provided an explanation of the potential benefits and known harms as well as the processes that will occur. Participants must be told that they have the right to withdraw from the study at any time for any reason. They do not have a right to know their treatment group assignment while in the study and may not be eligible to receive compensation through the investigation for adverse side effects of therapy.

Individuals entered into randomized clinical trials are often a relatively homogeneous group because they share inclusion and exclusion criteria. They are not usually representative of all those with the disease or all those for whom the therapy is intended (i.e., the target population). In addition, they often do not have the type of complicating factors encountered in practice. That is, they usually do not have multiple disease and multiple simultaneous therapies, and they usually do not have compromised ability to metabolize drugs as a result of renal or hepatic disease. Thus, it is important to distinguish between the study population and the target population.

Randomized clinical trials usually have a table that indicates the characteristics of those who were included as participants in the investigation. They should also indicate the characteristics of those assessed for eligibility following the CONSORT format. This table usually provides useful information for better understanding the characteristics of the study group and the control group and how they may differ from the target population.

Once an individual becomes a participant in the investigation, they may not immediately undergo randomization. Investigators may follow patients before randomizing them to a study or a control group. They may do this to determine whether they are likely to take the treatment, return for follow-up, or in other ways be compliant with the protocol of the investigation. Investigators may use what is called a *run-in period* to exclude patients who do not take prescribed medication, do not return for follow-up, or demonstrate other evidence that they are not likely to follow the study protocol. Because this is an increasingly frequent procedure, it is important to recognize that randomized clinical trials often use patients who are especially likely to adhere to treatment.

The randomization of patients to study and control groups is the hallmark of randomized clinical trials. An important feature of randomization is called *allocation concealment*. Allocation concealment implies that those assigning participants to groups are not aware of which group the next participant will be assigned to until the moment of assignment. That is, randomization implies unpredictability. The process of allocation concealment is intended to preserve unpredictability. This prevents the person making the assignment from consciously or unconsciously influencing the assignment process. That is, it prevents selection bias.

Randomization implies that any one individual has a predetermined probability of being assigned to each particular study group and control group. This may mean an equal probability of being assigned to one study and one control group or different probabilities of being assigned to each of several study and control groups. The proportion of the participants intended for each study and control group is called the *allocation ratio*.

Randomization is a powerful tool for eliminating selection bias in the assignment of individuals to study and control groups. In large studies, it greatly reduces the possibility that the effects of treatment are due to the type of individuals receiving the study and control therapies. It is important to distinguish between randomization, which is an essential part of a randomized clinical trial, and random sampling, which is not usually a part of a randomized clinical trial. *Random sampling* implies that the individuals who are selected for a study are selected by chance from a larger group or population. Thus, random sampling is a method aimed at obtaining a representative sample, one that, on average, reflects the characteristics of a larger group.

Randomization, on the other hand, says nothing about the characteristics of a larger population from which the individuals in the investigation are obtained. It refers to the mechanism by which individuals are assigned to study and control groups once they become participants in the investigation. The following hypothetical study illustrates the difference between random sampling and randomization:

> An investigator wishes to assess the efficacy of a new drug known as Surf-ez. Surf-ez is designed to help improve surfing ability. To assess the value of Surf-ez, the investigator performs a randomized clinical trial among a group of volunteer championship surfers in Hawaii. After randomizing half the group to Surf-ez and half the group to a placebo, the investigators measure the surfing ability of all surfers using a standard scoring system. The scorers do not know whether a particular surfer used Surf-ez or a placebo. Those taking Surf-ez have a statistically significant and substantial improvement compared with the placebo group. On the basis of the study results, the authors recommend Surf-ez as a learning aid for all surfers.

By using randomization, this randomized clinical trial has demonstrated the efficacy of Surf-ez among these championship surfers. Because its study and control groups were hardly a random sample of surfers, however, we must be very careful in drawing conclusions or extrapolating about the effects of Surf-ez as a learning aid for all surfers.[9]

Randomization does not eliminate the possibility that study and control groups will differ according to factors that affect prognosis (confounding variables). Known prognostic factors must still be measured and are often found to be different in study and control groups as a result of chance alone, especially in small studies. If differences between groups exist, these must be taken into account through an

---

[9] Care must be taken even in extrapolating to championship surfers because we have not randomly sampled all championship surfers. This limitation occurs in most randomized clinical trials, which select their patients from a particular hospital or clinical site.

adjustment process as part of the analysis.[10] Many characteristics affecting prognosis, however, are not known. In larger studies randomization tends to balance the multitude of characteristics that could possibly affect outcome, even those that are unknown to the investigator. Without randomization, the investigator would need to take into account all known and potential differences between groups. Because it is difficult, if not impossible, to consider everything, randomization helps balance the groups, especially for large studies.[11]

Masking or blinding of study subjects and investigators is a goal of assignment in a randomized clinical trial. *Single masking* implies that the participants are unaware of their group assignments; *double masking* implies that neither the patient nor the investigator is aware of the group assignment. The impact of not masking occurs in the assessment process.

Assessment

Assessment in randomized clinical trials, as in other types of investigations, requires us to carefully examine the outcome measures being used. Errors in assessing the outcome or endpoint of a randomized clinical trial may occur when the patient or the individual making the assessment is aware of which treatment is being administered. This is especially likely when the outcome or endpoint being measured is subjective or may be influenced by knowledge of the treatment group, as illustrated in the following hypothetical study:

> A randomized clinical trial of a new breast cancer surgery compared the degree of arm edema and arm strength among patients receiving the new procedure versus the traditional procedure. The patients were aware of which procedure they underwent. Arm edema and arm strength were the endpoints assessed by the patients and surgeons. The study found that those receiving the new procedure had less arm edema and more arm strength than those undergoing the traditional mastectomy.

In this study, the fact that the patients and the surgeons who performed the procedure and assessed the outcome knew which patients received which procedure may have affected the objectivity of the way strength and edema were measured and reported. This effect may have been minimized but not totally eliminated if arm strength and edema were assessed with a standardized scoring system by individuals who did not know which patients received which therapy. This system of masked assessment and objective scoring would not entirely remove the impact of patients and surgeons knowing which surgery was performed. It is still possible that patients receiving the new procedure worked harder and actually increased

---

[10] Many biostatisticians would recommend using a multivariable analysis technique such as regression analysis even when no substantial difference exists between groups. Multivariable analysis then permits adjustment for interaction. Interaction occurs, for instance, when both groups contain an identical age and sex distribution, but one group contains predominantly young women and the other contains predominantly young men. Multivariable analysis then allows one to separate out the interacting effects of age and sex.

[11] Randomization as defined by the CONSORT statement may be divided into simple randomization and restricted randomization. Simple randomization implies that each participant has a known probability of receiving each treatment before one is assigned. Restricted randomization describes any procedure used to achieve balance between the group either in terms of size or characteristics. Blocking may be used to ensure that the groups are of approximately the same size. Stratification may be used to ensure balance based on characteristics.

their strength and reduced their edema. This could occur, for instance, if the surgeon performing the new surgery stressed postoperative exercises or provided more physical therapy for those receiving the new therapy.

In practice, masking is often impractical or unsuccessful. Randomized clinical trials without masking are called *open* or *open-label trials*. Surgical therapy cannot easily be masked. The taste or side effects of medications are often a giveaway to the patient or clinician. The need to titrate a dose to achieve a desired effect often makes it more difficult to mask the clinician and in some cases the patient. Strict adherence to masking helps to ensure the objectivity of the assessment process. It helps to remove the possibility that differences in compliance, follow-up, and assessment of outcome will be affected by awareness of the treatment received.

Even when objective assessment, excellent compliance, and complete follow-up can be ensured, masking is still desirable because it helps control for the placebo effect. The placebo effect is a powerful biological process that can bring about a wide variety of objective as well as subjective biological effects. The placebo effect extends far beyond pain control. A substantial percentage of patients who believe they are receiving effective therapy obtain objective therapeutic benefits. When effective masking is not a part of a randomized clinical trial, it leaves open the possibility that the observed benefit in the study subject is actually the result of the placebo therapy.

Thus, when masking is not feasible, doubt about the accuracy of the outcome measures usually persists. This uncertainty can be reduced but not eliminated by using objective measures of endpoints, careful monitoring of compliance, and complete follow-up of patients.

In addition to attempting masking, the investigators are encouraged by the CONSORT statement to make an effort to determine whether masking was actually successful. This may be done by simply asking participants which treatment they believe they received and comparing their response to their actual treatment.

An assessment of outcome requires measures of outcome that are appropriate, precise and accurate, complete, and unaffected by the process of observation. The requirements are as important in a randomized clinical trial as in case-control and cohort studies, as we discussed in Chapter 5.

There are some special consideration that apply to randomized clinical trials. Investigators often wish to use outcome measures or endpoints that occur in a short period of time rather than waiting for more clinically important but longer-term outcomes, such as death or blindness. Increasingly, changes in laboratory tests are substituted for clinical endpoints. We call these surrogate endpoints or surrogate markers. Surrogate endpoints can be very useful if the test is an early indicator of subsequent outcome. If that is not the situation, however, the surrogate endpoint can be an inappropriate measure of outcome, as suggested in the following scenario:

> Researchers note that individuals with severe coronary artery disease often have multiple premature ventricular contractions and experience sudden death, often believed to be caused by arrhythmias. They note that a new drug may be able to reduce premature ventricular contractions. Thus, they conduct a randomized clinical trial that demonstrates the new drug has efficacy in reducing the frequency of premature ventricular contraction in patients with severe coronary artery disease. Later evidence indicates that despite the reduction in arrhythmias, those with severe coronary artery disease taking the drug have an increased frequency of death compared with similar untreated patients.

The investigator has assumed that reducing the frequency of premature ventricular contraction in the short run is strongly associated with a better outcome in the longer run. This may not always be the situation, as has been demonstrated with treatment for premature ventricular contractions in this type of setting. The fact that treatment seems like a logical method for reducing deaths caused by arrhythmia may have allowed investigators to accept a surrogate endpoint. They were assuming without evidence that reduction in arrhythmia would be strongly associated with the endpoint of interest, which was death in this case.

An additional problem can occur when individuals are lost to follow-up before the study is completed. Even moderate loss to follow-up can be disastrous for a study. Those lost may move to a pleasant climate because of failing health, drop out because of drug toxicity, or fail to return because of the burdens of complying with one of the treatment protocols.

Well-conducted studies take elaborate precautions to minimize the loss to follow-up. In some cases, follow-up may be completed by a telephone or mail questionnaire. A search of death records should be conducted in an effort to find participants who cannot be located. When outcome data cannot be obtained, re-sulting in loss to follow-up despite these precautions, it is important to determine, as much as possible, the initial characteristics of patients subsequently lost to follow-up. This is done in an attempt to determine whether those lost are likely to be different from those who remain. If those lost to follow-up have an especially poor prognosis, little may be gained by analyzing the data regarding only those who remain, as suggested by the following hypothetical study:

> In a study of the effects of a new alcohol treatment program, 100 patients were randomized to the new program, and 100 patients were randomized to conventional treatment. The investigators visited the homes of all patients at 9 P.M. on a Saturday and drew blood from all available patients to measure alcohol levels. Of the new treatment group, 30 patients were at home, and one-third of these had alcohol in their blood. Among the conventionally treated patients, 33 were at home, and two-thirds of these had alcohol in their blood. The results were statistically significant, and the investigators concluded that the new treatment reduced alcohol consumption.

Whenever loss to follow-up occurs, it is important to ask what happened to those lost participants. In this study, if those lost to follow-up were out drinking, the results based on those at home would be especially misleading. This is important even if loss to follow-up occurs equally in the study and control groups.

One method for dealing with loss to follow-up is to assume the worst regarding the lost participants. For instance, the investigator could assume that the partici-pants not at home were out drinking. It is then possible to redo the analysis and compare the outcome in the study and control groups to determine whether the differences are still statistically significant. When the loss to follow-up is great, this procedure usually indicates no substantial or statistically significant difference between the study and control groups. However, for smaller loss to follow-up, a statistically significant difference may remain. When statistically significant dif-ferences between groups remain after assuming the worst case for those lost to follow-up, the reader can be quite confident that loss to follow-up does not explain the observed differences.

In an ideal randomized clinical trial, all individuals would be treated according to the study protocol and monitored over time. Their outcome would be assessed from their time of entry until the end of the study. In reality, assessment is rarely so perfect or complete. Patients often receive treatment that deviates from the predefined protocol. Investigators often label these individuals as *protocol deviants.* Deviating from the protocol, as opposed to loss to follow-up, implies that data on subsequent outcomes were obtained.

Results

In a randomized clinical trial it is important to consider what to do with the outcomes from the protocol deviants. Let us see how this might occur by looking at the following hypothetical study:

> In a randomized clinical trial of surgery versus angioplasty for single-vessel coronary artery disease, 100 patients were randomized to surgery and 100 to angioplasty. Before receiving angioplasty, 30 of the patients deviated from the protocol and had surgery. The investigators decided to remove those who deviated from the protocol from the analysis of results.

It is likely that many of the patients who deviated from the protocol and underwent surgery were the ones doing poorly. If that is the situation, then eliminating those who deviated from the protocol from the analysis would leave us with a group of individuals doing especially well.

Because of the potential bias, it is generally recommended that deviants from the study protocol remain in the investigation and be subsequently analyzed as if they had remained in the group to which they were originally randomized. This is known as *analysis according to intention-to-treat.* By retaining the protocol deviants, the study question, however, is changed slightly. The study now asks whether prescribing the study therapy produced a better outcome than prescribing the standard therapy recognizing that patients may not actually take prescribed treatments. This allows the investigator to better address the effectiveness of the therapy as actually used in clinical practice.

Investigators may perform additional calculations excluding those who deviate from the protocol. These analyses are called *as-treated analysis.* While these analyses may be useful, especially if the intention-to-treat analysis is statistically significant, it is not considered proper methodology to use only an as-treated analysis. Deviations from the protocol are relatively common in randomized clinical trials because it is considered unethical to prevent deviations when the attending physician believes that continued adherence is contraindicated by the patient's condition or when the patient no longer wishes to follow the recommended protocol. Thus, in evaluating a randomized clinical trial, the reader should understand the degree of protocol adherence and determine how the investigators handled the data regarding those who deviated from the protocol.

Two other analysis questions face the investigator in a randomized clinical trial: when to analyze the data and how to analyze the data.

The seemingly simple question of when to analyze the data of a randomized clinical trial has provoked considerable methodological and ethical controversy. The more times one looks at the data, the more likely one is to find a point when the *P*-value reaches the 0.05 level of statistical significance using standard statistical techniques.

When to analyze is an ethical problem because one would like to establish that a true difference exists at the earliest possible moment. This is desirable to avoid subjecting patients to therapy that has less benefit. In addition, it is desirable that other patients receive a beneficial therapy at the earliest possible time.

A number of statistical methods called *sequential methods* have been developed to attempt to deal with these problems. When multiple times for analysis of data are planned, these sequential statistical techniques are available to take into account the multiple analyses.

Life Tables

Another issue that arises in randomized clinical trials is the method for presenting data. *Life tables or longitudinal life tables* are the most commonly used method for presenting data in randomized clinical trials.[12]

Let us begin by discussing why life tables are often, but not always, necessary in randomized clinical trials. Then we will discuss the assumptions underlying their use and demonstrate how they should be interpreted.

In most randomized clinical trials, individuals are entered into the study and randomized over a period of time as they present for care. In addition, because of late entry or loss to follow-up, individuals are actually monitored for various periods of time after entry. Therefore, many of the patients included in a study are not followed for the full duration of the study.

If all individuals were monitored for the desired length of observation, the probability of death in a study group or a control group can be calculated simply as the number of those dead at the end divided by the number of those initially enrolled in the group. All individuals, however, are not usually monitored for the same length of time. Life tables provide a method for using the data from those individuals who have been included in a study for only a portion of the possible study duration.[13] Thus, life tables allow the investigator to use all the data that they have so painstakingly collected.

The life-table method is built on the important assumption that those who were in the investigation for shorter periods would have had the same subsequent experience as those who were actually followed for longer periods of time. In other words, the short-termers would have the same results as the long-termers if they were actually followed long term.

This critical assumption may not hold true if the short-termers are individuals with a better or worse prognosis than the long-termers. This can occur if the entry requirements for the investigation are relaxed during the course of a study. Let us see how this might occur by looking at the next hypothetical study:

A new hormonal treatment designed to treat infertility secondary to severe endometriosis was compared with standard therapy in a randomized clinical trial. After initial difficulty recruiting patients and initial failures to get pregnant among the study patients, one woman in the study group became pregnant. News of her delivery became front-page news. Subsequent patients recruited for the study were found to

---

[12] Life-table methods can also be used in cohort studies thus they are often called longitudinal life-tables. Longitudinal life-tables should be distinguished from cross-school life table that we will encounter in Chapter 25. In this discussion, the adverse effect under study is referred to as death. However, life tables can be used for other effects, such as permanent loss of vision or the occurrence of pregnancy after infertility therapy.

[13] Variations of this type of life table are known as a Kaplan-Meier or Cutler-Ederer life table. Note that this type of life table assumes the endpoint can occur only once. Thus, it is not appropriate for studies of diseases such as strep throat, which may recur.

have much less severe endometriosis, but the investigators willingly accepted those patients and combined their data with data from their original group of patients.

As this study demonstrates, the same eligibility criteria may not be maintained throughout the investigation. It is tempting to relax the inclusion and exclusion criteria if only severely ill patients are entered into an investigation at the beginning. As the therapy becomes better known in the community, at a particular institution, or in the literature, a tendency may occur for clinicians to refer, or patients to self-refer, the less severely ill.

In this case, the short-term study participants are likely to have less severe illness and thus have better outcomes than the long-termers. This problem can be minimized if the investigators clearly define and carefully adhere to a protocol that defines the type of patients who are eligible for the study on the basis of inclusion and exclusion criteria related to prognosis.

Loss to follow-up may also result in differences between the short-termers and the long-termers. This is likely if loss to follow-up occurs preferentially among those who are not doing well or who have adverse reactions to treatment. We have already discussed the importance of loss to follow-up and stressed the need to assess whether those lost are similar to those who remain.

Life-table data are usually presented as a *survival plot*. This is a graph in which the percentage survival is plotted on the vertical axis, ranging from 100% at the top of the axis to 0% at the bottom. Thus, at the beginning of the investigation, both study and control groups start at the 100% mark at the top of the vertical axis. Life-table data may represent outcomes other than death, such as recurrence or blindness.[14] The horizontal axis depicts the time of follow-up. Time is counted for each individual beginning with their entry into the study. Thus, time zero is not the time in which the investigation began.

Survival plots should also include the number of individuals who have been monitored for each time interval. These should be presented separately for the study and the control groups. Thus, a typical life table comparing the 5-year data on study and control groups might be examined graphically in a survival plot like Fig. 9.2. The top row of numbers represents the number of study group subjects monitored through the corresponding length of time since their entry into the study, and the bottom row represents the same for control group subjects. The survival plot can be used directly to estimate the percentage death or survival at, for instance, 5 years; this probability of survival is known as the 5-year *actuarial survival*. For instance, in Fig. 9.2, the 5-year actuarial survival read directly from the graph is approximately 60% for the study group and 40% for the control group.

Life tables are often tested for statistical significance using the log rank or Mantel-Haenszel statistical significance tests. For these tests, the null hypothesis states that no difference exists between the overall life table results for the study and control groups. Notice that the statistical significance tests do not address the question of which treatment achieves better results at 5 years. In performing these tests, one combines data from each interval in time, using a method called *weighting* to take into account the number of individuals being observed during

---

[14] Alternatively, a graphic presentation of life tables may display the percentage who experience the adverse effect and start at the 0% point on the bottom of the vertical axis. When assessing a desirable outcome, such as pregnancy in an infertility study, a life table may also begin at 0%, indicating no pregnancies.

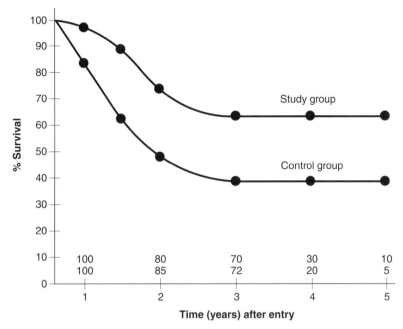

Figure 9.2. A typical study and control group survival plot demonstrating plateau effect, which typically occurs at the right end of life-table plots.

that time interval. Thus, these methods combine data from different time intervals to produce an overall statistical significance test. The combination of data from multiple intervals means that the statistical significance test asks this question: If no true difference exists between the overall effects of the study group and control group treatments, what is the probability of obtaining the observed or more extreme results?

In other words, if a statistically significant improvement in a study group has been demonstrated on the basis of life-table data, it is very likely that a similar group of individuals receiving the therapy will experience at least some improvement compared with the control group therapy.

As we have seen, life tables can be used directly to obtain estimates of the magnitude of difference in outcome between treatments. Inference can be performed using a statistical significance test that addresses the overall differences. In addition (as we will discuss in Section VI, Selecting a Statistic) adjustment for potential confounding variables may be incorporated into the life-table analysis using a technique known as *Cox regression* or *proportional hazards regression*. Thus, life tables can address all three basic questions of statistics: estimation, inference, and adjustment.

Interpretation

As we saw in Chapter 2, randomized clinical trials have the potential to demonstrate all three criteria need to definitively establish contributory cause or efficacy. However, data from life tables are prone to a number of misinterpretations. When displaying life-table data, it is important to display the number of individuals being monitored at each interval of time in the study group and in the control group. Usually only a small number are monitored for the complete duration of a study. For instance, in Fig. 9.2 only 10 individuals in the study group and 5 individuals in the control group are monitored for 5 years. This is not surprising because considerable time is often required to start up a study, and those individuals monitored for the longest time were usually recruited during the first year of the study.

A 5-year probability of survival can be calculated even when only one patient has been observed for 5 years. Thus, one should not rely too greatly on the specific 1-year, 5-year, or any other probability of survival observed unless a substantial number of individuals is actually observed for the full length of the study.

In interpreting randomized clinical trial results, it is important to understand the limitations in the reliability of the estimates obtained from the life-table. Failure to recognize this uncertainty can result in the following type of misinterpretation:

> A clinician looking at the life-table curves in Fig. 9.2 concluded that 5-year survival with the study treatment is 60% versus 40% for the control group. After extensive use of the same treatment on similar patients, he was surprised that the study treatment actually produced a 55% survival versus a 50% survival among control group patients.

If the clinician had recognized that life-table curves do not reliably predict exact 5-year survival, he would not have been surprised about his experience.

Knowledge of the procedures and assumptions underlying life tables also helps in understanding their interpretation. Many survival plots have a flat or plateau phase for long time periods at the right-hand end of the plot. These may be misinterpreted as indicating a cure once an individual reaches the flat or plateau area of the survival plot. Actually, this plateau phase usually results because few individuals are monitored for the entire duration of the study. Among those few individuals who are observed for longer periods, the deaths are likely to be fewer and more widely spaced. Because the survival curve moves lower when an outcome such as death occur, a plateau is likely when fewer deaths are possible. Thus, an understanding of this *plateau effect* is important in interpreting a life table. We should not interpret the plateau as demonstrating a cure unless large numbers of patients have been observed for long periods of time.

In addition to the dangers of relying too heavily on the 5-year probability of survival derived from life-table data and of misinterpreting the plateau, it is important to fully appreciate the interpretation of a statistically significant difference between survival plots, as illustrated in the next example:

> In the study depicted in Fig. 9.2, a statistically significant difference occurred in outcome between the study and control groups on the basis of the 5-year follow-up. The study was subsequently extended for 1 more year, resulting in the survival plot depicted in Fig. 9.3, in which the 6-year actuarial survival was identical in the study and control groups. On the basis of the 6-year data, the authors stated that the 5-year actuarial study was mistaken in drawing the conclusion that the study therapy prolonged survival.

Remember that a statistically significant difference in survival implies that patients receiving one treatment do better than patients receiving another treatment when taking into account each group's entire experience. Patients in one group may do better only early in the course, midway through, or at the end. Patients who received the better overall treatment may actually do worse early in the treatment

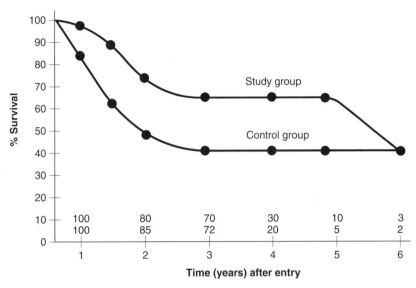

Figure 9.3. Survival plots may meet after extended periods of follow-up. The difference between the overall plots may still be statistically significant.

because of surgical complications, or at a later point in time as secondary complications develop among those who survive.

Thus, when conducting a study, it is important to know enough about the natural history of a disease and the life expectancy of the individuals in the investigation to choose a meaningful time period for follow-up. Differences in outcomes are unlikely if the time period is too short, such as one that ends before an extended period of therapy is completed.

Similarly, follow-up periods that are too long may not allow the study to demonstrate statistically significant differences if the risks of other diseases overwhelm the shorter-term benefits. For instance, a study that assesses only the 20-year outcome among 65-year-olds given a treatment for coronary artery disease might show little difference at 20 years even if differences occur at 5 and 10 years.

We have repeatedly emphasized the distinction between a statistically significant association and a cause-and-effect relationship. In randomized clinical trials, we use the same criteria to establish that a treatment has efficacy, meaning that it works for those in the investigation. Efficacy or a cause-and-effect relationship requires the existence of an association. Second, it requires a demonstration that the cause precedes the effect. Third, it requires that altering the cause alters the effect. One of the practical and intellectually satisfying aspects of randomized clinical trials is that they incorporate methods for helping to establish all three criteria for contributory cause and thus can establish the efficacy of a therapy as follows:

1. The investigators are able to produce study and control groups that are comparable except for the effects of the treatment being given. Thus, when substantial and statistically significant differences in outcome occur, the investigator can usually conclude that these differences are associated with the treatment itself.
2. By randomizing individuals to study and control groups at the beginning of the study, the investigators can provide strong evidence that the treatment precedes

the effect and is, therefore, a prior association, fulfilling the second criterion of contributory cause.

3. By providing a treatment that alters the disease process and comparing the study and control groups' outcomes, the investigators can provide evidence that the treatment itself (the "cause") is actually altering the outcome (the "effect"), thus fulfilling the third and final criterion for contributory cause.

Randomized clinical trials, therefore, can help to establish the existence of an association between treatment and outcome, can establish the existence of a prior association, and can demonstrate that altering the treatment alters the outcome. These are the three criteria necessary for establishing that the new treatment is the cause of the improved outcome. These criteria establish the efficacy of treatment. However, even after establishing that a treatment has efficacy, we need to ask what it is about the intervention that is working. The efficacy may not result from the intervention the investigator intended to study, as suggested in the following study:

> A randomized clinical trial of a new postoperative recovery program for posthysterectomy care was performed by randomizing 100 postsurgery women to a standard ward and 100 postsurgery women to a special care ward equipped with experimental beds and postoperative exercise equipment and staffed by extra nurses. Women on the special care ward were discharged with an average length of stay of only 7 days compared with 12 days for women randomized to the regular ward. The results were statistically significant. The investigators concluded that the experimental beds and a postoperative exercise program resulted in a substantially reduced length of stay.

This investigation established that the intervention had efficacy: It worked to produce more rapid recovery and thus to reduce length of stay. However, it is still not clear what actually worked. Before concluding that the experimental beds and postoperative exercise made the difference, do not forget that extra nurses were also provided. The availability of the extra nurses may have been the cause of the early discharge rather than the beds and exercise. In an unmasked or open study such as this one, it is possible that the effect of observation itself helped to bring about the observed effect.

The interpretation of safety data on adverse effects, side effects, or harms is an important part of randomized clinical trials, along with its emphasis on efficacy. Randomized clinical trials should display the frequency of adverse effects in both the study and control groups. The number of individuals who experience the adverse effects in the study and control groups is usually small. Statistical significance testing is not usually performed because the statistical power is low. That is, the results would not usually be statistically significant even when they have clinical importance. Failure to appreciate this approach to adverse effects may lead to the following interpretation problem:

> A randomized clinical trial of a hair-growth medication was conducted by randomizing 100 severely balding men to the new medicine and 100 severely balding men to a placebo. Ninety percent of the men randomized to the medication experienced substantial return of hair versus none in the placebo group. The results were statistically significant. Among the medication group, five experienced elevated liver function tests and one acquired clinical hepatitis. Among the placebo group, three experienced elevated liver function tests and none acquired clinical hepatitis. The investigators concluded that the therapy had efficacy and the increase in adverse effects was due to chance since it was not statistically significant.

It is very tempting to dismiss the occurrence of side effects as due to chance, especially when there is no statistical significance testing and the side effect occurs in both groups. Unfortunately, this is often the situation in randomized clinical trials because of their limited size. This investigation can only provide a suggestion that the new medication is associated with liver function abnormalities. The presence of other causes for liver disease in both study and control groups must be kept in mind. In conducting this investigation, it would be very important to further investigate the cause of the elevated liver function tests to rule out other common causes, such as viral infections. In addition, the response of the liver function abnormalities to discontinuation of the treatments would provide some help in determining whether altering the potential cause alters the effect.

Demonstrating cause-and-effect relationships for adverse effects is very difficult. One approach relies on the consequences of starting and stopping treatment in a single individual. This type of investigation has been called an *n-of-1* study. In an n-of-1 study, each patient serves as his or her own control. The treatment is administered to one individual who develops a side effect such as a rash, then the therapy is discontinued and the patient is observed to see whether and when the presumed side effect resolves. The final step is to readminister the treatment to see whether the side effect occurs again.

This approach incorporates the concepts of association, prior association, and altering the cause alters the effect to help establish a cause-and-effect relationship. The potential danger to individual patients has limited the use of this technique.

Data on adverse effects are often limited to establishing the frequency of the side effect in study and control groups without expecting definitive data establishing statistical significance or contributory cause. These less definitive data, however, cannot be simply dismissed as being due to chance. Because of the small numbers and the resulting low statistical power, it is often necessary to assume that an increase in the adverse events is caused by the study treatment. Thus, the approach to safety and efficacy is very different.

With randomized clinical trials, as with other types of investigations, questions of subgroups are often of great interest. In randomized clinical trials, tests of interaction are often performed that ask whether there is evidence that the effect of treatment differs from one subgroup to another. When interaction is present, close examination of the subgroups can provide important information, as illustrated in the next example.

> A randomized clinical trial of a new cancer treatment for Stage III or IV breast cancer found a modest but statistically significant improvement in outcome. A statistical test for interaction found interaction between the stages and the treatment to be statistically significant. The investigator then examined the data for Stage III and Stage IV separately and found substantial improvement for those who received the treatment during Stage III and slightly poorer average outcome for those who received the treatment during Stage IV.

Thus, at times interaction and the close examination of subgroups can add important clinical information to the interpretation of randomized clinical trials.[15]

---

[15] Unfortunately, the size of most randomized clinical trial provides only low statistical power for demonstrating interactions.

Extrapolation

An effort to extrapolate the results of an investigation should begin by reexamining the characteristics of the study's population. The strict inclusion and exclusion criteria established in the protocol to ensure uniformity in a randomized clinical trial often become a limitation when extrapolating to those not included in the investigation.

Patients included in many randomized clinical trials are chosen because they are the type of patients most likely to respond to the treatment. In addition, considerations of time, geography, investigator convenience, and patient compliance are usually of paramount importance in selecting a particular group of patients for an investigation. Pregnant patients, the elderly, the very young, and those with mild disease are usually not included in randomized clinical trials unless the therapy is specifically designed for their use. In addition to these inclusion and exclusion criteria that are under the control of the investigator, other factors may lead to a unique group of patient who become participants in a randomized clinical trial. Every medical center population has its own referral patterns, location, and socioeconomic patterns. A patient population referred to the Mayo Clinic may be quite different from one drawn to a local county hospital. Primary-care health maintenance organization (HMO) outpatients may be very different from the hospital subspecialty clinic outpatients. These characteristics, which may be beyond the investigator's control, can affect the types of patients included in a way that may affect the results of the study.

The fact that the group of patients included in randomized clinical trials is different from a group of patients whom clinicians might treat with the new therapy often creates difficulty in extrapolating the conclusions to patients seen in clinical practice. If the individuals in the investigation are not representative of the target population, extrapolation requires additional assumptions. This does not invalidate the result of a randomized clinical trial; however, it does mean the clinician must use care and good judgment when adapting the results to clinical practice.

Thus, despite the power and importance of randomized clinical trials, the process of extrapolation is still largely speculative. The reader needs to examine the nature of the study institutions and the study patients before applying the study results. Practitioners need to determine whether their own setting and patients are comparable to those in the study. If they are not, the differences may limit the ability to extrapolate from the study.

Patients and study centers involved in an investigation may be different from the usual clinical setting in many ways. For instance:

- Patients in an investigation are likely to be carefully followed up and very compliant. Compliance and close follow-up may be critical to the success of the therapy.
- Patients in the study may have worse prognoses than the usual patients seen in clinical practice. For this reason, the side effects of the therapy may be worth the risk in the study patients, but the same may not be true for patients seen in another clinical setting.
- The study centers may have special skills, equipment, or experience that maximize the success of the new therapy. This may not be true when the therapy is used by clinicians without experience with those techniques.

Despite a clear demonstration of a successful therapy using a randomized clinical trial, clinicians must be careful to account for these types of differences in extrapolating to patients in their own practices. Randomized clinical trials are capable of establishing the efficacy of treatment performed on a carefully selected group of patients treated under the ideal conditions of an experimental study. They must be used carefully when trying to assess the effectiveness of treatment for clinical care. Thus, well-motivated and conscientious clinicians providing usual care with usual facilities probably cannot always match the results obtained in randomized clinical trials.

Randomized clinical trials, at their best, are capable only of establishing the benefit of treatment under current conditions. Not infrequently, however, the introduction of a new treatment can itself alter current conditions and produce secondary or dynamic effects. Randomized clinical trials have a limited ability to assess the secondary effects of treatment. This is especially true for those effects that are more likely to occur when the therapy is widely applied in clinical practice. Consider the following hypothetical study:

> A new drug called Herp-Ex was shown to have efficacy in a randomized clinical trial. It was shown to reduce the frequency of attacks when used in patients with severe recurrent herpes genitalis. It did not, however, cure the infection. The investigators were impressed with the results of the study and advocated use of Herp-Ex for all individuals with herpes genitalis.

If Herp-Ex is approved for clinical use, several effects may occur that may not have been expected on the basis of a randomized clinical trial. First, the drug would most likely be widely used, extending its use beyond the indications in the original trial. Patients with mild attacks or who present with first episodes would most likely also receive the therapy. This often occurs because once a drug is approved, clinicians have a right to prescribe it for other indications. The efficacy shown for recurrent severe attacks of herpes genitalis may not translate into effectiveness for uses that extend beyond the original indications. Second, the widespread use of Herp-Ex may result in strains of herpes that are resistant to the drug. Thus, long-term efficacy may not match the short-term results. Finally, the widespread use of Herp-Ex and short-term success may reduce the sexual precautions taken by those with recurrent herpes genitalis. Thus, over time the number of cases of herpes genitalis may actually increase despite, or because of, the short-term efficacy of Herp-Ex.

Randomized clinical trials are a fundamental tool for assessing the efficacy of therapy. When carefully used, they serve as a basis for extrapolations about the effectiveness of therapy in clinical practice. Randomized clinical trials, however, are not specifically designed to assess the safety of therapy.

Safety of therapy is more difficult to extrapolate than efficacy. Patients, in practice, may be on complicated treatments for multiple diseases or may have reduced renal or hepatic function, which results in exclusion from the randomized clinical trial. Thus, side effects may be more common in practice than in the randomized clinical trial. A special problem exists for rare but serious side effects. The heart of the problem stems from the large number of individuals who need to receive the treatment before rare but serious side effects are likely to be observed.

The number of exposures required to ensure a 95% probability of observing at least one episode of a rare side effect is summarized in the *rule of three*. According to this rule, to achieve a 95% chance of observing at least one case of penicillin anaphylaxis, which occurs on average about 1 time per 10,000, one needs to treat 30,000 individuals. If the investigator wishes to be 95% certain to observe at least one case of irreversible aplastic anemia from chloramphenicol, which occurs about 1 time per 50,000 uses, the investigator would need to treat 150,000 patients with chloramphenicol. In general terms, the rule of three states that to be 95% sure we will observe at least one case of a rare side effect, we need to treat approximately three times the number of individuals that is expected to produce one case of a side effect.[16]

It is possible to use the rule of three in reverse to draw safety conclusions from a randomized clinical trial when there is no evidence in the investigation of rare but serious side effects. Imagine that 3,000 patients have received the new treatment and there is no evidence of a rare but serious side effect such as anaphylaxis. Then we can be 95% confident that if anaphylaxis occurs, its frequency of occurrence, on average, is no more than 1 per 1,000 uses. Most randomized clinical trials use fewer than 3,000 individuals in each group. If only 300 receive the new medication and no anaphylaxis is observed, then we can conclude with 95% confidence that if anaphylaxis occurs, its frequency of occurrence, on average, is no more than 1 per 100 uses. This may not be a very reassuring conclusion.

These numbers demonstrate that randomized clinical trials cannot be expected to detect many rare but important side effects. To deal with this dilemma, we often rely on animal testing. High doses of the drug are usually administered to a variety of animal species on the assumption that toxic, teratogenic, and carcinogenic effects of the drug will be observed in at least one of the animal species tested. This approach has been helpful but has not entirely solved the problem.

Long-term consequences of widely applied preventive treatments may be even more difficult to detect. Diethylstilbestrol (DES) was used for many years to prevent spontaneous abortions. It took decades before investigators noted greatly increased incidence of vaginal carcinoma among teenage girls whose mothers had taken DES.

It is only in clinical practice that a great number of patients are likely to receive the therapy. Therefore, in clinical practice we are likely to observe these rare but serious side effects. Alert clinicians and clinical investigators have been the mainstay of our current postmarketing surveillance. We currently do not have a fully developed systematic approach for detecting rare but serious side effects once a drug is released for clinical use. The FDA still relies heavily on the reports received from clinicians through what is called a *spontaneous reporting system.* Thus, clinicians must remember that FDA approval should not be equated with complete safety or even with clearly defined and well-understood risks.

Randomized clinical trials are central to our current system for evaluating the efficacy of drugs and procedures. They represent a major advance. However, as practitioners reading the health literature, we must understand their strengths and limitations. We must be prepared to draw our own conclusions about the application of the results to our own patients, institution, or community. We must also recognize that randomized clinical trials can provide only limited data on the safety and effectiveness of the therapy being investigated.

---

[16] These numbers assume there is no spontaneous or background incidence of these side effects. If these diseases occur from other causes, the numbers needed are even greater.

10 Database Research: Retrospective Cohort Studies

The immense growth in computer capacity and the rapid acceleration of data collection in the health care system in recent years have expanded potential approaches to health research. Long-term databases collected for research or other purposes such as billing are potentially available for research. In addition, it is now possible for investigators to use databases collected for the primary purpose of ongoing clinical care.[1]

Data that are collected as long-term research databases or collected in the course of health care can be used to conduct case-control studies.[2] More often they are used to conduct cohort studies. The type of cohort study done on an existing database is called a *retrospective cohort study* or a *nonconcurrent cohort study*. Sometimes, this type of research is called *outcomes* research since it is often used to evaluate the effectiveness as well as the safety of interventions.

Remember that a cohort study is defined by the fact that study and control groups are identified or observed before determining the investigation's outcome. Thus, at the time the investigators determine the assignment to study and control groups, they are not aware of the individual's endpoint or outcome.

In preceding chapters, we discussed cohort studies in which individuals are observed over time to determine their outcomes. We call this a concurrent cohort study or prospective cohort study because individuals are monitored concurrently or prospectively over time. In concurrent or prospective cohort studies, the treatment an individual received, or their observed assignment, is ideally identified at the time they first receive the treatment. For example, we might observe one group of patients who underwent surgery, the study group, and another group of patients who received medical treatment, the control group, in 2000. Then the study and the control groups would be observed over time to determine their outcome. The surgical and the medical patients might be monitored to assess their outcome from immediately after they were identified in 2000 until 2005.

With the availability of computerized databases on patients recorded during the course of their health care, it is possible to conduct a second type of cohort study, the nonconcurrent or retrospective cohort study. In this type of cohort study, it is not necessary to identify the treatment individuals received at one point in time and then to monitor them over time to determine the outcomes. In retrospective cohort studies, the information on treatment that an individual received in 2000 can be obtained from a database in 2005. By the time an investigation is

---

[1] HIPAA regulations have restricted the use of data that can be traced back to the individual, which has made it more difficult to use data that was not developed for research purposes.

[2] Case-control studies in which the cases and controls are identified from a database created for a cohort study or a randomized clinical trial are often called a *nested case-control study*. When the database used is representative of a population, the case-control study is called A *population-based case-control study*.

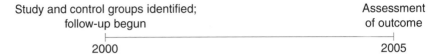

Figure 10.1. Time sequence of a concurrent or prospective cohort study.

begun in 2005, for instance, the assessment of outcome is already recorded in the computer database. To conduct a retrospective cohort study, the investigators could proceed as follows:

> In February 2005, investigators begin a study. The investigators search the database for all patients who underwent surgery and for all patients who received medical treatment for recurrent otitis media in 2000. Those who underwent surgery become the study group and those who received medication become the control group. After performing this observed assignment, the investigators search the database to determine the outcomes that occurred from the time of the assignment to study and control groups through January 2005.

A retrospective cohort study is still a cohort study because the study and control groups are assigned before the investigators become aware of the individuals' outcomes. It is not legitimate for the investigators to search the database for the outcomes until they have completed the assignment process, even though these outcomes have already occurred by the time the investigation is begun in February 2005.

Figures 10.1 and 10.2 demonstrate the conduct of concurrent (prospective) and nonconcurrent (retrospective) cohort studies. Both types of studies may be used to investigate either the cause of disease or the benefits and harms of therapy. Increasingly, retrospective cohort studies are being used to study the outcome of therapies, their effectiveness and safety. When the data comes from actual clinical practice, it can often complement the information that can be obtained from randomized clinical trials. That is, information from randomized clinical trials and information based on collection of data in the course of clinical practice can be used together to provide a fuller picture than can be obtained from either one alone.

Thus are a variety of potential uses of database research, including:

- Investigating potential improvements in outcomes that are expected to be too small to warrant a randomized clinical trial.
- Providing evidence for "altering the cause alters the effect," the third criteria of contributory cause, when randomized clinical trials are not ethical or practical.

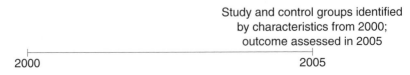

Figure 10.2. Time sequence of a nonconcurrent or retrospective cohort study.

- Investigating the impact of a therapy in a practice setting to establish effectiveness after efficacy has been established by randomized clinical trials.
- Investigating issues of safety after a new therapy has been approved for clinical use based on short term and/or relative small randomized clinical trials.

In this chapter, we will discuss costs, resource use, and other administrative issues that cannot be adequately addressed in randomized clinical trials. We will use the M.A.A.R.I.E. framework to examine retrospective cohort studies. We will look at how the information they provide is often different from and often complements the information obtained from randomized clinical trials. We will also examine the limitation of these types of investigations.

Method

The study's population chosen for retrospective cohort studies differ from randomized clinical trials in two important respects. First, randomized clinical trials are designed to include a homogeneous group of individuals who meet clearly defined inclusion and exclusion criteria. The study and control groups often are not designed to reflect the target population. That is, patients in a randomized clinical trial are not generally selected to reflect the entire spectrum of patients who would receive the treatment if applied in clinical practice.

Retrospective cohort studies that are conducted on the basis of data from ongoing clinical care are quite different from randomized clinical trials. By definition, they include those individuals who have received the treatment in clinical practice. Thus, everything else being equal, the result of a retrospective cohort study is a better reflection of the result that we could expect for patients in clinical practice. Thus retrospective cohort studies can often produce important information on the effectiveness and safety of the treatment as actually used in practice. Failure to appreciate this distinction can lead to the following type of error:

> A randomized clinical trial of nasal polyp surgery for individuals with recurrent sinusitis, aspirin allergy, and asthma demonstrated the efficacy of surgery. A retrospective cohort study using a database from ongoing clinical care was also conducted. It identified all patients who had undergone the same type of nasal polyp surgery and a comparable control group who had not undergone the surgery. The retrospective cohort study did not demonstrate effectiveness. Reviewers of these studies relied on the randomized clinical trial exclusively because of its inherently superior study design.

The randomized clinical trial and the retrospective cohort study address different questions and investigate different populations. Randomized clinical trials are the gold standard for determining efficacy for a specific indication. Efficacy for one clear-cut, narrowly defined indication for treatment such as the patient with recurrent sinusitis, aspirin allergy, and asthma may tell us very little about the outcomes the therapy produces when applied to a broader target population in clinical practice. The outcomes of a therapy for a target population in clinical practice defines its effectiveness. Efficacy is defined by the results of a randomized clinical trial.

Thus, the results of a retrospective cohort study, everything else being equal, may add to or complement the result of a randomized clinical trial by providing information on effectiveness in clinical practice.

Databases from clinical practice can be especially useful for investigating safety issues. As we have seen, patients in randomized clinical trials are often carefully chosen because they have only one or a limited number of diseases and are taking few, if any, medications other than the treatment being investigated. Once approved, these same treatments are often prescribed to patients with multiple diseases who are taking multiple medications. Thus data from clinical practice can be more dependable in detecting side effects due to interactions between treatments and between the treatment and other diseases. The ability of database research to detect these types of adverse effects is illustrated in the next example.

> A randomized clinical trial of a new medication for treatment of type 2 diabetes was used on newly diagnosed type 2 diabetics without other disease and who were not taking other medication. The treatment was very successful and no severe side effects were found. When approved and used in practice, the treatment was found to worsen kidney function among diabetics who were also being treated for hypertension with a wide range of antihypertensive medications.

The interaction between medications can easily be missed in randomized clinical trials when patients are only taking one medication for one disease. This type of side effects can often be detected using databases that more fully reflect clinical experience with the medication.

In addition to the advantages of investigating a study population of patients derived from clinical practice, retrospective cohort studies may include data on a much larger number of patients than randomized clinical trials. The number of patients included in randomized clinical trials is limited by time, money, and availability of patients. The sample sizes chosen, in fact, are often designed to be the smallest number that will provide acceptable statistical power (i.e., the largest acceptable Type II error, usually 10% to 20%) in addressing efficacy using what is called the primary endpoint. As discussed in the preceding chapter on randomized clinical trials, these numbers usually vary from less than 100 in both the study group and the control group to several thousand in each group.

The sample size in retrospective cohort studies is limited mainly by the availability of patient data in the database. Thousands or even millions of patients may be included. Thus, the potential sample size for retrospective cohort studies may dwarf that of randomized clinical trials. This difference in sample sizes may have important implications, as illustrated in the next example:

> A randomized clinical trial was conducted comparing removal of colon polyps versus observation. The study and control groups each included 500 patients. The investigation demonstrated a small but not statistically significant reduction in the subsequent rate of colon cancer. A retrospective cohort study using 10,000 patients who had polyp removal and 10,000 patients who underwent observation demonstrates a small difference in the subsequent rate of colon cancer, but the P-value was 0.00001 and the confidence limits were very narrow.

This type of discrepancy between the results of a randomized clinical trial and those of a retrospective cohort study is expected. If the retrospective cohort study is able to avoid the biases to which it is susceptible, we would expect the retrospective cohort study to have a far greater statistical power. That is, it would have a much greater chance of demonstrating statistical significance if a true difference exists in the population being sampled.

The advantages of large numbers are not limited to questions of effectiveness. Large numbers also allow us to address questions of safety, especially issues of rare but serious side effects. As we saw in our look at randomized clinical trials, the rule of three indicates that when a rare but serious side effect occurs on average once in 10,000 uses, we need to observe 30,000 exposures before we can be 95% certain that we will see at least one episode of the side effect. Numbers of this magnitude are rarely available in randomized clinical trials, but they may be available through database research. Thus, for small but real differences, everything else being equal, retrospective cohort studies often have a much greater probability of demonstrating statistical significance.

Assignment

When discussing retrospective cohort studies and comparing them with randomized clinical trials, we have repeatedly used the phrase "everything else being equal." "Everything else" is not usually equal when we compare these two types of studies because retrospective cohort studies are susceptible to a variety of potential biases. These potential biases are most dramatic in the area of assignment.

Randomized clinical trials by definition use randomization for their assignment process. The process of randomization is the hallmark of a randomized clinical trial. Remember that the process of randomization is designed to take into account not only the factors that are known to affect outcome but also those factors that have an effect on outcome we do not anticipate.

In retrospective cohort studies, assignment of patients to study and control groups is based on clinicians' treatment of patients. Clinicians try to tailor the treatment to the patient. When clinicians are successful in tailoring treatment to individuals, selection biases are created. Selection bias occurs, for instance, when clinicians assign patients with different prognoses to different treatments. In fact, we can regard the job of clinical care as one of creating biases by tailoring the treatment to the patient. The job of the clinician, then, is to create selection biases, and the job of the researcher is to untangle these selection biases. Selection bias created in database research has been called *case-mix bias.* Let us see how this type of confounding variable may influence the results:

> A randomized clinical trial of a smoking-cessation drug demonstrated a small, statistically significant reduction in smoking among those randomized to the drug. A large, retrospective cohort study identified those prescribed the drug and compared success in quitting among smokers who were prescribed the drug versus smokers who were not prescribed the drug. The investigation demonstrated a much larger reduction in smoking among those prescribed the drug.

The patients prescribed the drug in the retrospective cohort study may have been those who were especially motivated to stop smoking. Clinicians may have tailored their treatment by perhaps giving more intensive treatment to the patients they thought would benefit the most. This is a natural and often desirable tendency in clinical care. However, from the researcher's perspective, selecting motivated patients to receive the treatment results in the type of confounding variable we have called selection bias. This is the situation, since those who receive the treatment are the same individuals who are especially likely to quit smoking.

Recognizing the confounding variables created by the process of clinical care is important so these confounding variable can be taken into account in the analysis.[3]

Randomized clinical trials are often precluded by ethical issues and practical issues. Once it is suspected that a treatment benefits patients, clinicians and patients will often be unwilling to randomize patients to receive or not to receive the treatment. Thus, a retrospective cohort study may be the best available study design even when a randomized clinical trial would, in theory, be preferable.

In addition to randomized assignment, an ideal randomized clinical trial is also double-masked. That is, neither the patient nor the investigator is aware of the treatment being received. However, as we saw in Chapter 9, double-masked studies are often either unethical, impractical, or unsuccessful. Patient masking is not possible in a retrospective cohort study of a database from ongoing clinical care. In addition, the clinician who prescribes the treatment is not masked. Thus, for both randomized clinical trials and retrospective studies, we often need to ask what the implications are of a lack of masking. To do this, we usually need to examine how the method of assignment affects the results of the assessment process.

Assessment

The process of follow-up and assessment in well-conducted randomized clinical trials and retrospective cohort studies is very different. In a randomized clinical trial, patients in the study group and the control group are followed up at predetermined intervals, which are the same for the two groups. The same data are collected on individuals in each group at the predetermined follow-up intervals. The goal of randomized clinical trials is to investigate efficacy. The length of follow-up is usually determined by the minimum length of time needed to establish efficacy. Thus randomized clinical trials are often short-term trials designed to establish short-term efficacy. Longer-term efficacy may not be well studied in randomized clinical trials. In addition, side effects that take longer periods to develop may be missed entirely by randomized clinical trials but detected by retrospective cohort studies, as illustrated in the next example.

> The new diabetic medication was tested for six months to determine whether it could reduce and maintain a reduction in hyperglycemia. The drug was found to have efficacy and to satisfy the safety requirements for approval. When used in practice, however, it was found that despite its continued efficacy, after 6 months it was associated with a frequency of severe liver disease far above that expected on the basis of the 6-month study.

As illustrated in this example, retrospective cohort studies may help to extend the results of randomized clinical trials over longer periods of time and may help to detect longer-term safety problems that randomized clinical trials are not capable of identifying.

The process of follow-up and assessment in a retrospective cohort study is very different because it occurs as part of the course of health care. Data are collected if and when the patient returns for care. This return visit may be initiated by the clinician or the patient. Thus, the frequency of data collection, the type of

---

[3] Unfortunately, databases obtained from clinical care may lack the data needed to measure some important variables that should ideally be taken into account in the analysis.

data, and even the accuracy of the data collected are likely to be quite different in randomized clinical trials and retrospective cohort studies. These differences in follow-up may actually make it more difficult to detect certain types of side effects of treatment, as illustrated in the next example:

> A randomized clinical trial comparing surgery versus medication for benign prostate hypertrophy found that surgery produces far more retrograde ejaculation and impotence than medication. A retrospective cohort study using records from ongoing medical care found no difference in these adverse effects, as recorded in the patients' charts.

Unless patients are specifically asked or tested for these side effects, they may not recognize them or report them to clinicians. Thus, in retrospective cohort studies, the type of outcome measure that can be reliably used may be much more limited than in a randomized clinical trial, in which these side effects can be assessed in the same way for each group at the same time intervals.

Results

In randomized clinical trials, as we saw in Chapter 9 analysis is conducted using the principle of intention-to-treat. Thus, individuals are analyzed according to their assignment group even if they deviated from the protocol and never actually received the treatment. Remember that this is done so individuals with good prognosis are not disproportionately represented among those who are left after many participants with a poorer prognosis drop out of the study.

It is possible to aim for a comparable technique in retrospective cohort studies by making the assignment to groups, on the basis of the prescribed treatment and analyzing patients in their original groups including those who do not continue on the treatment. However, this may not be successful in database research because the only patients who appear in the database may be those who actually take the treatment and obtain follow-up, as illustrated in the next example:

> Radiation therapy for a specific type of metastatic brain cancer was studied using a retrospective cohort study. Radiation required premedication and could be started only after a month of pretreatment. The database recorded only patients who received the treatment and those who did not. Among those receiving the radiation therapy, survival was two months longer on average. The results were statistically significant. The investigators concluded that the retrospective cohort study had demonstrated the short-term effectiveness of radiation therapy.

The fact that the radiation therapy could not be undertaken for at least a month after it was prescribed may mean that those with the worst prognosis had already died or become too ill to receive the radiation therapy. Thus, the retrospective cohort study may have examined a study group with a better prognosis than the control group, indicating the groups may not actually have been analyzed using a method analogous to the intention-to-treat method.

In randomized clinical trials, adjustment is used as a way to account for the known prognostic factors that, despite randomization, differ between the study and control groups. Randomization itself often results in known prognostic factors being similar in the study and control groups. In addition, randomization has the aim to produce similarity even for unknown prognostic factors. Adjustment is still used in a randomized clinical trial; however, its role is only to take into account the differences that occur despite randomization.

In a retrospective cohort study, adjustment has a much larger role. It attempts to recognize and take into account all the differences between the study and control groups that may affect the outcome being measured. Adequate adjustment requires recognizing all potential confounding variables and taking them into account in the adjustment process, even though differences between groups are not substantial or statistically significant.[4]

Interpretation

As a type of cohort study, retrospective cohort studies are best designed to demonstrate that the treatment is associated with an improved outcome and that the treatment precedes the outcome. Even when this is successful, however, we are often left with some doubt as to the third criterion of contributory cause, or efficacy, of therapy: altering the "cause" alters the "effect."

A special type of retrospective cohort study, however, may help to establish that altering the cause alters the effect. This type of investigation recognizes that a change has occurred in one group over a period of time but not in another comparable group. The probability of a particular outcome before and after the change in each group is then calculated to determine whether the outcome was altered in the group that experienced the change. This type of investigation has been called a *natural experiment* since we are observing changes that occur in the natural course of events, not due to an investigator's intervention. Let us see how a natural experiment may enable us to draw the conclusion that altering the cause alters the effect:

> Cigarettes were smoked with nearly equal frequency among male physicians and attorneys in the 1960s, and they had a similar probability of developing lung cancer. During the 1970s, a large proportion of male physicians quit smoking cigarettes, whereas a smaller proportion of male attorneys quit smoking cigarettes. The investigators observed that both male physicians and male attorneys who stopped smoking had a reduction in their probability of developing lung cancer and that the probability of developing lung cancer among male physicians in subsequent years was far lower than among male attorneys.

A randomized clinical trial of cigarette smoking would have been the ideal method for establishing that altering the cause alters the effect. This type of natural experiment is the next best method. It is often, as in this situation, the only ethical and feasible method for establishing this cause-and-effect relationship.

After analysis of the results and interpretation are completed using all the individuals included in either a randomized clinical trial or a retrospective cohort study, the investigators are often interested in examining the meaning of the results for special groups included in the study. This process is referred to as *subgroup analysis*.[5] The large numbers of patients included in a retrospective cohort study may allow the investigators to subdivide the study group and control group into smaller subgroups and examine the therapy's effectiveness for these groups.

---

[4] Adjustment may also aim to consider the interactions that occur between confounding variables.

[5] Subgroup analysis, in general, should only be conducted after obtaining statistically significant results using all the data. In addition it should only be conducted to examine relationships hypothesized prior to collecting the data.

Because of the larger numbers, the data from the retrospective cohort studies' subgroups may be more reliable than those from subgroups derived from randomized clinical trials. This may have important implications, as illustrated in the next example:

> A randomized clinical trial of one-vessel coronary artery disease demonstrated that angiography had greater efficacy, on average, than drug treatment. Subgroup analysis performed by creating groups that differed in their extent of myocardium served by the vessel, age of the patients, and gender of the patient was not able to demonstrate statistically significant differences between these groups. A large retrospective cohort study demonstrated overall effectiveness of angiography, but also demonstrated that this effectiveness was limited to younger men and to patients with a lesion supplying a large area of myocardium.

This type of result illustrates the principle that the larger number of patients who may be available in a retrospective cohort study enables the study to better address issues among subgroups than even most well-designed, randomized clinical trials. This use of randomized clinical trials and retrospective cohort studies demonstrates the potential to use the results of one type of study to supplement the results of the other.

Extrapolation

Extrapolation of the results of a randomized clinical trial always requires making assumptions about the population that will receive the treatment (i.e., the target population). Remember that randomized clinical trials are usually conducted using homogeneous patients. That is, they often exclude patient who are not on multiple treatments, who do not have liver or kidney disease complicating their management, and who often do not have other diseases. In addition, special precautions may be used in randomized clinical trials to exclude patients who have special characteristics, such as those who are not likely to follow up or who are likely to become pregnant. Thus, the patients included in randomized clinical trials are often quite different from those included in retrospective cohort studies. Therefore, the results of a randomized clinical trial and those of a retrospective cohort study may look very different, even when the new therapy is administered using the same implementation procedures, as illustrated in the next example:

> A randomized clinical trial of a new method of home dialysis for newly diagnosed renal failure patients demonstrated substantial improvement in outcome compared with outpatient hemodialysis. The new dialysis method was then made available using the same implementation procedures to all dialysis patients throughout the country in two stages. During the first stage, all those using the new technique were compared with all those using standard outpatient hemodialysis in a retrospective cohort study. The investigators found no difference in outcome between the new home dialysis method and standard outpatient hemodialysis.

A randomized clinical trial on a small homogeneous group of new dialysis patients may show very different results compared with a retrospective cohort study involving a larger number of more heterogeneous patients. For instance, patients who are accustomed to outpatient hemodialysis may have difficulty switching to the new treatment. Patients with more complications or long-standing outpatient hemodialysis may not do as well on the new therapy.

Thus, we cannot necessarily expect that the results of a randomized clinical trial and those of a retrospective cohort study will be the same even when both are well designed and the therapy is administered using the same implementation procedures. It is still likely that for carefully selected patients, like those in the randomized clinical trial, the new method of home dialysis is better than the standard therapy.

As we discussed, randomized clinical trials are limited to assessing outcomes or endpoints at one point in time. They actually represent a snapshot view of the therapy's effects. After they are introduced into practice, dynamic effects may occur that may alter the longer-term effectiveness of the therapy. Resistance may occur; the treatment may be used for new indications, producing more or less effectiveness; or patient behavior may change, altering the effectiveness of treatment.

Retrospective cohort studies may be more successful in detecting these changes in effectiveness that occur over time. The large number of patients in a database may allow the investigator to compare the outcomes that occurred when the treatment was prescribed in different years. Alternatively, the degree of effectiveness can be followed over extended periods, and an assessment can be made of the persistence of a benefit. This advantage of retrospective cohort studies is illustrated in the next example:

> A new high-energy treatment for kidney stones has been demonstrated in a randomized clinical trial to have efficacy in the treatment of obstruction of a ureter compared with surgery when patients are observed for 3 years. A retrospective cohort study was performed on obstruction of a ureter caused by kidney stones treated with the new technique and followed for up to 10 years. The results demonstrated less efficacy for the new treatment compared with surgery. Those undergoing surgery actually did better after 3 years.

These two results may both be true. They may complement each other. This could be the case if the new treatment increases the rate of recurrence of kidney stones. The relatively short-term follow-up that is usually possible in randomized clinical trials leaves an important role for retrospective cohort studies using databases obtained from ongoing clinical care in the longer-term assessment of safety and efficacy.

Remember that randomized clinical trials are the gold standard for assessing efficacy, but they have severe limitations when assessing effectiveness for the target population, when assessing the occurrence of rare but serious side effects, and when examining the longer-term results of the treatment. Retrospective cohort studies can complement randomized clinical trials and compensate for some or all of these deficiencies.

11 Meta-analysis

Thus far, we have examined the three basic types of investigations in the health research literature which are designed to compare study and control groups: case-control studies, cohort studies, and randomized clinical trials. Each study type can be used to address the same relationship such as the relationship between strokes and birth control pills that we illustrated in Chapter 2. These investigations often provide consistent results. At times, however, studies published in the health research literature seem to conflict with one another, making it difficult to provide definitive answers to important study questions.

It is often desirable to be able to combine data obtained in a variety of investigations and to use all the information to address a study question. *Meta-analysis* is a collection of methods for combining information from different investigations in order to reach conclusions or address questions that were not possible on the basis of a single investigation.

Meta-analysis aims to produce its conclusion by combining data from two or more existing investigations. Traditionally, this process of research synthesis has been the review article's role. In recent years, it has been increasingly recognized that the informal and subjective process of literature review has not always produced accurate conclusions. Let us examine one extreme example indicating why this might occur.

Assume that we are interested in examining a recent innovation in the treatment of coronary artery disease known as transthoracic laser coronaryplasty (TLC). TLC is designed to treat coronary artery disease through the chest wall without using invasive techniques. The first two studies of TLC produced the following results:

Study 1

	Die	Live	Total
TLC	230	50	280
Control	530	210	740

$$\text{Relative risk} = \frac{230/280}{530/740} = \frac{0.821}{0.716} = 1.15$$

$$\text{Odds ratio} = \frac{230/50}{530/210} = \frac{4.60}{2.52} = 1.83$$

$$\text{Risk difference} = 0.716 - 0.821 = -0.105$$

$$\text{Number needed to treat} = \frac{1}{0.716 - 0.821} = -9.5$$

Study 2

	Die	Live	Total
TLC	190	405	595
Control	50	210	260

$$\text{Relative risk} = \frac{190/595}{50/260} = \frac{0.319}{0.192} = 1.66$$

$$\text{Odds ratio} = \frac{190/405}{50/210} = \frac{0.469}{0.238} = 1.97$$

$$\text{Risk difference} = 0.192 - 0.319 = -0.127$$

$$\text{Number needed to treat} = \frac{1}{0.192 - 0.319} = -7.9$$

Investigators were discouraged and feared that this new procedure would not have a bright future. Before relegating this technique to history, however, they decided to combine the results of the two studies and see what happened. Combining the data from the two studies produced the results shown below.

Notice that the differences in outcomes now favor TLC as measured by the odds ratio, the relative risk, or the number needed to treat almost as strongly as the single studies argued against the efficacy of TLC. Thus, combining studies may produce some surprising results.[1]

This process set into motion a widespread effort to evaluate the use of TLC in a variety of settings and for a variety of indications worldwide. Most studies focused on single-vessel coronary artery disease as assessed by new noninvasive procedures. Over the next several years, dozens of studies resulted in apparently conflicting results. Thus, it was considered important to conduct a full-scale meta-analysis evaluating the effects of TLC on single-vessel coronary artery disease.

Combined Studies 1 and 2

	Die	Live	Total
TLC	420	455	875
Control	580	420	1,000

$$\text{Relative risk} = \frac{420/875}{580/1,000} = \frac{0.480}{0.580} = 0.827$$

$$\text{Odds ratio} = \frac{420/875}{580/420} = \frac{0.923}{1.381} = 0.668$$

$$\text{Risk difference} = 0.580 - 0.480 = 0.10$$

$$\text{Number needed to treat} = \frac{1}{0.580 - 0.480} = 10$$

[1] This is known as *Simpson's Paradox*. It is a very unusual situation illustrated here because of its dramatic impact. Its occurence requires large differences between the numbers of study and control group participants in the two studies.

Method

The process of combining information using meta-analysis can be best understood if we regard each of the studies included in the analysis as parallel to one study site in a multiple-site investigation. In a multiple-site investigation, the investigator combines the data from multiple sites to draw conclusions or interpretations. In meta-analysis, the investigator combines information from multiple studies to draw conclusions or interpretations. This parallel structure allows us to learn about meta-analysis using the M.A.A.R.I.E. framework.

As with our other uses of the M.A.A.R.I.E. framework, we start by defining the study question or study hypothesis. Meta-analysis can be used to accomplish a variety of purposes. It may begin by defining a hypothesis related to the specific purpose for conducting the meta-analysis. Meta-analysis might be used to accomplish any of the following purposes:

- Establish statistical significance when studies are conflicting
- Establish the best possible estimate of the magnitude of the effect
- Evaluate harms or safety when small numbers of side effects are observed in studies
- Examine subgroups when the numbers in individual studies are not large enough

As with our other types of investigations, the investigators ideally begin with a study hypothesis and proceed to test that hypothesis and draw inferences. When they do this for a therapy, for instance, they may hypothesize that the treatment has been shown to have efficacy.

The studies that should be included in a meta-analysis depend on the purpose of the analysis. Thus, the study hypothesis of the meta-analysis helps to determine the inclusion and exclusion criteria that should be used in identifying relevant studies. The following example shows how the hypothesis can help to determine which studies to include:

> In preparation for a meta-analysis, researchers searched the world's literature and obtained the following 25 studies of TLC for single-vessel coronary artery disease. These investigations had characteristics which allowed them to be grouped into the following types of studies:
>
> A. Five studies of men with single-vessel disease treated initially with coronary bypass surgery versus medication versus TLC
> B. Five studies of men and women treated initially with TLC versus bypass surgery
> C. Five studies of men and women treated initially with TLC versus medication
> D. Five studies of men treated with TLC versus medication after previous bypass surgery
> E. Five studies of women treated with repeat TLC versus medication after previous TLC

If the meta-analysis is designed to test a hypothesis, then the studies to be included are chosen because they address issues relevant to the hypothesis. For instance, if the investigator wanted to test the hypothesis that men do better than women when TLC is used to treat single-vessel coronary artery disease, then studies B and C should be used in the meta-analysis. These investigations include comparisons of the outcomes in both men and women.

If the investigators were interested in testing the hypothesis that initial TLC is better than surgery for single-vessel coronary artery disease, then studies A and B should be used in the meta-analysis because these studies compare TLC versus surgery as the initial therapy. Alternatively, if the researcher hypothesized that medication was the best treatment for single-vessel coronary artery disease, then studies A, C, D, and E would be used. In general, the studies that are used are determined by purpose of the investigation as defined by the study hypothesis of the meta-analysis.

Despite the many similarities between meta-analysis and a multi-site investigation, there is one important difference. In original research, in theory the investigator may define the study question, then find settings and study participants that are suited to addressing the question, and determine the desired sample size. In meta-analysis, the questions we may ask are often limited by the availability of previous studies. Thus, the study population and the sample size are largely outside the investigator's control.

To try to circumvent this problem, meta-analysis researchers often define a question or issue broadly and begin by identifying all investigations related to that issue. When this is done, the investigators are conducting an *exploratory meta-analysis* as opposed to a *hypothesis-driven meta-analysis*.

In conducting an exploratory meta-analysis of TLC, for instance, the investigator might initially include all 25 studies just mentioned. Thus, the meta-analysis researcher would define the study group as consisting of those who received TLC, and the control group would consist of all the individuals receiving other therapy.

This process of using all available studies without a specific hypothesis is parallel to the process of conducting a conventional investigation without defining a study hypothesis. This type of exploratory meta-analysis can be useful, but must be conducted carefully and interpreted differently from hypothesis-driven meta-analysis. Despite the potential dangers of combining studies with very different characteristics, the limited number of available studies makes it important for meta-analysis to include techniques for combining very different types of studies.

Meta-analysis attempts to turn the diversity of studies into an advantage. Combining studies with different characteristics may allow us to harness the benefit of diversity. By including apples and oranges, we can ask whether it makes a difference if a fruit is an apple or an orange, or whether it is enough that it is a fruit.

The approach for harnessing the benefit of diversity is discussed later. For now, we must recognize that there are actually two types of meta-analysis, hypothesis-based and exploratory.

It is important to remember that the fundamental difference between meta-analysis and other types of investigations is that the data have already been collected and the researcher's choice is limited to including or excluding an existing study from the meta-analysis. Thus, the sample size in meta-analysis is limited by the existence of relevant studies.

Other types of investigations usually start by defining the question to be investigated. This question determines the types of individuals who should be included in the investigation. Similarly, the question to be addressed by a meta-analysis determines the types of studies that should be included in the meta-analysis. Thus, in hypothesis-driven meta-analysis, the first question we need to ask is whether a particular study is relevant to the meta-analysis's hypothesis.

Assignment

Process of Assignment

Once the study question is defined, the investigators can determine which studies to include in a meta-analysis. This identification of studies to include is the assignment process, requires us to ask: Have all the relevant studies been identified?[2]

Identifying all relevant studies is an essential step in the assignment process of a meta-analysis. It is important that the investigator describe the method used to search for research reports, including enough detail to allow subsequent investigators to obtain all the identified literature.[3] This can even include unpublished data. Doctoral dissertations, abstracts, grant reports, and registries of studies are other possible ways to locate previous research.

Confounding Variable: Publication Bias

An extensive search for research reports as part of the assignment process in a meta-analysis is important due to the potential for a special type of selection bias known as *publication bias*. Publication bias occurs when there is a systematic tendency to publish studies with positive results and to not publish studies that suggest no differences in outcome. Small investigations are frequently not submitted or are rejected for publication. The next example illustrates publication bias:

> After identifying the studies available through a computerized search of published articles, the TLC meta-analysis researchers identified 20 studies of the relationship between TLC and single-vessel coronary artery disease. There was a wide variation in the sample sizes of the studies and in the outcomes, as shown in Table 11.1.

One technique that can be used to assess the presence and extent of possible publication bias is known as the *funnel diagram*. The funnel diagram can be understand by examining Table 11.1 and Fig. 11.1.

The funnel diagram is based on the principle that smaller studies, by chance alone, are expected to produce results with greater variation. A funnel diagram that does not suggest the presence of publication bias should look like a funnel, with larger variation in results among smaller studies. Cases in which the lower side of the funnel is incomplete, as in Fig. 11.1A, suggest that some studies are missing.[4]

Now imagine that the TLC meta-analysis researchers searched further and came up with five additional studies. They redrew their funnel diagram plotting the

---

[2] Efforts are underway to ensure registration of all randomized clinical trials thus preventing the withholding of negative results.

[3] In performing this search, it is important to avoid double counting. Studies originally presented as abstracts, for instance, will often subsequently appear as original articles. Including the same data two or more times jeopardizes the accuracy of the results of a meta-analysis by violating the assumption that the data obtained in each of the studies are independent of the other studies.

[4] Note that the scale for the odds ratio is defined so that it is equally spaced above and below 1. Thus a study with an odds ratio less than 1 is converted to its reciprocal and then plotted below the horizontal line, for instance study numbers 5, 16 and 19 are converted from 0.5 to their reciprocal 2 and then plotted.

Table 11.1. *Data from 20 studies of transthoracic laser coronaryplasty*

Study number	Odds ratio	Sample size (each group)
1	4.0	20
2	3.0	20
3	2.0	20
4	1.0	20
5	0.5	20
6	3.5	40
7	2.5	40
8	1.5	40
9	2.5	60
10	1.5	60
11	1.0	60
12	1.5	80
13	1.0	80
14	1.5	100
15	1.0	100
16	0.5	100
17	1.5	120
18	1.0	120
19	0.5	120
20	1.0	140

additional studies and obtained Fig. 11.1B. From this funnel diagram, which has a more complete funnel appearance, they concluded there was no longer evidence of publication bias and they had likely obtained all or most of the relevant studies.

Even after extensive searching, it is possible that investigations will be missed. This does not preclude proceeding with a meta-analysis. It is possible, as we will see, to take into account this potential publication bias as part of the analysis.

Another important part of the assignment process in a meta-analysis is to determine whether there are differences in the quality of studies that justify excluding low-quality studies from the meta-analysis.

There are two potential approaches to this issue. It has been argued that study types with the potential for systematic biases should be excluded from a meta-analysis. For this reason, some meta-analysis researchers have favored the exclusion of all studies except randomized clinical trials, arguing that this type of study is the least likely to produce results that have a systematic bias in one direction or the other.

If randomized clinical trials and other types of studies are available, however, an alternative approach is to include all types of studies, at least initially. All investigations are then evaluated to determine their quality. Quality scores are usually obtained by two readers of the research report, each using the same standardized scoring system without knowledge of the other reader's score or the authors' identities. Then it is possible to compare the results of high-quality studies with those of low-quality studies to determine if the results, on average, are similar. Let us examine what might happen when we combine high-quality and low-quality studies:

A meta-analysis of the strength of the relationship between TLC and the outcome of single-vessel coronary artery disease included all known studies, including case-control, cohort, and randomized clinical trials. The investigators had two readers score each investigation using the same standardized scoring system without knowledge of the other reader's score or the authors' identities. The outcomes on average for the

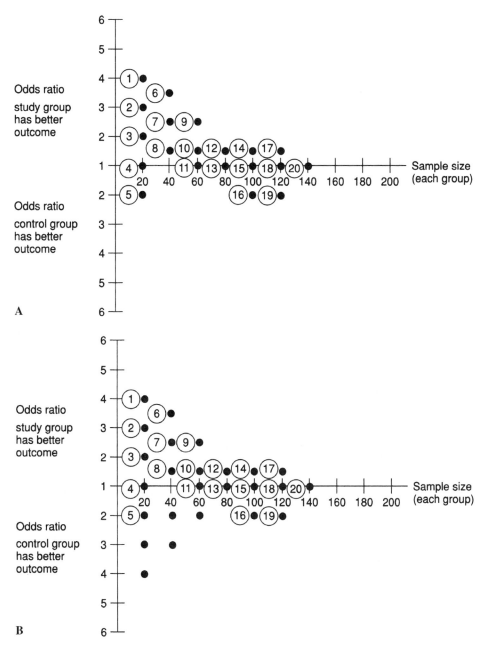

Figure 11.1. A: Funnel diagram of 20 studies of transthoracic laser coronaryplasty. **B:** Funnel diagram after adding five additional studies.

low-quality studies were approximately equal to those for the high-quality studies. Thus, the investigators decided to retain all studies in their meta-analysis.

A variety of other potential confounding variables can affect the outcome. As with conventional investigations, it is important that the investigator recognize these characteristics in order to take them into account. The usual approach is to recognize the differences as part of the assignment process and take them into account as part of the analysis.

For instance, in the TLC studies, we should know whether some studies used only older patients, more severely ill patients, or those with other characteristics or prognostic factors that often result in a poorer outcome in coronary artery disease. In addition, we would want to know whether there were important variations in the treatment given, such as different TLC techniques or different adjunct therapy, such as duration of anticoagulation. Thus, in the assignment process in a meta-analysis, we need data on the degree of uniformity of the patients and of the procedures used.

Masking

Masking of assignment in meta-analysis has a somewhat different meaning than in other types of investigations. In one sense, the meta-analysis relies on the methods used in the individual studies to mask the participants and investigators. In meta-analysis, masking of assignment can also be achieved by preventing the investigators from being biased by knowledge of the results, the authors, or other characteristics of an investigation when determining whether a particular investigation should be included in the meta-analysis. More than one individual may be asked to judge whether an investigation meets the predefined criteria for inclusion in the meta-analysis.

Assessment

In conventional investigations, whether they are case-control, cohort, or randomized clinical trials, the investigators define the techniques used to measure the outcome and collect the data to assess the outcome. In meta-analysis, the researcher is usually limited to the techniques used by the primary investigator for assessing the study outcome.

The meta-analysis is also limited by the extent of data presented and the statistical methods used in the original article. However, it is increasingly possible to go back and obtain the original data. Some journals are beginning to ask investigators who submit research articles to make available a complete data set from their study for later review by other investigators or for use in a meta-analysis. In the future, this may allow meta-analysis researchers to reexamine and redefine the various studies' outcomes so that each investigation uses the same measurement.

Precision and Accuracy

Currently, the meta-analysis researcher usually must live with what is available in existing articles. Because of the differences in the definitions and measurements of outcomes in different studies, the researcher performing a meta-analysis is faced with a series of unique issues. First, the meta-analysis researcher must determine which outcome to use in comparing studies. This may pose a serious problem, as illustrated in the next example:

In the studies of TLC, the following outcome measures were assessed. Ten studies used time until a positive stress test, time until evidence of occlusion on noninvasive angiography, and time until myocardial infarction as the outcomes. Ten other studies used only time until a positive stress test as their measure of outcome. Five studies used time until a positive stress test and evidence of occlusion on noninvasive angiography as their measures of outcome. As a result of the different outcome measurements used, the researcher concluded that a meta-analysis could not be performed.

The need to use precise and accurate measures of outcomes do pose major issues in meta-analysis.

The researcher may be interested in an accurate and early measure of outcome, which, in this case, may be a positive noninvasive angiography indicating closure of the treated vessel. Despite the desirability of using this outcome measure, if it is used to assess outcome, 10 of the 25 studies would need to be excluded. Thus, the researcher performing this meta-analysis may be forced to use time until a positive stress test as the measure of outcome if he wishes to include all the studies.

Even after determining that the measure of outcome will be time until a positive stress test, the meta-analysis researcher's problems are not solved, as shown in the following example:

The 25 studies define a positive stress test in several different ways. Some require greater duration and extent of ST depression on ECG than others. The meta-analysis researcher decides to use only studies that use the same definition of a positive stress test. Unfortunately, only 12 studies can be included in the meta-analysis.

It is important to find a common endpoint for a meta-analysis, but it is not essential that the endpoint be defined in the same way in all the studies. This is a common problem that is not generally dealt with by excluding studies. Rather, all studies with data on follow-up testing are included. The results of studies that use a common definition of a positive stress test can then be compared with studies that use other definitions. If the results are similar, regardless of the definition of a positive stress test, then all the studies can be combined in one analysis using their own definitions of a positive stress test. If there are substantial differences that depend on the definition of a positive stress test, then separate analyses can be performed for studies that used different definitions.

Completeness and Effect of Observation

The completeness of the investigations included in a meta-analysis depends on the completeness of the particular studies chosen for inclusion. The effect of observation also depends on the particular type and characteristics of the investigations that are included. Because of the large number of factors that can influence the quality of the assessment process, it is tempting for the meta-analysis investigator to eliminate studies that do not meet quality standards. As we have seen, some meta-analyses are conducted using only studies that meet predefined quality standards. Other meta-analysis researchers attempt to achieve this end by including only randomized clinical trials, presuming that they constitute the preferred type of investigation. While these are accepted approaches, others argue that both high- and low-quality studies should be included and that an analysis should be conducted to determine if they produce similar or different results.

Results

The goals of analysis of results in meta-analysis are the same as those in other types of clinical investigations. We are interested in the following:

- **Estimation.** Estimating the strength of an association or the magnitude of a difference. This is often called *effect size* in meta-analysis
- **Inference.** Performing statistical significance testing to draw inferences about the population on the basis of the data in the sample
- **Adjustment.** Adjusting for potential confounding variables to determine whether they affect the strength or statistical significance of the association or difference

Estimation

The strength of an association in meta-analysis can be estimated by using any of the estimation measures used in conventional studies. Most meta-analyses in the health literature use odds ratios, differences in probabilities, or number needed to treat. Odds ratios are often used because they can be calculated for case-control studies, cohort studies, and randomized clinical trials.[5]

When the number of patients in each group and the number who experience a particular outcome in each group are reported, it may be possible to convert one outcome measurement to another. At times, there are not enough data presented in an article to convert one estimation technique to another. Thus, it is not always possible to produce a useful estimation, even though several relevant studies are available in the literature.[6]

Inference

Even when different estimation techniques prevent calculation of an overall estimation of the strength of the association or the size of the difference, it is usually possible to perform an overall statistical significance test. As long as the type of statistical significance test used, the number of patients in each of the groups, and the p value are available, it is possible to combine the results and produce an overall statistical significance test.

When we combine a large number of studies and perform statistical significance testing, the results may be statistically significant even when the individual studies are not statistically significant. Remember from our previous discussion that when the number of patients is large, it is possible to demonstrate statistical significance even for small differences that have little or no clinical importance. Thus, in meta-analysis, it is especially important to distinguish between statistically significant and clinically important.

Statistical significance testing in meta-analysis can use two types of techniques, often called *fixed effects model* and *random effects models*. Fixed effect models assume that all the studies come from one large population and only differ by chance. Random effects models assume that there are differences between the study populations that made a difference in outcome. It is easier to demonstrate statistical significance using a fixed effect model. That is, fixed effect models have greater statistical power. However, it is useful in meta-analysis to perform both

---

[5] Continuous dependent variables such as weight or diastolic blood pressure can also be used in meta-analysis, though they require different techniques. These techniques are more frequently used in the social science literature and rarely appear in the medicine and public health literature.

[6] The increasing availability of the actual data from studies may make it easier to combine data from different studies that use different estimation techniques.

types of statistical significance tests. If their results are nearly identical, one can be confidence about combining the different studies.

Adjustment

When there is a difference between the results of a random effects and a fixed effects statistical significance test, it suggests that there are differences between the studies' populations that make a difference in their outcomes. This is a form of confounding variable.

Adjustment in meta-analysis, like adjustment in the other types of studies we have examined, is designed to take into account potential confounding variables. In meta-analysis, adjustment also has additional goals. Adjustment aims to determine whether it is legitimate to combine the results of different types of studies. It also examines the effects of including investigations with particular characteristics in the combined results. Thus the process of adjustment allows us to determine whether including studies with different characteristics, such as different types of patients or different approaches to treatment, affects the results. Looking at the impacts of those types of factors is what we mean by harnessing the benefits of diversity.

To combine investigations, we need to establish that the results are what we call *homogeneous*. This concept is illustrated in the following example:

> Assume that the randomized clinical trials and cohort studies of TLC for single-vessel coronary artery disease in Table 11.2 were identified for a meta-analysis. Look at the graph in Fig. 11.2, which compares the results of the study and control groups in these studies with respect to their outcome measure.

The two curves in Fig. 11.2 are constructed by connecting the points represented by randomized clinical trials with one another, and the points represented

Table 11.2. *Studies of transthoracic laser coronaryplasty in randomized clinical trials and cohort studies*

Study number	Adverse outcomes	Study type
1	5/100 ST	RCT
	10/100 C	
2	80/1,000 ST	RCT
	100/1,000 C	
3	25/100 ST	RCT
	20/100 C	
4	2/100 ST	RCT
	10/100 C	
5	40/1,000 ST	RCT
	120/1,000 C	RCT
6	5/100 ST	RCT
	20/100 C	RCT
7	10/100 ST	Cohort
	10/100 C	Cohort
8	20/100 ST	Cohort
	20/100 C	
9	30/1,000 ST	Cohort
	90/1,000 C	
10	60/1,000 ST	Cohort
	150/1,000 C	

ST, study; C, control; RCT, randomized clinical trial.

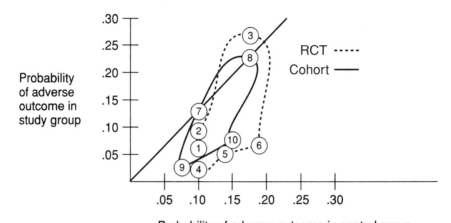

Figure 11.2. Homogeneity demonstrated by the inability to separate randomized clinical trials (RCT) from retrospective cohort studies.

by retrospective cohort studies with one another. They demonstrate a homogeneous effect because the curves overlap to a large extent. A homogeneous effect allows the meta-analysis investigator to combine the two types of studies into one analysis.

Table 11.3 and Fig. 11.3, on the other hand, show that when studies including patients with more severe illness are compared with studies including patients with less severe illness, the outcome measures are not homogeneous. The curve connecting the studies of patients with a high severity of illness can be separated from the curve connecting studies of patients with a low severity of illness. Studies

Table 11.3. *Studies of transthoracic laser coronaryplasty with high and low severity of illness*

Study number	Adverse outcomes	Severity of illness
1	5/100 ST 10/100 C	Low
2	80/1,000 ST 100/1,000 C	Low
3	25/100 ST 20/100 C	Low
4	2/100 ST 10/100 C	High
5	40/1,000 ST 120/1,000 C	High
6	5/100 ST 20/100 C	High
7	10/100 ST 10/100 C	Low
8	20/100 ST 20/100 C	Low
9	30/1,000 ST 90/1,000 C	High
10	60/1,000 ST 150/1,000 C	High

ST, study group; C, control group

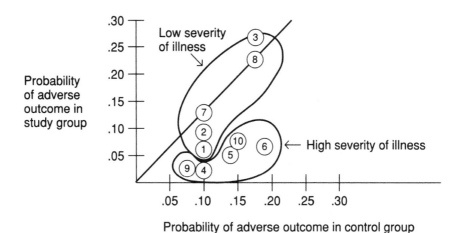

Figure 11.3. Lack of homogeneity demonstrated by the ability to separate low and high severity of illness.

of more severe illness in general tend to have a high proportion of bad outcomes in the control group. This lack of homogeneity implies that separate analyses should be conducted, with one analysis for studies of patients with low severity of illness and a separate analysis for studies of patients with high severity of illness. The results of these meta-analyses may demonstrate that TLC is has greater efficacy for patients with a high severity of illness.[7]

Interpretation

In a meta-analysis the investigator often tries to determine whether contributory cause or efficacy has been demonstrated. As with other types of investigation, the interpretation begins by asking whether the definitive criteria of (a) association, (b) prior association, and (c) altering the cause alters the effect been fulfilled?

In establishing associations using meta-analysis, it is important to recognize that meta-analysis aims to increase the sample size by combining studies. This has the potential advantage of increasing the statistical power. Increases in statistical power improve the probability of demonstrating statistical significance. Thus, even small but real differences may be demonstrated to be statistically significant, although they may not have clinical importance.

The ability of a meta-analysis to establish the criteria of prior association and altering the cause alters the effect often depends on the type and quality of the individual investigations included in the meta-analysis. When randomized clinical trials are included, these have the potential for definitively establishing all three criteria.

The large number of individuals included in a meta-analysis may give it advantages in accomplishing the other goals of interpretation—that is, looking at

---

[7] The degree of overlap in the curves needed to label the effect as homogeneous is subjective. This is an inherent limitation of the graph technique. Statistical significance testing is also available to examine the homogeneity of studies. These statistical significance tests, such as the Q-statistic, have low statistical power. However, a P-value <0.1 is often used to justify use of a fixed-effect model.

adverse effects and at subgroups. The greater number of individuals that may be included in a meta-analysis allows us to interpret the data on safety or harms with greater reliability. The rule of three in reverse is still a useful tool for helping us to interpret the implications of the absence of an adverse effect. Thus, if a meta-analysis includes 30,000 patients and there is no evidence of anaphylaxis, we can be 95% confident that if anaphylaxis occurs, its true frequency is less than 1 per 10,000.

When there is an increase in frequency of side effects among those in the treatment group, combining the data from many investigations may enable the investigators to draw conclusion about the frequency of side effect in the study groups compared to the control groups.

In meta-analysis as opposed to other types of investigations, we do not need to wait until statistically significance is established using all of the data before we can examine subgroups.[8] When the analysis of results suggests the presence of heterogeneity, the meta-analysis researcher can examine the individual investigations to see what can be learned about subgroups, as illustrated in the following example.

> A meta-analysis of the efficacy of a treatment for Alzheimer's disease suggested heterogeneity according to the severity of the disease and the extent of family support. The studies suggested that the treatment had the greatest efficacy when used on groups with early disease who had the highest level of family support. This data was used as the basis for planning a randomized clinical trial using only patients with early Alzheimer's disease who had high levels of family support.

This example illustrated the way the meta-analysis can be interpreted and used as the basis for drawing conclusions. Even when conclusions about statistical significance are not possible, the interpretation may be useful in planning future studies.

The large numbers of subjects included in a meta-analysis is an advantage when examining subgroups.

For instance, if an exploratory meta-analysis of TLC used all 25 available studies, the investigator might be able to examine subgroups such as men versus women and repeat TLC versus initial TLC, especially if differences between these groups were hypothesized at the beginning of the investigation. If the data were available, the investigator might also examine a subgroup such as types of anticoagulation used to examine the hypothesis that this factor makes a difference. Unfortunately, data are often not presented in a way that allows the investigator to combine the subgroups from different investigations. As with other types of investigations, even when the data are available, it is important to perform a limited number of subgroup analyses on the basis of predetermined study questions.

In the process of interpretation for meta-analysis, the investigators may want to consider removing *outliers*. Outliers are studies that produce results that are very different from the majority of studies. It is very tempting to merely exclude all outliers from an analysis, but this should be done only if there is very good reason. Often, in fact, additional information can be obtained by looking carefully at the

---

[8] Remember that at times, a small number of subgroups identified at the beginning of an investigation can be examined even in the absence of a demonstration of statistical significance using the overall data.

outliers as part of the interpretation and asking why the results are different. This is demonstrated in the next example:

> Among the 25 studies of TLC, one demonstrated that the results of TLC were sub-stantially worse than those associated with medication or surgery. This study was performed at the beginning of the TLC era, using obsolete procedures and no antico-agulation. A second outlier demonstrated that the best results for TLC were achieved using the newest technique at a medical center that has the largest volume and longest experience with TLC.

Here, the exceptions help to prove the rule that TLC is an effective treatment. At other times, outliers may challenge the conclusion, producing new hypotheses for further investigations. In general, outliers should not be excluded from a meta-analysis. If one outlier is excluded, the others should also be excluded. Here, examination of these two studies supports the efficacy of TLC.

Finally, when interpreting the results of a study, we need to reexamine the issue of publication bias. Publication bias is so important in meta-analysis that we often examine its potential impact as part of the interpretation. In doing so, we can estimate the number of studies showing no effect that would need to be missing from the meta-analysis in order for the results to no longer be statistically significant.[9] This number of studies is called the *fail-safe n*. The following example illustrates how to interpret the fail-safe n:

> A meta-analysis of TLC for single-vessel coronary artery disease using all 25 studies has a fail-safe n of 100. Thus, the authors concluded that publication bias is very unlikely to affect the meta-analysis results.

It is unlikely that there exists 100 completed but unpublished studies that on average showed no difference between TLC and standard therapy. This degree of publication bias is unlikely to occur. Thus, we can be reasonably confident that if publication bias exists, it does not explain or have a dramatic effect on the conclusions.

Extrapolation

To Similar Populations

Meta-analysis is capable of providing an estimate of the average strength of an association i.e., the effect size. It can also help us with statistical significance testing, allowing us to infer efficacy in the larger population from which the study samples were obtained. Average strength of an association can be very useful when making extrapolations designed for groups of individuals. However, when trying to make decisions for a particular patient, the results of a meta-analysis may not be as useful as examining the results of a particularly relevant study, as demonstrated in the next example:

> A patient at the medical center with the longest experience using TLC, the newest techniques, and the largest volume is being considered for TLC. The results of the meta-analysis comparing TLC with other therapies for this type of high-risk patient indicate very little difference. However, the data from this medical center

---

[9] The investigator actually calculates the fail-safe n assuming that the missing studies are, on average, the same size as the studies included in the meta-analysis, and that the studies, on average, show no effect (i.e., they have a zero difference or a ratio of 1).

unequivocally support the use of TLC for this type of high-risk patient at this medical center.

Data available from the same institution based on similar patients are often more informative than using the average strength of an association obtained from a meta-analysis. Thus, despite the important role that meta-analysis can play in research and clinical care, it does not automatically produce the most useful results for a particular patient.

Beyond the Data

Issues of extrapolation are not limited to how well the therapy works. Issues of harm or safety also need consideration and require extrapolation beyond the data. The large number of patients that are often included in a meta-analysis can produce more reliable extrapolation about harms or safety of therapies. The assessment of safety, however, is still limited to the duration, dosage, and types of outcomes assessed by the studies included in the meta-analysis, as illustrated in the next hypothetical example:

> The meta-analysis of TLC demonstrated efficacy of TLC for single-vessel coronary artery disease. It also demonstrated short-term harms similar to medication or surgery. More than a decade after the widespread use of TLC began, it was recognized that late effects on the coronary artery made it more likely to suddenly close, producing a higher incidence of late myocardial infarction.

Studies can only draw conclusions about what they measure. The ability to assess long-term consequences requires long-term follow-up. Long-term safety or effectiveness considerations are no better assessed by meta-analysis than by conventional studies.

To Other Populations

Extrapolating results from a meta-analysis to practice poses the same dangerous consequences as with other types of investigations. When extrapolating to populations that are not included in the meta-analysis, it is important to recognize and make explicit the assumptions that are being made. For instance, imagine the following situation:

> A large, well-conducted meta-analysis of TLC concluded that TLC was safe and effective and better than standard treatment for single-vessel coronary artery disease. The authors concluded that TLC should be used for treatment of coronary artery disease in two- and three-vessel disease. Subsequent studies demonstrated the superiority of TLC for single-vessel disease but found that the extensive exposure to laser treatment needed for two- and three-vessel disease was associated with side effects not previously recognized when using TLC to treat single-vessel coronary artery disease.

Whenever an extrapolation is made to new situations, it must be assumed that the new circumstances will not be associated with new side effects. In this example, this assumption was not correct. Thus, regardless of the type of investigation, the reader of the health research literature must be aware of the dangers of extrapolation to new populations and situations.

Meta-analysis has gained an important role in health research. It has helped to halt continued study of issues for which there are already adequate data. It has helped us gain more accurate measures for the magnitude of effects and the degree of safety of therapies. By harnessing the benefits of diversity, meta-analysis has also helped us better understand what factors affect the outcomes of a therapy.

Despite the many advantages of meta-analysis, it requires the same type of attention to quality study design that is required for other types of research. In addition, because it relies on the existing literature, meta-analysis incorporates special techniques and is often limited in what it attempts to do and what conclusions it can draw.

The classic literature review article has been dramatically restructured by the introduction of meta-analysis. If we are to obtain the maximum amount of information from the existing literature, the principles of meta-analysis must be understood and applied.

12 Questions to Ask and Flaw-Catching Exercises

Questions to Ask when Studying a Study

Throughout this "Studying a Study" section, we have examined the use of the M.A.A.R.I.E. framework to organize our review of research articles, including case-control studies, cohort studies, and randomized clinical trial, as well as meta-analyses. For all of these types of investigations we found that the same basic questions needed to be addressed. Now we are ready to organize these questions into a set of Questions to Ask when Studying a Study.

These Questions to Ask can be used as a checklist when reading the health research literature. For additional practice using the M.A.A.R.I.E. framework, please go to the Studying a Study Online Web site at www.StudyingaStudy.com.

The following are the Questions to Ask when Studying a Study:

Method: The purpose and population for the investigation

1. **Study hypothesis:** What is the study question being investigated?
2. **Study population:** What population is being investigated and what are the inclusion and exclusion criteria for the subjects of the investigation?
3. **Sample size and statistical power:** How many individuals are included in the study and in the control groups and what is the statistical power?

Assignment: Selection of participants for the study and control groups

1. **Process:** What method is used to identify and assign participants to study and control groups?
2. **Confounding variables:** Are there differences between study and control groups, other than the factor being investigated, that may affect the outcome of the investigation?
3. **Masking or blinding:** Are the participants and/or the investigators aware of the participants' assignment to a particular study or control group?

Assessment: Measurement of outcomes or endpoints in the study and control groups

1. **Appropriate:** Does the measurement of outcomes address the study's question?
2. **Accurate and precise:** Is the measurement of outcomes an accurate and precise measure of the phenomenon that the investigators seek to assess?
3. **Complete and unaffected by observation:** Is the follow-up of participants nearly 100% complete and is it affected by the participants' or the investigators' knowledge of the study group or control group assignment?

Results: Comparison of outcomes in the study and control groups

1. **Estimation:** What is the magnitude or strength of the association or relationship?
2. **Inference:** What statistical technique(s) are used to perform statistical significance testing?
3. **Adjustment:** What statistical technique(s) are used to take into account or control for potential confounding variables?

Interpretation: Meaning of the results for those included in the investigation

1. **Contributory cause or efficacy:** Does the factor being investigated alter the probability that the disease will occur (contributory cause) or work to reduce the probability of undesirable outcomes (efficacy)?
2. **Harms and Interactions:** Are adverse effects and/or interactions that affect the meaning of the results identified?
3. **Subgroups:** Are the outcomes observed in subgroups within the investigation different from outcomes observed in the overall investigation?

Extrapolation: Meaning for those not included in the investigation

1. **To similar individuals, groups, or populations:** Do the investigators extrapolate or extend the conclusions to individuals, groups, or populations that are similar to those who participated in the investigation?
2. **Beyond the data:** Do the investigators extrapolate by extending the conclusions beyond the dose, duration or other characteristics of the investigation?
3. **To other populations:** Do the investigators extrapolate to populations or settings that are quite different from those in the investigation?

As we have seen, the use of the M.A.A.R.I.E. framework and the meaning of these questions varies by the type of investigation. To see this process in action, including modifications of the Questions to Ask for each type of investigation, please go to the Studying a Study Online Web site at **www.StudyingaStudy.com.** The Web site includes interactive exercises and practice using the checklist to read actual journal articles.

Flaw-Catching Exercises

The following hypothetical studies illustrate the potential errors that can occur in each component of the M.A.A.R.I.E. framework. These flaw-catching exercises are designed to test your ability to apply the framework in order to study a study critically. Examples of case-control, concurrent and retrospective cohort studies, randomized clinical trials, and meta-analysis are presented. A sample critique organized using the M.A.A.R.I.E. framework follows and points out important errors that occur.

Flaw-catching is a useful skill applicable to reading real research articles. While real investigations hopefully don't have as many flaws as are combined in the exercises that follow, flaws are inevitable. Flaw-catching is not an end in itself. It is important to recognize that not every flaw is fatal. The job of the reader of research is to recognize the flaws and then ask: How do they affect the meaning of the results?

For additional interactive flaw-catching exercises, please go to the Studying a Study Online Web site at **www.StudyingaStudy.com.**

Case-Control Study

FLAW-CATCHING EXERCISE NO. 1: FACTORS ASSOCIATED WITH CONGENITAL HEART DISEASE

A case-control study was undertaken to study the factors associated with the development of congenital heart disease (CHD). Two hundred women with first-trimester spontaneous abortions in which congenital heart abnormalities were found in the fetus on pathologic examination were used as the study group. The control group included 200 women with first-trimester voluntarily induced abortions in which no congenital heart defects were found.

An attempt was made to interview each of the 400 women within 1 month after her abortion to determine which factors in the pregnancy may have led to CHD. One hundred variables were studied. The interviewers gained the participation of 120 of the 200 study group women who experienced spontaneous abortions and 80 of the 200 control group women who underwent induced abortions. The other women refused to participate in the study.

The investigators found the following differences between women whose fetuses had CHD and those whose fetuses were not affected:

1. Women with CHD fetuses were three times more likely to have used antinausea medications during pregnancy than were women whose fetuses did not have CHD. The difference was statistically significant.
2. There was no difference in the use of tranquilizers between the study group and control group.
3. The women with CHD fetuses drank an average of 3.7 cups of coffee per day, whereas women whose fetuses did not have CHD drank an average of 3.5 cups of coffee per day. The differences were statistically significant.
4. Among the other 97 variables studied, the authors found that women with CHD fetuses were twice as likely to have blond hair and be taller than 5 ft. 6 in. Both differences were statistically significant using the usual statistical methods.

The authors drew the following conclusions:

1. Antinausea medications cause CHD because they are more often used by women whose fetuses have CHD.
2. Tranquilizers are safe for use in pregnancy because they were not associated with an increased risk of CHD.
3. Because coffee drinking increases the risk of CHD, coffee drinking should be eliminated completely during pregnancy, which would largely eliminate the risk of CHD.
4. Despite the fact that no one had hypothesized height and hair color as risk factors for CHD, these were proved to be important predictors of CHD.

CRITIQUE: EXERCISE NO. 1

Method

The investigators have not clarified the aims of their study. Are they interested in specific types of CHD? Congenital heart disease consists of a variety of conditions involving valves, septum, and blood vessels. By lumping all conditions under CHD, the investigators are assuming that a common cause exists for all these conditions. In addition, the specific hypotheses being tested are not clarified in this study. The groups chosen consist of a study group that underwent spontaneous abortions and a control group that underwent voluntarily induced abortions. These groups can be expected to differ in a variety of ways. It would have been preferable to choose more comparable groups of women, for instance, those who had induced abortions with and without CHD or those who had spontaneous abortions with and without CHD.

With this study design, remember that the population of women consisted only of those with abortions. This implies that the investigator must be cautious in drawing conclusions about live births. In addition the study group included only CHD that was severe enough to cause early spontaneous abortion. Although this may provide important information, the factors causing CHD severe enough to abort fetuses may be different from the factors causing CHD in full-term infants.

Assignment

To determine whether a selection bias exists, we first consider whether the study group and control group differ in some respect. Second, we ask whether these differences could have affected the results. The experiences of women having voluntarily induced abortions versus those having spontaneous abortions are likely to be different in many ways. The women probably also have different attitudes about their pregnancies, which may affect their use of medications during pregnancy. Such differences between the study group and control group could affect the outcomes, so selection bias may well be present.

Assessment

The high rate of subjects lost to follow-up because they refused to participate suggests the possibility that those who were lost to follow-up had different characteristics than those who participated in the study. A high rate of loss to follow-up weakens the conclusions that can be drawn from any observed differences. Recall bias by participants is possible, particularly when a traumatic event has occurred in a case-control study. In addition, participants were asked to recall events such as coffee consumption and medication use that are frequently occurring and subjectively remembered events. This suggests that the conditions are right for recall error. The accuracy of retrospective reporting of medication use, for instance, may be influenced by the emotions caused by losing the fetus among those women who experienced an unexpected spontaneous abortion. The consequence may be a closer scrutiny of the memory, leading to a more thorough recall of medication use among those who had a spontaneous abortion.

Results, Interpretation, and Extrapolation

The investigators' four conclusions may contain the following flaws:

1. Even if one assumes that the relationship between antinausea medications and CHD was properly derived, no cause-and-effect relationship has been shown. Case-control studies cannot definitively settle the question of which factor is the cause and which is the effect. It is possible that women with CHD fetuses have more nausea and, therefore, take more antinausea medications. Before a contributory cause is definitively established, investigators must show that the postulated cause precedes the effect and that altering the cause alters the effect. The authors of this study have made an interpretation that is not warranted by the data.

2. The absence of a difference between groups in terms of tranquilizer use does not necessarily ensure the safety of these drugs. The samples may be too small—that is, they have a low statistical power to determine the association between tranquilizer use and CHD. The rule of three tells us that we should not expect to observe rare but serious side effects in small studies. Even if there is no association between tranquilizers and CHD, this does not ensure the absence of other adverse effects on the fetus that make tranquilizers unsafe for use during pregnancy. The investigators have, therefore, extrapolated too far beyond the data.

3. The difference between the average amount of coffee consumed by women with a CHD fetus compared with the amount consumed by women without a CHD fetus is statistically significant, but it is not large. A statistically significant result is one with a low probability of occurring by chance if no true differences exist in the larger populations from which the sample data were drawn. However, it is clinically unlikely that such a small reduction in coffee consumption would have a substantial effect on the risk of CHD. Statistical significance must be distinguished from clinical importance and from contributory cause. Coffee drinking may have an effect, but with such small differences, one must be careful not to conclude too much.

4. By testing 100 variables, it is not surprising that the authors found associations that were statistically significant by chance alone. When using many variables, one cannot use the usual level of statistical significance to reject the null hypothesis of no association. The usual 5% level assumes one hypothesis is developed before the study. Because it was not anticipated that height and hair color would be associated with CHD, these differences are likely to be the results of chance. Thus, the authors cannot safely conclude that height and hair color are risk factors for CHD.

Concurrent Cohort Study

FLAW-CATCHING EXERCISE NO. 2: A STUDY OF SCREENING IN THE MILITARY

During their first year in the military service, 100,000 18-year-old male privates were offered the opportunity to voluntarily participate in a yearly health maintenance examination that included history, physical examination, and multiple laboratory tests. The first year, 50,000 participated and 50,000 failed to participate. The 50,000 participants were selected as a study group, and the 50,000 nonparticipants were selected as a control group. The first-year participants were then offered yearly health maintenance examinations during each year of their military service.

On discharge from the military, each of the 50,000 study group members and each of the 50,000 control group members were given an extensive history, physical examination, and laboratory evaluation to determine whether the yearly health maintenance visits had made any difference in the health and lifestyle of the participants.

The investigators obtained the following information:

1. On the basis of self-reporting, participants had half the frequency of alcohol consumption as nonparticipants.

2. Participants had twice as many examinations and twice as many diagnosed illnesses during military service as did nonparticipants.
3. Participants had advanced an average of twice as many ranks as nonparticipants.
4. No statistically significant differences in the rate of myocardial infarction (MI) occurred between the groups.
5. No differences were found between the groups in the frequency of development of testicular cancer or Hodgkin's disease, the two most common cancers in young men.

The authors then drew the following conclusions:

1. For frequency of alcohol consumption, since the relative risk is 2, the attributable risk percentage is 50%. Thus yearly examinations can reduce the frequency of alcoholism in the entire military by half.
2. Because participants had twice as many examinations and twice as many diagnosed illnesses during their military service, their illnesses were diagnosed at an earlier stage in the disease process, when therapy is more beneficial.
3. Because participants had twice the military advancement of nonparticipants, the screening program must have contributed to the quality of their work.
4. Because the groups did not differ in the rate of MI, screening and intervention for coronary risk factors should not be included in a future health maintenance screening program.
5. Because testicular cancer and Hodgkin's disease occurred with equal frequency in both groups, future health maintenance examinations should not include efforts to diagnose these conditions.

CRITIQUE: EXERCISE NO. 2

Method

This is a concurrent cohort study because assignment is observed and study and control groups are then followed up over time with subsequent assessment of an outcome. The investigators have stated only a general goal of studying the value of an annual health maintenance examination in the military. They do not identify the target population to which they wish to apply their results. They do not state specific hypotheses or clearly identify their specific study questions.

If the investigators' goal was to study the effects of an annual health maintenance examination, they have not accomplished this goal because no evidence exists that first-year participants actually took part in subsequent examinations.

Furthermore, the authors' choice of a population to be investigated may not have been appropriate. The study selected young men who already had been screened for chronic illness by virtue of passing the entry physical for military service. Being a young and healthy group, they may not have been an appropriate population for testing the usefulness of health maintenance for other older or higher-risk populations in which the frequency of pathologic conditions would be expected to be much higher.

Assignment

Individuals in this study were self-selected; that is, they decided for themselves whether or not to participate. The participants, therefore, can be considered volunteers. The researchers presented no evidence to indicate whether those who elected to participate differed in any way from those who elected not to participate. It is likely that participants had health habits and health risks that were different from those of the nonparticipants. These differences may well have contributed to the observed differences in the outcome. Because no baseline evaluation is available on the control group, it is not known whether or how they differed from the study group. Thus, it is not known whether the study group and control group were comparable.

The individuals in both the study and control groups were self-assigned on the basis of their participation in the first year of the health maintenance examinations. Because the examinations were conducted on a yearly basis, those who initially participated may not have continued to participate.

Assessment

Without a clear hypothesis, it is not possible to determine if the assessment is appropriate. Problems with precision and accuracy as well as reporting errors are likely when confidential and subjectively remembered measures such as alcohol consumption are used. Assessment of outcome was conducted only on those who were discharged from the military; thus, it was not complete. Those who remained in the military service would not have been included. Individuals who had died during military service would not have been included among those assessed at discharge. The individuals who had died from disease may have been the most important in terms of assessing the potential benefits gained by screening.

Individuals participating in multiple health maintenance examinations were under much more intensive observation than the nonparticipants. The unequal intensity of observation may have resulted in the greater number of illnesses diagnosed during their military service. Nonparticipants may have had the same number of conditions, without all of them resulting in a recorded diagnosis. The absence of masked assignment and masked assessment may have affected the measurement of outcomes.

Results, Interpretation, and Extrapolation

The five conclusions made by the investigators may contain the following flaws:

1. Participants had a lower rate of alcohol consumption than nonparticipants, perhaps due to differences between the groups before entry into the study. If heavy drinkers were less likely to participate in the health screening, then the examinations would only appear to have altered the frequency of alcohol consumption. Comparative baseline data on alcohol consumption and other variables and adjustment for these differences were lacking in the analysis. Potential assessment errors draw into question the validity of the measurement of outcome. Even if none of these potential errors existed, there is no evidence in the study that the examinations themselves were the causative factor in producing a lower rate of alcohol consumption. Extrapolating to the military in general went well beyond the range of the data.

2. The greater intensity of observation of participants compared with nonparticipants may explain the greater number of diagnoses. This greater number does not in and of itself ensure that the diseases were detected at an earlier stage or that their treatment benefits the patients.

3. If a higher level of motivation is associated both with participation in the study and advancement in the military, then motivation would be a confounding variable due to selection bias. Without the use of randomization or adjustment for this potentially confounding variable, no conclusion can be reached about the relationship between participation status and advancement.

4. Many of the participants with an MI may have died and thus were excluded from the assessment. In addition, one would expect a very low rate of MI in a young population. Even with the large numbers included in this study, the sample may not have been large enough to observe small differences between the groups. There is no evidence that despite the screening those who participated had either more recognized risk factors or more risk factors altered. Even if they had more altered risk factors, the effects of these alterations may not become apparent until years after the participants have left the military. Therefore, this study was incapable of answering the question of whether screening for risk factors for coronary artery disease alters prognosis.

5. The absence of differences in the frequency of testicular cancer and Hodgkin's disease cannot be assessed on the basis of those discharged alive. The frequencies of developing these diseases were identical, but this says little about the success or failure of the examination program. A cancer screening program aims to pick up disease at an early stage; it does not aim to prevent disease. Thus, the frequency of cancer cannot be used to evaluate the success or failure of a screening program. Therefore, one would expect nearly identical frequency of Hodgkin's disease and testicular cancer. The stage of illness at diagnosis and the prognosis for those who developed either of the conditions would be more appropriate measures for evaluating the success of the screening program. No such data are presented here; thus, no interpretation can be made.

Retrospective Cohort Study

FLAW-CATCHING EXERCISE NO. 3: CESAREAN VERSUS VAGINAL DELIVERY AFTER PREVIOUS CESAREAN

A large database was available to study all births that occurred after a previous cesarean section delivery. The investigators hypothesized that repeat cesarean section delivery would result in improved pregnancy outcomes compared to vaginal delivery during the next birth. During the time period of the study, it was up to individual physicians and individual patients to decide whether to perform repeat cesarean section or vaginal delivery.

Of 20,000 repeat cesarean section deliveries available in the database, 10,000 were included in the investigation. These repeat cesarean section deliveries were included because complete data were available on delivery, hospital course, and child's health and development at age 12 months. The vaginal deliveries included all 10,000 deliveries after a previous cesarean section that were available in the database even if the child did not return for a developmental assessment at 12 months.

Data from study and control group deliveries were collected on parity (number of children), mother's age, and mother's socioeconomic status. Outcome measures included the number of stillbirths, Apgar score for live births, mother's and child's length of hospital stay, child's health and developmental status at 12 months, and mother's health outcomes.

The parity was nearly identical between the groups; however, the repeat cesarean section group had an average age of 34 years versus an average age of 28 years for the vaginal delivery group. The repeat cesarean section patients were five times more likely to be in the top half of the socioeconomic scale.

There were 60 stillbirths in the repeat cesarean section delivery group versus 6 in the vaginal delivery group. Apgar scores for the repeat cesarean section deliveries were a mean of 8 compared with a mean of 7.8 for the vaginal deliveries. The length of hospital stay in the repeat cesarean section group was 5 days longer, on average, than the vaginal delivery group. The developmental indices at 12 months of children born by cesarean section were 1% better on average than children in the vaginal delivery group. All these differences were statistically significant. There were 100 cases of thrombophlebitis and one death among the women who underwent repeat cesarean section, and 10 cases of thrombophlebitis and one death among the women in the vaginal delivery group.

The authors drew the following conclusions:

1. Although this was not a randomized clinical trial, the large number of deliveries and the nearly identical parity ensure that the two groups were similar.
2. The relative risk is 10 and the attributable risk percentage is 90% for stillbirth among repeat cesarean section deliveries compared with vaginal deliveries. This implies that 90% of the stillbirths are caused by repeat cesarean section delivery and could be eliminated by vaginal delivery.
3. The difference in length of stay was expected because of the need to recover from surgery and was, therefore, not a relevant finding.
4. The increase in Apgar score and developmental scores at 12 months among repeat cesarean section deliveries was caused by the repeat cesarean section delivery.
5. Because the number of maternal deaths is equal in the two groups, the harms to the mothers do not need to be considered in making recommendations.
6. The authors concluded that repeat cesarean section deliveries result in better Apgar scores and improved child development at 12 months. This more than compensates for the increased thrombophlebitis and the longer length of hospital stay.

The authors recommended repeat cesarean section for all women who had previously delivered by cesarean section.

CRITIQUE: EXERCISE NO. 3

Method

This investigation is designed to be a large, retrospective cohort study. It intended to compare the results of a subsequent delivery vaginally or by repeat cesarean section after a previous cesarean section delivery. The investigation is a retrospective cohort study because the investigators started by identifying a study group with delivery by repeat cesarean section and a control group with delivery vaginally. This assignment occur before the investigators were aware of the outcomes.

The two groups are intended to be the same except for the method of delivery. This goal is difficult to achieve in the best of circumstances in a retrospective cohort study. However, the choice of method for identifying the study and control groups in this investigation has compounded this problem. The repeat cesarean section deliveries are a subgroup of all repeat cesarean section deliveries, chosen because of the availability of complete data. The vaginal deliveries include all available patients. When groups selected because they have complete data are compared with groups with incomplete data, we expect to find differences in the patient characteristics which may affect the outcomes being assessed.

In addition, the process of study design requires identifying a study population by defining inclusion and exclusion criteria for study and control group patients. This may not have been fully performed in this investigation because we do not know whether patients with more than one previous cesarean section delivery were included.

Assignment

The major problem with cohort studies is the need to recognize and address clinicians' tendency to tailor the therapy to their perceptions of what individual patients need. This often clinically beneficial tendency can create selection bias, which must be recognized and taken into account in research studies.

For instance, imagine that clinicians are willing to perform a vaginal delivery in women who have had a previous cesarean section only if the women were progressing very well in their deliveries. This would create a strong selection bias favoring the outcomes of vaginal delivery. In addition, it is possible that clinicians may only be willing to perform vaginal delivery on women in their 20s. This could explain the younger age of the women undergoing vaginal deliveries. This difference between groups may produce a selection bias if women in their 20s not only have a greater chance of having a vaginal delivery but also have a better outcome regardless of the form of deliveries. Thus the difference in average age needs to be recognized and taken into account or adjusted for as part of the analysis.

The investigators do record a number of baseline patient characteristics that are useful for comparison. However, the characteristics that are not recorded may affect the results. For instance, there are no data on the duration of pregnancy before delivery by either method. It is possible that repeat cesarean section deliveries were used predominantly for premature, or alternatively, for delayed delivery. These deliveries may be for pregnancies that were developing complications and required intervention. If this was the case, it would create a selection bias that would greatly affect the results by making stillbirths far more likely in the repeat cesarean section group.

Assessment

The investigators did not assess the perinatal deaths that occur in either group. This may be an endpoint that would reflect an important clinical outcome.

Retrospective cohort studies, like this one, may assess patients on the basis of data collected in the course of ongoing medical care. This leads to the potential for bias because those who return for follow-up may not be an accurate reflection of all those entered into the study. We know that the repeat cesarean section deliveries were all followed up to assess child development at 12 months, whereas the vaginal deliveries did not have complete follow-up. If the vaginal deliveries that returned for follow-up child development assessment had a worse outcome than those who failed to return, this difference could explain the small difference in results between the two groups.

The assessment process did not fully take into account adverse maternal effects of the cesarean section. To the extent that thrombophlebitis represents an adverse and costly effect, for instance, the authors did not recognize its importance and acted as though the only important adverse maternal effect was death.

Results

The investigators do not distinguish between differences in outcome that are large or substantial verus ones that are small and perhaps clinically of little or no importance. When the sample sizes are as large as in this investigation, many small differences may be statistically significant. These differences, however, are not likely to be clinically important.

The small difference in Apgar scores or the differences in child development at 12 months, for instance, are not likely to represent a clinically important difference. The use of multiple outcome measures requires additional caution.

Some of the differences are large enough to be of clinical importance, such as large differences in numbers of stillbirths, length of stay, and frequency of thrombophlebitis. The investigators, however, did not consider the possibility that these differences were the result of confounding variables that require adjustment.

Interpretation

The authors drew six conclusions that may contain the following flaws:

1. Similar parity and the large number of deliveries do not ensure that the two groups were similar. The failure to adjust for differences in the study and control groups for potential confounding variables, such as age and socioeconomic status, may have altered the results.
2. The relative risk is 10 for stillbirths because there were 60 stillbirths per 10,000 deliveries in the repeat cesarean section group compared with 6 per 10,000 deliveries in the vaginal delivery group. From this, the investigators correctly derived an attributable risk percentage of 90%. However, the relative risk and the attributable risk percentage can be calculated even in the absence of a cause-and-effect relationship. If repeat cesarean sections are performed when premature delivery is threatened, then stillbirths may cause repeat cesarean sections and not the other way around. That is, this could be an example of reverse causality. Attributable risk percentages can only be used to imply the potential to reduce the risk or to remove a percentage of the bad outcome if contributory cause has been demonstrated.
3. The length of stay is a relevant outcome even if it is completely expected on the basis of the type of delivery. The costs and harms associated with extended hospitalization are relevant to the decision whether or not to deliver by repeat cesarean section. This is true even if its impact is completely predictable.
4. It is not clear that the cesarean section delivery causes the slight increase in Apgar scores or the slightly improved development score at 12 months. These may have been the result of selective follow-up, differences in socioeconomic status, or multiple outcome measures.

5. The potential harms to the mother should not be limited to death. Death is typically a rare occurrence. More frequent events such as thrombophlebitis are important outcome measures. Thrombophlebitis produces considerable morbidity and cost in addition to any deaths that may result.

6. The conclusion that the benefits of repeat cesarean section outweigh the harms assumes that both the benefits and the harms are real. There is considerable doubt concerning the benefits. Even if the investigation's outcomes are valid, this is not the only possible conclusion. The small benefits may be viewed as less important than the substantial increase in the length of stay and the probability of developing thrombophlebitis.

Extrapolation

The uncertainties about the efficacy of repeat cesarean section among the women in the study make extrapolation even to other women like those in the investigation difficult. It is especially dangerous to make recommendations for a target population of all women who have undergone previous cesarean section. Even if the data established the benefits of cesarean section, including a modest increase in Apgar score and 12-month child development, these benefits would still need to be balanced against the potential harms of greatly increased thrombophlebitis risk and extended hospital stays before recommending cesarean section deliveries for all women who had previously delivered by cesarean section.

Randomized Clinical Trial

FLAW-CATCHING EXERCISE NO. 4: BLOOD SAFE—A NEW TREATMENT TO PREVENT AIDS

An investigator believed he discovered an improved method for preventing human immunodeficiency virus (HIV) infection through blood transfusions. His method required treating all transfusion recipients with a new drug called Blood Safe. At the time of his discovery, the rate of HIV transmission via blood transfusions was 1 per 100,000 transfusions.

Having gained approval to study this drug in humans, the investigator set out to design a randomized clinical trial for the initial use of the drug. He designed a study in which a random sample of all blood transfusion recipients in a major metropolitan area was asked whether they wished to receive the drug within 2 weeks after their blood transfusion.

The study enrolled 1,000 study group individuals who accepted the therapy. An additional 1,000 individuals who refused Blood Safe were used as the control group. Control group individuals had received an average of 1.5 blood transfusions compared with 3 for the average individual receiving Blood Safe. The investigators were able to obtain a follow-up HIV blood test on 60% of those receiving Blood Safe and 60% of those who refused approximately 1 month after their date of receiving a blood transfusion.

Those performing the follow-up blood testing were not aware of whether the patient did or did not receive Blood Safe. The investigator found that one patient in the study group was HIV-antibody-positive within 1 month after treatment with Blood Safe. In the control group, two individuals were HIV-antibody-positive.

The investigator did not find any evidence of side effects caused by Blood Safe during the 1-month follow-up period. The investigator concluded that the study established that Blood Safe was effective and safe. He advised administration of Blood Safe to all blood transfusion recipients.

CRITIQUE: EXERCISE NO. 4

Method

The investigator intended to conduct a randomized clinical trial to test the hypothesis that Blood Safe has efficacy in preventing HIV infection via blood transfusions.

Randomized clinical trials are best suited to assessing the efficacy of a therapy once a defined dose and method of administration have been developed during initial studies on humans. They are not well suited to the initial human investigations. The absence of HIV testing before entry into the study is a major error in defining the population because we cannot be sure that the HIV-antibody-positive patients converted from HIV negative to HIV positive after their blood transfusion.

The risk of HIV from blood transfusions at the time of the study was 1 per 100,000 transfusions, a very low risk. Randomized clinical trials that aim to reduce an already low risk require a very large number of individuals. Millions of individuals would be required to properly conduct a randomized clinical trial when the probability of occurrence of the disease is 1 per 100,000. A study of the size here does not have adequate statistical power—that is, it has a very large Type II error. In other words, this study would not be able to demonstrate statistical significance for this therapy even if Blood Safe were capable of substantially reducing the incidence of AIDS from blood transfusions, for instance, from 1 per 100,000 to 1 per 1,000,000.

Assignment

The investigator identified a random sample of patients comparable to those who might receive an effective therapy. Random sampling is not a requirement of randomized clinical trials, but it does make extrapolation to those in the target or the intended population who are not included in the trial more reliable.

However, the investigator did not randomize patients to the study and control groups. The control group consisted of those who refused administration of Blood Safe. Thus, despite the investigators intention to conduct a randomized clinical trial, they did not conduct randomization, the essential feature of a randomized clinical trial. The control group consisted of those who refused to participate. Thus the control group may be different from those who agreed to participate in a number of ways related to the potential for acquiring HIV infection. Randomization is considered a critical characteristic of a randomized clinical trial. Therefore, this study is not truly a randomized clinical trial. In addition, the assignment process was defective because: (a) The investigators made only limited efforts to establish the initial or baseline characteristics of their study and control groups; (b) they indicated that the study group received an average of 3 blood transfusions compared to 1.5 for the control group. This is an important difference because it may well be related to the risk of developing HIV infections. Once the investigators recognized this potential confounding variable, even if it were due to chance, it is expected that they would take it into account as part of the analysis of results. Finally, (c) the investigators did not mask the participants.

Assessment

It is important to remember that the study is actually measuring HIV status after the blood transfusion rather than conversion from HIV negative to HIV positive. This could be considered an inappropriate measure because the important issue is conversion. Those who assessed the outcome of this study were not aware of whether the patient had received Blood Safe. This masked assessment helps to prevent bias in the assessment process. The lack of masking in the assignment process, however, means that patients were aware of whether they received Blood Safe. This may have affected the precision or accuracy of assessment outcome; for instance, those who received Blood Safe may have believed they were protected from acquiring HIV infection.

The investigators assessed HIV-antibody status 1 month after the patients received a transfusion. This is too early to accurately assess whether an individual actually will convert to an HIV-antibody-positive status.

The large number of study and control patients who were lost to follow-up is an important assessment problem even though the percentages lost were equal in both groups. When the number of adverse outcomes is low, those lost to follow-up become especially important. Those lost to follow-up may disproportionately experience side effects or develop symptoms.

Results

The investigator did not report statistical significance testing or confidence intervals. The investigator in this study would not have been able to demonstrate statistical significance. This is not surprising because a single additional case of HIV infection would have made the outcome in the study and control groups equal.

The confidence interval in this study would be very wide, indicating that the results of this study are compatible with no difference or even a difference in the opposite direction.

As discussed under "Assignment," the higher number of blood transfusions among those who received Blood Safe is a confounding variable that should have been taken into account through an adjustment as part of the analysis of results.

Interpretation

The previous method, assignment, assessment, and results flaws means that the study must be interpreted with great care.

Although not performed in the study, the result of statistical significance testing and confidence intervals imply that the difference in HIV infections between the study and control groups could be due to chance.

The probability of developing an HIV infection from blood transfusion in the absence of administration of Blood Safe is so small that other means of acquiring the HIV infection may be much more likely. Therefore, any difference between a study group and a control group cannot automatically be attributable to Blood Safe. The difference may be due to other risk factors for AIDS or even in HIV status before the study. No data are presented that deal with these factors, which may be far more important risk factors than blood transfusions. Thus the investigation clearly does not achieve its goal of establishing all three criteria of efficacy through use of a well-designed randomized trial.

In terms of safety, the size of the investigation was too small to provide convincing evidence of safety. Remember that the rule of three in reverse indicates that if 1,000 individuals receive a treatment and there are no observed side effects, we can only say that if side effects exist, it is likely that they will occur no more often than once per 333 times on average. While this may provide some assurance of safety, rare but serious side effects may still occur even under the conditions of the investigation.

Extrapolation

Even if Blood Safe was shown to have efficacy in preventing transfusion-associated HIV infections, one could not draw conclusions about its effectiveness or safety in practice from this study.

Randomized clinical trials can draw conclusions about the efficacy of therapy under the ideal conditions of an investigation. Effectiveness implies that the therapy has benefit under the usual conditions of clinical practice.

Using Blood Safe in clinical practice would imply administering Blood Safe to very large numbers of individuals. Thus, rare but serious side effects are important. Despite the absence of side effects among those who received Blood Safe in this study, they may still occur. Practice conditions, in which patients may have multiple diseases or be taking multiple medications, lends itself to many more side effects than are usually observed in research studies.

Meta-analysis

FLAW-CATCHING EXERCISE NO. 5: MAGNESIUM CHANNEL BLOCKERS AND CORONARY ARTERY DISEASE

A meta-analysis was conducted to determine whether a class of medications called magnesium channel blockers used for the treatment of hypertension is associated at high dose with an increased frequency of coronary artery disease.

A total of 50 studies including 25,000 patients prescribed magnesium channel blockers were identified by searching for all articles published in the leading peer-reviewed journals. The authors initially sought to use only randomized clinical trials, believing that these would provide the highest quality data. Because of the inability to identify a sufficient number of randomized clinical trials, case-control and cohort studies were also used. Studies were used in the meta-analysis regardless of the specific magnesium channel blocker used by the study group or the antihypertensive medication used by the control group as long as the outcome being assessed was coronary artery disease. A funnel diagram revealed an incomplete funnel with missing small studies that were negative.

The studies examined the frequency of coronary artery disease regardless of the definition of coronary artery disease used in the studies. Graphic and statistical methods were used to evaluate homogeneity. Separate meta-analyses were conducted only when the results of a statistical significance test indicated that there was heterogeneity. Separate meta-analyses were conducted for high-dose verses low-dose treatment. Short- and long-acting medications were separable by graphical analysis, but the differences were not statistically significant.

Overall, the meta-analysis demonstrated an odds ratio of 1.5 for coronary artery disease comparing all patients on magnesium channel blockers with those on other types of antihypertensive medications. The results were not statistically significant even after two outlier studies were removed. For those on high-dose treatment, the odds ratio for coronary artery disease was 2.0; it was 1.2 for low-dose treatment.

The authors drew the following conclusions:

1. This meta-analysis included all appropriate investigations.
2. The methods used to search for relevant investigations were ideal.
3. The definition of coronary artery disease as assessed by each article was the only way to perform this meta-analysis.
4. As performed here, separate meta-analyses are appropriate only when statistical significance tests indicate that there is heterogeneity.
5. The fact that the results of the meta-analysis were not statistically significant implies that magnesium channel blockers does not cause coronary artery disease.
6. This meta-analysis establishes that magnesium channel blockers should not be removed from the market.

CRITIQUE: EXERCISE NO. 5

Method

This was a hypothesis-driven meta-analysis designed to test the hypothesis that magnesium channel blockers used at high dose for the treatment of hypertension are associated with coronary artery disease. In a hypothesis-driven meta-analysis, articles may be selected to meet the specific features of the hypothesis. The authors attempted to use only randomized clinical trials and exclude other types of investigations. This is a common approach, but an alternative approach is to include all types of investigations, as was eventually done in this investigation. When there is a question of the quality of the investigations included in a meta-analysis, it may be possible to compare the results of different types of studies.

The large numbers of patients included in this meta-analysis means that it may be possible to examine rare side effects. However, since serious side effects are rare, we cannot always expect to be able to establish statistical significance.

Assignment

This meta-analysis included only studies published in leading peer-reviewed journals. Thus, other published articles and unpublished research was excluded. Even if the authors argue that leading peer-review articles are the hallmark of quality, they should search for all relevant articles before deciding which to use. The incomplete funnel with missing small studies with negative results suggests the existence of publication bias.

Assessment

When there are a variety of ways to define the outcome under investigation, the authors must decide how to measure it. At times, it may be desirable to use the outcome as measured by each investigation in the meta-analysis, even if each investigation measures the outcome differently as was done in this investigation. However, it is desirable to determine if the results depend on the way the outcome is defined. Thus, it is often desirable to use more than one measure of outcome and to determine if the results are different depending on the definition used. If the results do not depend on how the outcome is measured, then it is reasonable to use an outcome measure that allows the meta-analysis to use the largest number of relevant studies. Using the measure employed by each study as done here accomplishes this goal of increasing the number of usable studies.

Results

Using statistical significance testing to assess homogeneity has become a common practice in meta-analysis. However, when the number of investigations is relatively small, these tests have limited statistical power to demonstrate statistical significance. Graphical measures, on the other hand, give a better sense of the relationship between the results of the investigations. When doubt exists, it is preferable to perform separate meta-analysis using homogeneous groupings of studies. For instance, in this example it might have also been important to perform a meta-analysis separately for short-acting and long-acting magnesium channel blockers. It is permissible to perform separate analyses if there is graphical evidence that the results are heterogeneous even if heterogeneity cannot be established by a statistical significance test. Differences between short-acting and long-acting magnesium channel blockers might have helped to define the nature of the relationship.

Interpretation

This investigation focus on unusual harms rather than on efficacy or effectiveness. Statistically significant results are possible for side effects in a large meta-analysis but should not be expected even in a large meta-analysis. As with any investigation, it is important to look at the magnitude of the effect and not just at whether it is statistically significant.

Outliers should be included in a meta-analysis of the overall data. Close examination of outliers as part of the interpretation is often useful in gaining new insights. While the investigators examined the results with and without inclusion of the outliers, they failed to closely look at the outlier studies themselves to see what they could learn.

An incomplete funnel diagram suggests publication bias. When publication bias exists, it can be helpful to calculate a fail-safe n.

The most impressive finding here is the existence of a dose-response relationship suggesting that use of a high-dose magnesium channel blocker is associated with an increased risk of developing coronary artery disease. While this dose-response relationship is not in and of itself enough to establish a cause-and-effect relationship, it does fulfills one of the ancillary criteria. While this meta-analysis does not definitively demonstrate the existence of even an association between magnesium channel blocker and coronary artery disease, it does provide additional supportive evidence.

Extrapolation

If removal from the market requires meeting the criteria of cause and effect it would be difficult to meet these criteria even using meta-analysis. Meta-analysis may provide a more complete picture of the benefit and the harms allowing judgments on benefits vs. harms based on the available data. Assuming an association exists, assumptions still must be made in order to compare the relative benefits and harms. To address this, one needs to ask such questions as: Are there other equally effective alternatives? Can the harm be eliminated by limiting the dose or duration? Are there other important indications for magnesium channel blockers?

Summary

Having critiqued the flaw-catching exercises in this chapter, you may feel that there are too many errors in research to draw useful conclusions. Of course, most health research studies have far fewer errors than the hypothetical exercises presented here. However, it may help you to remember that a certain number of errors are unavoidable and that identifying errors is not the same as invalidating research.

The practice of clinical medicine and public health requires that practitioners act on probabilities. A critical reading of the health research literature helps the practitioner to define these probabilities more accurately. The art of reading the literature is based on the ability to draw useful conclusions from uncertain data. Learning to detect errors not only helps the practitioner to recognize the limitations of a particular study, but also helps to temper the tendency to automatically put the newest research results immediately into practice.

Testing a Test

II

13 Method

Using the information obtained from tests to make decisions has become an integral part of the practice of medicine and public health. Thus it is not surprising that studies designed to measure the information provided by diagnostic tests is an increasingly important form of investigation. We will examine these types of investigations in the Testing a Test section by using the M.A.A.R.I.E. approach to look at method, assignment, assessment, results, interpretation, and extrapolation. Let us begin by taking a look at method and asking the question, what is the purpose of testing? The application of the M.A.A.R.I.E. framework to research on tests is illustrated in Fig. 13.1.

Purpose of Testing

Testing can be seen as the collection of information that provides the basis for decision making. When looked at this way, much of what is done in medicine can be regarded as testing, from the history and physical examination to trials of treatment. Not all purposes of testing are currently subject to the same degree of scrutiny; therefore, it is helpful to begin by categorizing the basic purposes of testing.

The use of testing to assist in or make the diagnosis of disease is often considered synonymous with testing. When testing is used as part of diagnosis, it assumes a preliminary step, that of making an educated guess as to the probability of disease prior to performance of the test. As we will see, the probability of the disease after the test results are known is very much affected by what is called the *pretest probability* or the *prior probability* of the disease. The pretest probability of the disease is the best estimate, or "guestimate," of the probability of disease before obtaining the results of the test.

The pretest probability of disease is derived from four basic types of inputs. To understand the sources of these four types of inputs imagine the following individuals:

A 23-year-old woman
A 65-year-old male diabetic

The first type of input is derived from the frequency of disease in populations or groups of individuals similar to a particular patient. This is called the *prevalence* of the disease. Prevalence indicates how common or probable the disease is in a particular population as defined by demographics and the presence of other diseases.

These two patient profiles represent very different probabilities of coronary artery disease. The 23-year-old woman has a very low pretest probability of clinically important coronary artery disease, well under 1%. The 65-year-old male diabetic, on the other hand, has a considerably higher pretest probability of clinically important coronary artery disease, most likely more than 20% by virtue of his gender, age, and diagnosis of diabetes, regardless of any other risk factors or symptoms.

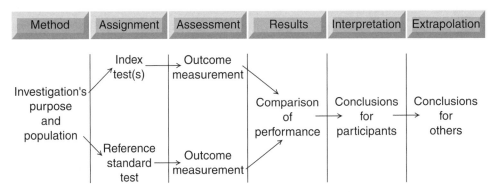

Figure 13.1. M.A.A.R.I.E. framework for investigations of tests.

Thus, what we know about the frequency of coronary artery disease in particular populations, including the influence of demographic factors such as age and gender, and the impact of other diseases such as diabetes provides the starting point for establishing a pretest probability of the disease.

The second input into the pretest probability is the risk factor exposure of the individual. Let us imagine the following pattern of risk factors in our 23-year-old woman and 65-year-old man.

The 23-year-old woman with a strong family history of early coronary artery disease exercises regularly, does not smoke cigarettes, and has a blood pressure of 110/70 and an LDL level of 100.

The 65-year-old male diabetic has no known family history of early coronary artery disease but does not exercise regularly, is 30% over his ideal body weight, has smoked 1 pack of cigarettes per day for 45 years, and has a blood pressure of 150/95 and an LDL level of 160.

Now we know much more about the pretest probability of disease. This information from risk factors may modestly increase the probability that the 23-year-old woman has clinically important coronary artery disease, while the presence of multiple risk factors raises the pretest probability for the 65-year-old man, most likely to the range of 40–60% or more.

Notice that the pretest probability itself often utilizes the results of previous testing. Here, the blood pressure obtained on physical examination as well as LDL level from laboratory testing are used to develop a pretest probability of disease. Thus, one important purpose of testing is to help establish a pretest probability prior to performance of another test.

The third input into the pretest probability is the pattern of symptoms presented by the patient. Imagine the following in our patients:

The 23-year-old woman experiences chest pains radiating to her left arm when she exercises strenuously.

The 65-year-old man with diabetes has not experienced chest pains or pressure, including when walking slowly, which is his most strenuous form of exercise.

This information substantially raises the probability that the 23-year-old woman has clinically important coronary artery disease but has little effect on the probability for the 65-year-old man. Despite the presence of symptoms in the 23-year-old woman, she still is far less likely to have clinically important coronary artery disease than the 65-year-old man.

Imagine that our 23-year-old woman and our 65-year-old man each undergo exercise stress testing. The use of exercise stress testing on the 23-year-old woman in this setting may be called a *diagnostic test* because it is conducted in the presence of symptoms. The same test conducted on the 65-year-old man would be called a *screening test*, implying that it was conducted as part of a diagnostic process but on a patient who was asymptomatic, that is, free of symptoms of coronary artery disease.[1]

Now imagine the results of the exercise stress testing.

The 65-year-old man has an exercise test with strongly positive electrocardiographic evidence of coronary artery disease. The results of the exercise stress test for the 65-year-old man greatly increases the probability of coronary artery disease. Testing would generally not stop here. In fact, the results of the test would be used to revise the probability of disease prior to more definitive testing, such as a coronary arteriogram.

Thus, the results of a test such as a screening test may be used to estimate the pretest probability prior to conducting another test such as the coronary arteriogram. Use of a prior screening test is a fourth source of data that may contribute to our estimation of the pretest probability of a disease.

Imagine the results of a coronary arteriogram were as follows:

Coronary artery narrowing was present in all major vessels, with one vessel having over 90% narrowing. On the basis of the coronary arteriogram, one-vessel angioplasty is recommended.

This coronary arteriogram has been used as a definitive diagnostic test. That is, it is being used to definitively define the presence or absence of the disease. Notice, however, that the coronary arteriogram also serves as the basis for evaluating the severity of the disease as well as the assisting in planning the therapy. These two purposes of testing might be called *testing for severity* and *testing for planning therapy.*

Now let us return to our 23-year-old woman.

When she exercised strenuously on a treadmill during her stress test, she reproduced her chest pain. The pain occured at the time she was experiencing an episode of atrial fibrillation without electocardiographic evidence of ischemia. Her atrial fibrillation was subsequently controlled through medication. A follow-up exercise stress test was negative during strenuous exercise and she did not experience any chest pain or discomfort.

This test was very helpful because it reproduced the patient's symptoms and allowed a correlation between the symptoms and the finding on the test. The results helped to reduce the probability of coronary artery disease, but more importantly, they provided what can be called a *test for causation.*

Testing to correlate symptoms and diseases is becoming an important form of testing. The use of the follow-up test not only confirms the diagnosis but serves as a test of the success of the treatment. This example illustrates one additional use of testing that we will call *monitoring the results of treatment.*

---

[1] Note that a patient may have symptoms and still be asymptomatic from the perspective of the disease for which the screening test is being conducted. Also note that the term "screening" is also used to imply that testing is being conducted in the presence of symptoms to provide information on which of a number of conditions might be causing the condition such, as drug screening in the presence of symptoms suggestive of drug abuse. This use of the term "screening" can be confusing and should be distinguished from a screening test as used here.

The examples of these two patients demonstrates most of the basic uses of testing. Note that one test such as an exercise stress test or a coronary arteriogram may be used for more than one of the following purposes.

- Testing for risk factors for disease
- Screening test: testing patients without symptoms for a particular disease
- Diagnostic testing: testing patient with symptoms for a particular disease
- Definitive testing: testing to define the presence or absence of a disease in a patient with previous positive test results on a screening or diagnostic test
- Testing for causation: testing to establish the relationship between symptoms and disease
- Testing for severity of the disease
- Testing for planning treatment
- Testing to monitor the results of treatment

Thus testing can be used for a wide variety of purposes.[2] The multiple uses of testing can cause confusion when reading the results of a research article. Most of the time research articles on tests address screening tests or diagnostic tests—that is, testing for diagnosis on individuals who are either asymptomatic (screening) or symptomatic (diagnostic testing) for a particular disease.

The research articles that we will focus on in the "Testing a Test" section examine diagnostic and screening tests. Tests for other purposes are not often subjected to the same degree of evaluation that are increasingly required for adoption of diagnostic and screening tests.[3]

In order to identify the test that is being evaluated, the term *index test* is used. Thus the first question to ask when reading an investigation on tests is: What is the purpose for investigating the index test?

Until recently, research on diagnostic and screening tests has not been published in a consistent format, often leaving the reader with many unanswered and unanswerable questions. Recently, a set of standard and comprehensive methods for reporting investigations of diagnostic tests known as STARD (Standards for Reporting Diagnostic Accuracy) have been adopted by many journals.[4] These criteria have been incorporated into the components of the M.A.A.R.I.E. framework for Testing a Test.

Study Population

In examining the study population, we need to ask: Were the participants similar to the population for which the test is intended i.e., the target population?

---

[2] There are other possible uses of testing, including environmental testing to determine possible exposure to a risk factor and testing to provide a baseline for subsequent diagnostic testing. Environmental testing will not be discussed here. Baseline testing can be considered a method for substituting individual data for population data.

[3] Tests of prognosis, for instance, have traditionally only required biological plausibility. Increasingly, methods known as prediction rules are being used to evaluate the ability of tests to predict the future for individuals. Prediction rules differ from other types of evaluations of testing in that they require good *calibration* as a measure of outcome, not just good performance. Calibration is a measurement of how well the test performs not only for the average participant in an investigation but also for those that have characteristics far removed from the average. Use of tests for monitoring safety and effectiveness are not usually expected to be rigorously evaluated.

[4] STARD Initiative: checklist and flowchart, first official version, January 2003, www.consort-statement.org/stardstatement.htm (May 20, 2004).

The investigation's setting as well as specific inclusion and exclusion criteria provide the basis for understanding the population from which the participants come. Ideally, the participants should reflect the range of severity and other characteristics of the disease that are expected when the test is used on its target population.

Let us see what can happen when the participants used for evaluation of a test are quite different from the people for which the test is intended.

> A test is intended to be used to make an early diagnosis of myocardial infarction. It was evaluated on patients who presented with chest pain in a cardiologist's office. The patients were included even if they had a previous myocardial infarction. The results of the test indicated excellent diagnostic performance in early diagnosis of myocardial infarction. When the same test was used in emergency rooms on all patients with chest pain compatible with myocardial infarction, the test did not perform nearly as well.

The patients being followed by cardiologists are likely to have had a previous myocardial infarction. These patients are at high risk of a recurrent episode. Patients presenting in the ER are most likely at lower risk of MI. Therefore, it is important the we consider whether the setting for the test and the indications for the test are the same in the target population in the ER as they are in the investigation's setting in a cardiologist's office. If the intent is to use the test on ER patients, it is important that the investigation be conducted in ERs or a similar setting.

In order to describe the participants, the STARD criteria expects that investigators will indicate their inclusion and exclusion criteria. In addition, as we will see in the Assignment chapter, considerable detail is expected on the process of patient recruitment that along with the inclusion and exclusion criteria ultimately determine whether the participants are representative of the target population for whom the index test is intended.

Sample Size and Statistical Power

Participants in an investigation of diagnostic accuracy undergo the test under evaluation, i.e., the index test, as well as a second test. This second test is the best available or agreed-upon method for definitively diagnosing the presence or absence of the disease. This definitive test is called the *reference standard* or the *gold standard*. As we will see, the data for evaluating tests comes from comparing the results of the index test and the reference standard test.

We need to ask: How may participants need to undergo the index test and the reference standard test to provide adequate statistical power? That is, what is the expected sample size?

It may be surprising to learn that sample size for evaluating diagnostic and screening tests have not been agreed upon. The STARD recommendations do not make specific recommendation for the number of participants.[5]

---

[5] Despite the absence of clear-cut recommendations for the number of participants, as we will discuss in the Results chapter, investigators are now expected to report the confidence intervals around their results. This has the effect of encouraging larger sample sizes. Often investigators will utilize a sample in which half of the patients have the disease as defined by the reference standard test and half have been shown to be free of the disease according to the reference standard test. This approach is attractive because it helps minimize the total size of the sample that needs to be included in the investigation.

Despite the absence of specific recommendations for sample size, some general guidelines are useful. For diagnostic tests in which the pretest probability is moderately high, 100 to 200 participants are usually adequate. When we are dealing with screening tests with a low pretest probability of disease, 1,000 or more participants are often required to adequately evaluate an index test.[6]

Now we have addressed the basic issues of the method component. We have focused on the purpose of the testing, the study population, and the sample size. Now we can take a look at the Assignment chapter and examine the characteristics of the participants and the conduct of tests.

[6] The issue of statistical power in evaluating diagnostic tests is different from hypothesis-testing investigations since there is no hypothesis that the index test differs from the reference standard test. The clinically relevant question is, what is the confidence interval around the measurement of results such as the sensitivity and specificity? Hypothesis testing may be relevant when tests are being compared to one another. In this situation large numbers of participants are often required in order to produce substantial statistical power to demonstrate statistically significant difference between the performance of two tests. Sample size for case-control studies might be used as a guide for sample size in evaluating diagnostic tests. The use of from 100 to several hundred patients with and also without the disease can serve as general guidelines for appropriate sample size for investigations of diagnostic tests, especially when the pretest probability of the disease among those who receive the test are in the range of 50%. The evaluation of screening tests require a considerably larger sample size. Their sample size often parallels that of cohort studies or randomized clinical trials.

14 Assignment

The assignment process in investigations of diagnostic tests describes the recruitment of patients, how they were assigned to comparison groups, and how the index test and the reference standard test were conducted.

Recruitment

It is important that the investigators report and the reader understand how the participants included in the testing sample was recruited. Recruitment is the process of identifying individuals who fulfill the inclusion and exclusion criteria and turning them into study participants. Recruitment can occur through a variety of mechanisms, from advertising to inviting all eligible patients coming to an ER to become participants. The mechanism used may affect the types of individuals who become participants, as illustrated in the next example.

> One investigator conducted a study of a new test for cardiac output by recruiting patients in a tertiary care (referral) hospital who had a history of myocardial infarction. A second investigator studied the new test by recruiting participants from a retirement community. The performance of the test was very different in these two populations despite the fact that all participants in both studies fulfilled the inclusion and exclusion criteria.

Patients recruited in a tertiary care hospital may differ from those recruited in a retirement community in subtle and not so subtle ways. Even when efforts are made to take into account the severity of disease, these two studies are likely to include very different types of participants. It may be useful to investigate the new test on different types of populations, but we should not be surprised to find quite different results.

According to the STARD recommendations, the investigator needs to indicate the beginning and end dates of recruitment as well as the setting(s) and location(s) where the data were collected. The clinical and demographic characteristics such as age, sex, spectrum of presenting symptoms, and other conditions and treatments need to be reported. The reader should be especially interested in whether the participants' severity of disease is likely to be similar to that of the target population.

Assignment Process

Investigations need to report the method of assignment of participants. Participants may be assigned in three basic ways:

1. Recruit all patients from a particular setting who fulfill entry and exclusion criteria, such as having specific signs or symptoms, before they have had either the index test or the reference standard test.

2. Identify individuals with the disease and without the disease as defined by the results of the reference standard test. Those who are identified are then recruited to subsequently undergo the index test.
3. Identify individuals who have already undergone the index test and who then are recruited to subsequently undergo the reference standard test.

The first of these methods is considered the best way to assign participants. It helps ensure that the participants are representative of all those who fulfill the inclusion and exclusion criteria. Methods number 2 and 3 are also used and can each produce errors in investigations.

When using method 2, we need to ask whether those chosen reflect the full spectrum of the disease that we are interested in. It is tempting for the investigator using this approach to include only those with clear-cut disease and those in good health. When those in the gray area, such as those with other diseases of the same organ system, are included, the results may be very different, as illustrated in the next example.

> An investigation of a new test for prostate cancer began by identifying those with prostate cancer and age-matched men who had no evidence of prostate cancer according to the reference standard test and no evidence of other prostate disease. Those with and without prostate cancer then received the new test. The investigator found that the new test was as good as the reference standard test. When used in practice, the new test did not perform as well because it was often positive for those with moderate to severe benign prostate hypertrophy.

This failure to include those with other diseases that might also be positive on the test is called *spectrum bias.*

Method 3 is also prone to bias. When participants are identified based on having already undergone the index test, there is the possibility for what is called *verification bias.* Let us see how verification bias can occur and its potential consequences in the next example.

> A new test for coronary artery disease was evaluated by obtaining data on all patients who underwent the new test and were then recruited to undergo the reference standard coronary arteriogram. Only a small percentage of those who underwent the new test were willing to volunteer to undergo the invasive reference standard test. The new test performed extremely well against the coronary arteriogram. When another investigator evaluated the new test by obtaining the new test and also a coronary arteriogram on all those who were eligible for an investigation, the new test did not perform well.

In this example, only those who already had undergone the new test and agreed to undergo the reference standard test are included in the investigation. Those who underwent the new test but not the reference standard test may not volunteer for a variety of reasons. For instance, they may have had such an unequivocally negative test that they did not want to accept the potential harm of the coronary arteriogram. Alternatively, they may have had such a positive test that it was decided to act on the basis of the results of the patients' condition and the new test.

Thus, whenever patient are assigned based on having already had either the index test or the reference standard test, there is the potential for bias. Ideally, participants are recruited who meet inclusion and exclusion criteria and have not undergone either the index test or the reference standard test. That is method number 1.

Even when method number 1 is used, the STARD criteria require reporting the number of eligible individuals who are excluded and the reasons for exclusion. Let us see how exclusion of patients might affect an investigation in the next scenario.

Investigators offer a new test along with a reference standard test to all patients who presented with hematuria. The test requires transurethral insertion of a fiberoptic scope. Most of the patients who agreed to the test had gross hematuria, while most of those who met the inclusion and exclusion criteria but refused the test had microscopic hematuria. The test performed very well among those recruited for the investigation. However, when used in practice, the test failed to detect the types of pathology often associated with microscopic hematuria.

When an investigation is conducted on only a subset of the intended population of participants, it should not come as a surprise when its performance on the patients like those excluded from the investigation is not as good as on the types of patients included. Thus, it is important to understand not only the inclusion and exclusion criteria but to appreciate the types of participants that were actually included in the investigation.

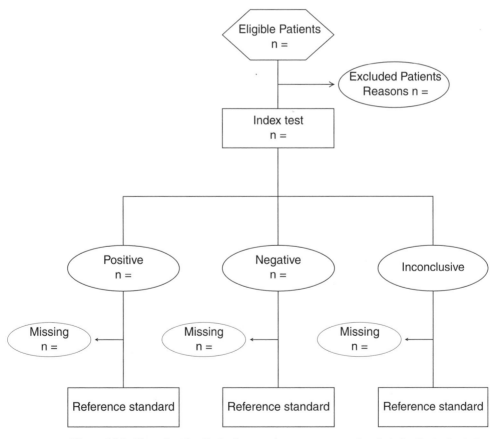

Figure 14.1. Flow chart for displaying recruitment process and excluded patients plus index and reference standard tests and missing patients. (Adapted from STARD Initiative checklist and flow diagram. www.consort-statement.org/stardstatement.htm (May 20, 2004).

Because of the importance of understanding the characteristics of participants, the STARD criteria strongly encourage investigators to include a flowchart which indicates the characteristics of not only the participants but also indicates the reasons for exclusion of those who met the eligibility criteria. Figure 14.1 illustrates the type of flowchart that should be included in a journal article to provide data on recruitment as well as any participants missing from the reference standard test.

Investigations of tests may be conducted by comparing one index test to a reference standard. Alternatively, an investigation may compare two or more index tests. When comparing two or more tests we need to ask how the participants were assigned to groups.

As with the types of investigations we examined in the Studying a Study section, it is possible to assign participants to study and control groups by observing their condition, or it is possible for an investigator to intervene and assign the patients using a process of randomization. When ethical and practical, randomization is a better method because it helps ensure that the participants in each group will be similar. This can have important implications for the results, as illustrated in the next example.

> Two methods for detection of coronary artery disease were compared to the same reference standard test. One method required invasive testing and the other required only blood tests. The patients' physicians advised each patient on which group to enter. The investigation found that the invasive test performed better.

The investigators have observed the assignment rather than use a process of randomization. Thus we can regard this as a special type of cohort study that investigates a test. It is likely that those who received the blood tests were different than those who chose the more invasive test. For instance, one group may have had more advanced or more clear-cut disease. These differences may affect the results of the test.

Conduct of Tests

The technical details of the conduct of the index test and the reference standard test need to be described in sufficient detail, or citations provided, to allow for replication of the investigation. According to the STARD criteria, these details should include:

- Technical specifications of materials and methods used, including how and when measurements were taken
- The training and expertise of individuals conducting and reading the test

In addition, the investigator needs to provide information on the reference standard test indicating the rationale for its use to establish a definitive diagnosis. The selection of the reference standard test may not be straightforward. In order to compare the results of the reference standard test with the index test, the reference standard test needs to definitively diagnose those with and those without the disease.

To accomplish this goal, invasive tests such as biopsies may need to be used. Determining the best reference standard test can itself be an important issue, since to paraphrase Will Rogers, nothing is certain except biopsy and autopsy, and even these may miss the diagnosis. Let us see the type of problem that may be encountered in selecting an appropriate reference standard test in the next example.

> One hundred individuals who were admitted to a hospital with diagnostic Q waves on their electrocardiograms (ECGs) and who died within 1 hour of admission were autopsied for evidence of myocardial infarction (MI). The autopsy was used as the reference standard test for MI. Autopsy revealed evidence of MI in only 10 patients. The authors concluded that the ECG was not a useful method of making the diagnosis of an MI. They insisted on the reference standard test of pathologic diagnosis.

The usefulness of all index tests is determined by comparison to a reference standard test that has previously been shown by experience to definitively diagnose the disease under study. Autopsy diagnoses may be used as the reference standard test. However, even an autopsy may be a less-than-perfect measure of disease, as illustrated in this example, because the pathologic criteria for MI may take considerable time to develop. It is possible that the diagnostic Q waves on an ECG are a better reflection of a MI than pathologic changes at autopsy. The investigator should be sure that the reference standard test selected has, in fact, been shown to be the definitive standard for diagnosis.

Two specific relationships between the conduct of the index test and the reference standard test should be examined:

1. Were the investigators masked as to the results of the other test?
2. Were there any interventions that occurred between the conduct of the index test and the reference standard test?

Those who conduct the index test and the reference standard test should ideally be masked as to the results of the other test. That is, neither those who conduct nor read either test should be aware of the outcomes of the other test. Let us see how this expectation might be violated in the next example.

> A gastroenterologist was investigating a new test for gastric cancer. He properly identified and recruited the participants. He then conducted the new test during the course of an endoscopy. He compared the results of the new test to the results of the endoscopy, using the endoscopy as the reference standard test.

Though convenient, having the endoscopist perform and read both the reference standard test and the index test does not result in masking. The investigator here is aware of the results of the endoscopy when obtaining and reading the results of the new test. To avoid this problem would have required two investigators to participate in the endoscopy process, one performing the endoscopy itself and the other performing and reading the new test, each without knowledge of the other's findings.

In addition to reporting whether masking occurred, the STARD criteria expect the investigators to indicate the time interval between the tests and whether any treatment was administered between conducting the tests. The following example illustrates how intervening time and treatment might affect the results.

> An investigator properly identified and recruited patients to investigate a new test for asthma. Participants were initially administered the new test. Two weeks later, after having received whatever treatments were provided by their attending physicians, they underwent a reference standard test. The new test did not perform as well as expected when compared to the reference standard test.

Ideally, the index test and the reference standard test should be performed within a brief period of time. The administration of treatment between the two tests may make it more difficult for the subsequent test to detect the disease. This is especially important in a disease such as asthma, where the treatment can hide the existence of the disease even when tested by a reference standard test.

Thus the process of assignment requires the investigator and the reader to look closely at how the individuals were recruited and assigned to receive the index and reference standard tests and how these tests were conducted. Once this is accomplished, the next step is to look at the measurements made as part of the assessment process.

15 Assessment

The assessment process in studies of testing, like the assessment process in other types of investigations, addresses the issues of measurement. When performing the measurements, we usually aim to establish whether the diagnostic test is positive or negative. Thus we first need to examine how positives and negatives are defined.

Definition of Positives and Negatives

The STARD criteria expect the investigators to report the definition and rationale for defining positive and negative test results. As we will see, there are several methods that may be used to define positive and negative results for the index test.

When the test claims to either detect or fail to detect a condition, defining positives and negatives may be quite straightforward, such as when a test is positive or negative for growth of an organism or presence of a drug.[1]

However, this in not the situation when tests provide numerical data such as the prostate-specific antigen test, pulmonary function testing, or even such basic tests as the hemoglobin level. The investigators then need to define what they mean by a positive and a negative. This often requires the use of *cutoff lines* or *cutoff points* that separate negative from positive measurements.

In order to utilize a test that produces quantitative results, the authors need to report the procedure used to establish these cutoff lines. Often this entails development of what is called the *reference interval* or *range of normal*. The reference interval often divides test results into below the reference interval, within the reference interval, and above the reference interval.[2]

Most clinical laboratory results are reported using the concept of a reference interval. Laboratory reports often express this reference interval as, for example, 30 ± 10 or 60 ± 40.

The first reference interval should be interpreted as 20 to 40 and the second as 10 to 100. [3]

---

[1] Even for tests that appear to have only positive and negative results, there may be levels below which the test is defined as negative and above which the test is defined as positive. This may be due to the presence of cross-reacting substances that may naturally be present, because the test is not reliable below a certain level, etc.

[2] Here we will proceed under the assumption that a negative test result is a result that is within the reference interval and a positive result is one that is above the reference interval. Low levels on a test may or may not be of importance, depending on the nature of the test and of the disease. When low levels are associated with a disease, the same basic principles apply for defining a positive and a negative test.

[3] It is important to distinguish the method for presenting reference intervals from the method used to present confidence intervals. Data may at times be presented as an observed value plus and minus the standard error, e.g., 30 ± 10. In this situation the confidence interval is approximately 30 ± 2 (10) or 10 to 50. To avoid this confusion, it is recommended that confidence intervals be presented as follows: 30 (95% confidence intervals 10, 50) where 30 represents the observed value, 10 represents the lower 95% confidence limit and 50 represents the upper 95% confidence limit.

Let us take a look at how a reference interval is obtained using the traditional approach. Then we will examine the limitations of this approach and outline other methods that are increasingly being used to define positives and negatives.

The reference interval values may be developed using the following steps:

1. The investigator locates a particular group of individuals who are believed to be free of the disease for which the test is being conducted. This group is known as the *reference sample group,* but for clarity we will call it the *disease-free group.* These individuals are frequently students, hospital employees, or other easily accessible volunteers. Usually they are merely assumed to be free of the disease, although at times they may undergo extensive testing to ensure they do not have the disease that the test attempts to diagnose.

2. The investigator then performs the test of interest, i.e., the index test, on all the individuals in the disease-free group and plots their test measurements.

3. The investigator then calculates a reference interval that includes the central 95% of the disease-free group. Strictly speaking, the reference interval includes the mean (average) measurement plus or minus the measurements within two standard deviations from the mean. Unless there is a reason to do otherwise,[4] the investigator chooses the central part of the range so that 2.5% of disease-free individuals have measurements above the reference interval and 2.5% of disease-free individuals have measurements below the reference interval.

To illustrate the development the reference interval, imagine that investigators have measured the heights of 100 male medical students and found numerical values that looked like those in Fig. 15.1.

The investigators would then define a reference interval that includes 95 of the 100 male medical students. Unless they had a reason to do otherwise, they would use the middle part of the range so that the reference interval for this "disease-free group" would be from 60 to 78 inches.

Let us look first at the implications of those principles for calculating the reference interval and illustrate the errors that can result from failure to understand these implications.

• By definition, 5% of a group without disease will have a measurement on a particular test that lies outside the reference interval.

As suggested by our reference interval for male medical students, individuals outside this range may not have any disease; they may simply be healthy individuals who are outside the reference interval. Thus, outside the reference interval and disease are by no means synonymous. The more tests that are performed, the more individuals there will be who do not have a disease but whose numerical values are outside the reference interval on at least one test.

Taking this proposition to its extreme, one might conclude that a "normal" person is anyone who has not been investigated sufficiently. Despite the absurdity of this proposition, it emphasizes the importance of understanding that the definition of the reference interval often intentionally places 5% of those without the disease

---

[4] One reason to do otherwise is when the distribution of the test measurements is not symmetrical. An alternative in this situation is to perform a transformation such as a logarithmic transformation which may produce a symmetrically distribution. Use of the central 95% or the mean +/− two standard deviations may then still be a useful approach. At times, levels beyond one end of the reference interval, often the lower end, may also be included in the definition of negative. For instance low levels of uric acid or cholesterol are not considered to be outside the reference level. When this is the situation, the 5% outside the reference interval may refer entirely to those with levels above the cut-off point of the reference interval.

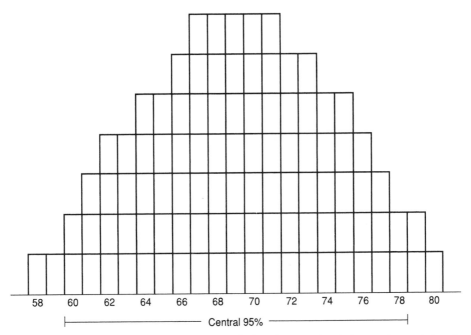

Figure 15.1. Heights of 100 male medical students used to derive a reference interval.

outside the reference interval. Thus, the phrase "outside normal limits" or "outside the reference interval" must not be equated with disease, and outside the reference interval should not be labeled "abnormal."

Let us see how the impact of violating this principle in the next example.

> In a series of 1,000 consecutive health maintenance examinations, a series of 12 laboratory tests was done on each patient even though no abnormalities were found on a history or physical examination. Five percent of the tests were outside the reference interval, a total of 600 tests. The authors concluded that these test results fully justified doing the 12-test panel on all health maintenance examinations.

A reference interval, by definition, usually includes only 95% of those who are believed to be free of the condition. If a test is applied to 1,000 individuals who are free of a condition, on average 5%, or 50 individuals, will have test results outside the reference interval. If 12 tests are applied to 1,000 individuals without evidence of disease, then on average 5% of 12,000 tests will be outside the reference interval. Five percent of 12,000 equals 600 tests.

Thus, even if these 1,000 individuals were completely free of disease, one could expect on average 600 test results that are outside the reference interval. These may merely reflect the method of determining the reference interval. Remember that test results outside the reference interval do not necessarily indicate disease and do not by themselves justify doing multiple laboratory tests on all health maintenance examinations.[5]

---

[5] In considering the implications of test results, it is important to realize that all levels outside the reference interval do not carry the same meaning. Numerical values well beyond the limit of the reference interval may be much more likely to be caused by disease than numerical values that are near the borderlines of the reference interval. Test results nearer the limits of the reference interval are more likely to be due to variation of the test or to biologic variation. For instance, if the upper limit of male hematocrit is 52, then a value of 60 is more likely to be associated with disease than a value of 53.

• The reference interval used needs to be derived from individuals like those on whom it is being used.

In general, the reference interval is calculated using one particular disease-free group. Therefore, when applying the reference interval to a particular individual, we need to ask whether a particular individual has a reason be different from those in the disease-free group.

For instance, if male medical students are used to obtain a reference interval for height, this reference interval may not be applied to women. One might even have to be careful applying it to older individuals or perhaps even students not in medical school. The type of problem that can result from using an inappropriate reference interval is illustrated in the next example.

> A group of 100 male medical students was used to establish the reference interval for granulocyte counts. The reference interval was chosen so that 95 of the 100 granulocyte counts were included in the range of normal. The reference interval for granulocyte count was determined to be 2,000 to 5,000. When asked about an elderly black man with a granulocyte count of 1,900, the authors concluded that this patient was clearly outside the reference interval and needed to be further evaluated to identify the cause of the low granulocyte count.

It is unlikely that there are many elderly black men among the group of medical students used to establish the reference interval. In fact, elderly black men have a different reference interval for granulocyte count than elderly white men. Thus, the reference interval established for the medical students may not have reflected the reference interval applicable to this elderly black man. This gentleman was well within the range of normal for an individual of his age, race, and sex. Because elderly black men are known to have a lower reference interval for granulocyte counts, this must be taken into account when interpreting the test results.

• Changes within the reference interval may be pathologic.

Because the reference interval includes a wide variation in numerical values, an individual's measurement may change considerably and still be within the reference interval. For instance, the reference interval for the liver enzyme AST is 8 to 20 U/L, the range of normal serum potassium may vary from 3.5 to 5.4 mEq/L, and the reference interval for serum uric acid may vary from 2.5 to 8.0 mg/dL.

It is important not only to consider whether an individual's measurement lies within the reference interval but also whether the individual's test result has changed over time. The concept of a reference interval is most useful when no historic data are available for the individual. When previous results are available, however, they should be taken into account, as illustrated in the next example.

> Among 1,000 asymptomatic Americans with no known renal disease and with no abnormalities showing on urinalysis, the reference interval for serum creatinine was found to be 0.7 to 1.4 mg/dL. A 70-year-old woman was admitted to the hospital with a serum creatinine of 0.8 mg/dL and was treated with gentamicin. On discharge, she was found to have a creatinine value of 1.3 mg/dL. Her physician concluded that because her creatinine was within the reference interval on admission as well as on discharge, she could not have had renal damage secondary to gentamicin.

The presence of a result within the reference interval does not ensure the absence of disease. Each individual has a disease-free measurement that may be higher or lower than the average measurement for individuals without disease. In this example, the patient increased her serum creatinine over 60% but still fell within the reference interval. The change in the creatinine measurement suggests a pathologic process occurred. It is likely that the gentamicin produced renal damage. When historic information is available, it is important to include it in evaluating a test result. Changes within the range of normal may be a sign of disease.[6]

- The reference interval must not be confused with the desirable range of test results.

The reference interval is an empirical measurement of the way things are among a group of individuals currently believed to be free of the disease. It is possible that large segments of the community may have test results that are higher (or lower) than ideal and may be predisposed to develop a disease in the future, even though the results are within the reference interval. For instance, imagine the following example.

> The central 95% of total serum cholesterol level is determined among 100 American men aged 20 to 80 years who reported no evidence of coronary artery disease. The reference interval was found to be 200 to 300 mg/dL. A 45-year-old American man was found to have total serum cholesterol of 250 mg/dL. His physician informed him that because his cholesterol was within the traditionally defined reference interval, he did not have to worry about the consequences of high cholesterol.

Remember that the reference interval is calculated using data collected from a group currently believed to be free of the disease. It is possible that the disease-free group consists of many individuals whose results on the test are higher (or lower) than desirable. A result within the central 95% does not ensure that an individual will remain free of the disease.

Thus the reference interval defines the way things are, not the way they should be. American men as a group have higher than desirable cholesterol levels. Thus, an individual with a cholesterol of 280 mg/dL may well suffer the consequences of high cholesterol. When research data strongly suggests a range of desirable numerical values for a test, it is permissible to substitute the desirable range for the usual reference interval. This is now standard procedure for serum cholesterol. [7]

As this example illustrates, the reference interval approach to defining negative and positive is not the only approach. The use of the reference interval assumes that we do not know what an individual's level should be, and therefore we need to rely on the test level as determined for others who are believed to be free of the condition.

These limitations of the reference interval suggest other methods for defining a negative and a positive result. At times each of these may be useful clinically:

- Use of a different range of normal for different ages, gender, race or other characteristics

---

[6] This example also reflects the fact that older individuals have a different serum creatinine reference interval than young individuals, and women have a different creatinine reference interval than men because serum creatinine reflects the quantity of muscle mass. This example also suggest that previous levels for a test may also indicate the desirable level for an individual. This is the rationale for establishing and using baseline levels that establish an individual's level prior to the onset of a condition or disease.

[7] We can use evidence based on subsequent outcomes to define the reference interval. This approach requires long-term follow-up rather than comparing the results of the index test to the reference standard test. Thus, it is often not a practical approach to defining positive and negative results.

- Use of an individual's own baseline level on the test at a time when they are believed to be free of the disease—i.e., an individual's own desirable level
- Use of a desirable interval based on long-term follow-up of individuals with varying levels

For research purposes, another approach is increasingly being used. Using this approach, no definition of a positive or negative is used during the assessment component. The definition of positive and negative is established only after comparing the measurements obtained using the index test to the results of the reference standard test. In this approach a positive result and negative is later defining after first determining the cutoff point at which the index test's performance is the best. We will examine this approach in the next chapter.

Precision

In addition to establishing whether the measurement obtained from an index test is positive or negative, we also need to ask whether the test is precise. Precision, or reproducibility, implies that the results are nearly identical when repeated under the same conditions. Let us see how failure to repeat the test under the same conditions can mislead us, as illustrated in the following example.

> The precision and accuracy of a test of serum cortisol levels were evaluated by selecting 100 study subjects and drawing two blood samples from each individual. The first test was obtained at 6 A.M. and a second at noon. The authors found that, on average, an individual's second test result was twice the level found in the first test. They concluded that the large variation indicated that the test was not precise.

Precision, or reproducibility, implies the test produces nearly the same results when conducted under the same conditions. In this example, the investigators did not repeat the test under the same conditions. Throughout the day and night, a physiologic cycle occurs in individuals' cortisol levels in which they are lowest in the early morning. By drawing blood at 6 A.M. and again at noon, the investigators were testing at different points in this cycle. Even if the test itself was completely reproducible, the different conditions of the subjects would produce variation in the test results.

Studies that examines the reproducibility require that the test be read or interpreted twice. A reproducible test should produce nearly identical results when read by two readers or observers, or by the same observer when they are unaware of their own reading on the first attempt. This is called *interobserver* and *intraobserver reproducibility*.

Interobserver reproducibility is evaluated by have two investigators record their test results without knowing the results of the other investigator. Intraobserver error is evaluated by having the same investigator obtain results twice. The second reading occurs without the observer knowing their own measurement on the initial test.

Let us see how these conditions may be violated when evaluating precision, as illustrated in the next example.

> An investigator studying the reproducibility or precision of urinalysis asked an experienced laboratory technician to read a urinalysis sediment, to leave the slide in place, and then to repeat the reading in 5 minutes. The investigator found that the reading performed under the same conditions produced perfectly reproducible results.

In this example, the technician knew the results of the first test and was likely to have been influenced by the first reading when reexamining the urine 5 minutes later. Determining that a test's results are reproducible requires that the second measurement be performed without knowing the results of the first measurement.

Whenever an observer's assessment is needed to obtain the results of a test, there is potential for interobserver and intraobserver variations. Two radiologists frequently read the same x-ray film differently (i.e., interobserver variation). An intern may interpret an electrocardiogram differently in the morning than he or she did when reading the same test performed in the middle of the night (i.e., intraobserver variation).

Reproducibility of test measurements ensure us that the measurements obtained can be relied on to be the same if and when the test is repeated. Reproducibility is sometimes called reliability because when it is present, we can rely on the measurement obtained from using the test once.

Reproducibility of an index test can be expressed quantitatively.[8] The STARD criteria do not require a quantitative assessment of reproducibility. However the STARD criteria does require reporting the methods used and the estimates of reproducibility obtained if these were conducted.[9]

Completeness

When participants are recruited based on inclusion and exclusion criteria, the aim is for all patients to undergo both the index test and the reference standard test. It is possible that participants may undergo one of the tests, usually the index test, and then fail to have the other test. This is a form of loss to follow-up that, like other forms of loss to follow-up, can bias an investigation if those lost to follow-up are different from those who remain.[10]

Thus, at a minimum the investigators are expected to report the number and characteristics of those who are lost to follow-up. This is usually done as part of the overall flowchart of participation.

In addition to the issue of completeness, test results may at times be inconclusive or indeterminant. For instance, lung scans as a test for pulmonary embolism

---

[8] Notice that the question of precision is generally related to the index test and not to the reference standard test. Even though reference standard tests may not be completely reproducible, they are assumed to have perfect precision as well as perfect accuracy.

[9] Kappa scores are a widely used measurement of agreement between results of tests. Kappa scores vary from 0 to 100%, but it is important to recognize that a Kappa score of 50% or .5 represents only chance agreement. A statistic called Phi has been proposed as an alternative to Kappa. Phi $= [(\sqrt{\text{Odds ratio}^2}) -1)] / [(\sqrt{\text{Odds ratio}^2}) +1)]$. When the odds ratio is greater than 1, Phi=(Odds ratio $-1)/($Odds ratio $+1)$. Phi can vary from $+1$ to -1, with 0 indicating only chance agreement. Thus the magnitude of Phi as opposed to Kappa directly indicates the extent of agreement. It may be argued that Phi could also serve as a measurement of test performance instead of discriminant ability. This would allow use of the odds ratio to relate the measurements for reproducibility (or extent agreement), the performance of a test, and the estimate of the effect size.

[10] The reason for the absence of a test result may not be known and the measurement may be referred to as missing. When results are missing, it is tempting to assume that the measurements are on average the same as those for other similar participants. When this is done we say that the data is *interpolated*. Interpolation is a general term implying that data is filled in, usually between two points that are actually measured, as opposed to *extrapolation* that implies that data is extended beyond the points actually measured. The form of interpolation referred to here makes the assumption that missing data is missing by chance and therefore the measurement would have been on average the same as the data on those we were not missing. This assumption may often turn out to be incorrect. Thus when using interpolation, is it often important to also analyze the data by excluding participants with missing data.

are often reported as three potential outcomes: low probability or negative, high probability or positive, and intermediate probability or inconclusive.

A test may also be indeterminant because it was not possible to successfully complete the test for technical reasons; failure of the patient to be willing or able to fully cooperate; or a variety of other reasons.

When a large percentage of the results are indeterminant or inconclusive, this may greatly affect the value of the test, as illustrated in the next example

> A new index test for acute aortic rupture was shown to produce results very similar to the reference standard when it is positive and also when it is negative. However, over 50% of the time the test could not be completed because of its technical complexity. In addition 10% of the patients died while waiting for the results.

Tests that have a substantial number of indeterminant values may not be as useful as they first appear. As illustrated in this example, it is important not only to understand the probability of indeterminant results but also the reasons that they occur. If the results take considerable time, they may not be helpful for an emergency condition such as ruptured aortic aneurysm even if they are eventually shown to be just as good as the reference standard test.

We have now examined how the index test is measured and are ready to see how these measurements can be compared to the reference standard test. We are ready to move on to the results component of the M.A.A.R.I.E. framework.

16 Results

Estimates: Sensitivity, Specificity, and Discriminant Ability

The results component of the M.A.A.R.I.E. framework asks us to compare the index test and the reference standard test, and to produce summary measurements of their performance. The basic measurement that are used to perform this important job are called *sensitivity* and *specificity*. A single summary measurement can be produced by combining sensitivity and specificity to produce what is called *discriminant ability*. These are the estimates used in reporting the results of an investigation of tests. Let us see how we calculate sensitivity, specificity, and discriminant ability.

Sensitivity measures the proportion or percentage of the participants with the disease as defined by the reference standard test that are correctly identified by the index test. In other words, it measures how sensitive the test is in detecting the disease. It may be helpful to think of sensitivity as *positive in disease (PID)*.

Specificity measures the proportion or percentage of the participants who are free of the disease as defined by the reference standard test that are correctly labeled free of the disease by the index test. In other words, it measures the ability of the test to detect the absence of the disease. Specificity can be thought of as a *negative in health (NIH)*.

To calculate sensitivity and specificity, the investigator must:

1. Classify each participant as being disease positive or disease negative according to the results of the reference standard test.
2. Classify each participant as positive or negative according to the index test.
3. Relate the results of the reference standard test to the index test, often using the following 2×2 table:

	Reference Standard Positive = Disease	Reference Standard Negative = Free of the Disease
Index Test Positive	A = Number of participants with the disease and index test positive = **True Positives**	B = Number of participants without the disease and index test positive = **False Positives**
Index Test Negative	C = Number of participants with the disease and index test negative = **False Negative**	D = Number of participants without the disease and index test negative = **True Negative**
	A + C = Total with the disease	B + D = Total Free of the Disease

Sensitivity = Percentage of the participants with the disease as defined by the reference standard test who are correctly identified by the index test = $A/(A + C) \times 100\%$ = True Positives/(True Positive + False Negatives) $\times$ 100%

Specificity = Percentage of the participants who are free of the disease as defined by the reference standard test who are correctly labeled free of the disease by the index test = $D/(B + D) \times 100\%$ = True Negatives/(True Negatives + False Positives) $\times$ 100%

To illustrate this procedure using numbers, imagine that a new test is performed on 500 participants who have the disease according to the reference standard test and 500 participants who are free of the disease according to the reference standard test. We can now set up the 2×2 table as follows:[1]

	Reference Standard Positive = Disease	Reference Standard Negative = Free of the Disease
Index Test Positive	**400=True Positives**	**50=False Positives**
Index Test Negative	**100=False Negatives**	**450=True Negatives**
	500	**500**

Sensitivity = 400/500 × 100% = 80%

Specificity = 450/500 × 100% = 90%

A sensitivity of 80% and a specificity of 90% are in the range of many tests used clinically to diagnose disease.[2]

Notice that the sensitivity and specificity are always defined in comparison to the reference standard test. That is, the best that they can be do is produce the same results as the reference standard test. When there is a disagreement between the index test and the reference standard test, the index test is considered wrong and the reference standard test is considered correct.

What happens if the new test is actually better than the reference standard test? If the new test is safer, cheaper, or more convenient than the reference standard test, it may come to be used in clinical practice even if its performance is less than perfect. Clinical experience may eventually demonstrate the new test's superior performance, even allowing the new test to be used as the reference standard test. In the meantime, the best the test can do is to match the established reference standard test.

Discriminant Ability

As we have seen, sensitivity and specificity are our basic measures of how well the index test discriminates between those with the disease and those who are free of the disease.

---

[1] Notice that the index test being evaluated has been applied to a group of participants in whom 500 have the disease and 500 are free of the disease as defined by the reference standard test. This division of 50% with the disease and 50% free of the disease is a common distribution used for an investigation of a new test and provides the greatest statistical power. Notice, however, that is does not represent the population's prevalence of the disease except in the unusual circumstance in which the prevalence is 50%.

[2] The principles stressed here are most important when the sensitivity and specificity are in this range. When tests have a sensitivity and specificity close to 100%, issues such as Bayes' theorem and the relative importance of false positive and false negative take on less importance. However, issues such as safety, cost, and patient acceptance may then take on additional importance.

Sensitivity and specificity together provide us with the information we need to judge the performance of the index test relative to the reference standard test. Ideally, however, we would like to have one number that summarizes the performance of the test. Fortunately, there is a simple means to combine the sensitivity and the specificity to obtain a single measurement of what is called the *discriminant ability* of a test. Discriminant ability is the average of the sensitivity plus the specificity:

$$\text{Discriminant Ability} = (\text{Sensitivity} + \text{Specificity})/2$$

Thus in our example, the sensitivity equals 80% and the specificity equals 90% and the discriminant ability is calculated as follows:

$$(80\% + 90\%)/2 = 85\%$$

How do we interpret discriminant ability? The discriminant ability tells us how much information the index test provides compared to the reference standard test, which by definition provides perfect information. That is, we assume that the reference standard test does a perfect job of separating positive and negative results. Perfect discriminant ability is therefore 100%. That only occurs when both the sensitivity and the specificity are 100%.

Discriminant ability provides a means to understand the information content of a test. To understand this use of discriminant ability, let us take a look at what we call a *receiver operator characteristics* curve, or *ROC curve.* The ROC curve axes are illustrated in Fig.16.1.

The ROC curve compares the sensitivity on the y-axis to 100% − specificity (or the false positive rate) on the x-axis. Notice that for the ROC curve, a perfect test lies at the left upper corner where the sensitivity and specificity are both 100%. Thus the ROC curve allows us to compare the performance of a particular index test to this perfect test that lies in the left upper corner of the ROC curve.

The diagonal line that crosses from the lower left to the upper right of the ROC curve in Fig. 16.1 indicates the zero information line. That is, the combination of sensitivity and specificity that provides no additional information. If the discriminant ability is 50%, mere guessing or flipping a coin would do just as well as the index test.

Now let us plot our sensitivity of 80% and our specificity of 90% on the ROC curve. Figure 16.2 plots this test. It also has lines from this test to the left lower and right upper corners of the ROC curve. The area under these lines turns out to be the discriminant ability,[3] that is, the (sensitivity+specificity)/2.

Here, the discriminant ability is 85%. To understand the discriminant ability, it is important to recognize that the information provided by the index test is the difference between the discriminant ability and the diagonal no-information line.[4] Failure to appreciate this principle can lead to the following type of error.

> A new test has been shown to have a sensitivity of 60% and a specificity of 40%. The authors of the investigation conclude that while these results are less than ideal, they still indicate the new test has a discriminate ability of 50% and can therefore provide 50% of the information necessary for diagnosis. They thus advise routine use of the test.

[3] To convince yourself of this relationship draw lines connecting the 'dot' to the left lower and right upper corners. Then using geometry, calculate the area under these lines. The sum of these areas equals the discriminant ability.

[4] One way to think of the meaning of a discriminant ability of 85% is to think of the potential information obtainable from a test as 50%. Thus the discriminant ability of 85% provides 35% of the maximum 50%, or 70% of the perfect information provided by the reference standard test.

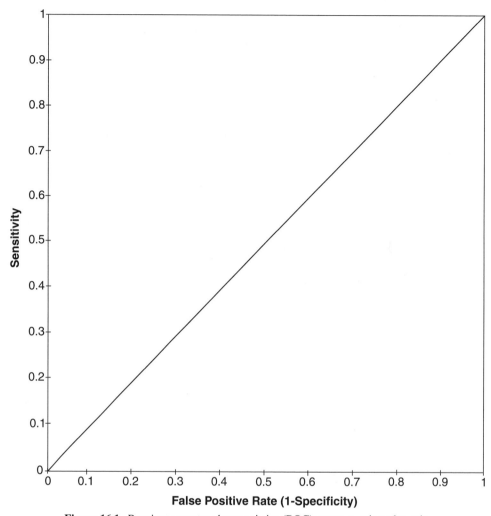

Figure 16.1. Receiver operator characteristics (ROC) curve, x-axis and y-axis.

The authors are correct that the discriminant ability equals 50%, since 40% plus 60% divided by 2 equals 50%. However, a discriminant ability of 50% indicates that the test provides no additional information beyond what could be obtained by chance—that is, by guessing. Thus when drawing conclusions about the discriminant ability, the area under the ROC curve, we need to compare this summary measurement to 50%, not to 0%.

As we have seen, discriminant ability and the ROC curve tells us how well an index test performs. Discriminant ability can also be helpful in determining the best cutoff points to use to define positive and negative for the index test. The aim is to set cutoff points that maximize the performance of the index test.

Remember that in the assessment chapter we stressed the need to define a positive and a negative result and indicated that other approaches are available other than the reference interval approach. One increasingly common approach is to wait to

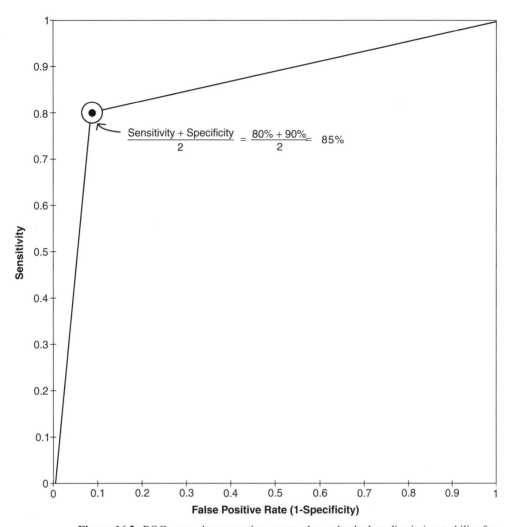

Figure 16.2. ROC curve demonstrating use to plot and calculate discriminant ability for test with 80% sensitivity and 90% specificity.

choose the cutoff points for positive and negative until after the measurements of both the index test and reference standard test are known.

To select the best cutoff points to define negatives and positives, the investigator chooses the cutoff points in which the discriminant ability will be maximized.[5] Thus, to determine cut-off point, the investigators may take the following steps:

1. Choose several sets of potential cutoff points.
2. Calculate the sensitivity and specificity for each set of potential cutoff points.
3. Calculate the discriminant ability for each set of potential cutoff points.
4. Choose the set of cutoff points that produces the greatest discriminant ability.

---

[5] Determining the maximum discriminant ability is the same as finding the point on the ROC curve that maximizes the area under the curve. Thus this method may also be referred to as maximizing the area under the ROC curve.

Thus we have now seen that sensitivity, specificity, and their average (their discriminant ability) are the most common measures of a test's performance. Once these measures are obtained, we need to examine how the results may have been affected by chance.

Inference

When drawing inferences from the results of an investigation of a test, we are interested in whether the results that we observed are likely to hold true in larger populations like those from which the sample was obtained. To address this question the, STARD criteria recommends that investigations of tests report not only the sensitivity and specificity but also the confidence intervals around the sensitivity and specificity.

Thus, the investigations will increasingly report a sensitivity and specificity and also their 95% confidence intervals. These confidence intervals, like those we encountered in the Studying a Study section, tell us how much confidence we should place on the results observed in our samples. They let us know that the true values in the population from which the samples were obtained may be higher or lower than the observed values.

It is important to recognize that one factor affecting the confidence interval is the number of participants included in the investigation. Everything else being equal, the larger the number of participants, the narrower the confidence interval. Large investigations will tend to have narrow confidence limits and will encourage us to place more confidence in the precision of their results.

Ideally confidence intervals for tests are converted into statistical significance levels. However, we do not expect to be able to conclude that one test's sensitivity or specificity is statistically significant compared to another. Thus, for tests, the question we ask is, what is the 95% confidence interval around the sensitivity and the specificity?

Diagnostic Ability

In investigations of testing, like other types of investigation, we need to ask whether there are other factors that need to be taken into account or adjusted for as part of the analysis of the results. When we discussed the measurement of discriminant ability, we assumed that a false negative and a false positive were equally undesirable. That is, we gave equal weight or importance to false negatives and false positives.[6]

False negative results and false positive results may not always be of equal importance. There are a variety of reasons why a false negative and a false positive may not be of equal importance, for instance:

- A false negative may or may not result in harm to the patient, depending on whether the disease may be detected later before there are adverse consequences.
- A false positive may or may not result in harm to the patient, depending on the probability of harm due to further testing and/or from treatment begun on the basis of the false positive test.

---

[6] Discriminant ability assumes that false positives and false negatives are of equal importance. Thus, when maximizing discriminant ability to set the cutoff points, one is assuming that false positives are equal to false negatives.

To better understand what we mean by the relative importance of false negative and false positive results, we can examine testing for glaucoma and ask: What factors influence the importance of false negative and false positive results?

- Factors that may influence the importance of false negative results for glaucoma include: Vision loss from glaucoma is largely irreversible and may develop before it is apparent to the patient. Treatment is generally safe but not completely effective in preventing progressive visual loss. Repeat routine testing may still detect the glaucoma in time for treatment to prevent substantial visual loss.
- Factors that influence the importance of false positive tests include: Follow-up of initial positive results requires multiple tests and follow-up visits that may create patient anxieties and costs. Follow-up tests pose little danger of harm to the patient.

Thus for glaucoma testing, let us assume that you came to the conclusion that a false negative is worse than a false positive. Let us see how this conclusion can influence the use of tests, as illustrated in the next example.

> Test A for glaucoma has a sensitivity of 70% and a specificity of 90%, giving it a discriminant ability of 80%. Test B for glaucoma had a sensitivity of 80% and a specificity of 80% giving it the same discriminant ability. The investigators concluded that these two tests were interchangeable in terms of diagnostic ability.

These two tests are interchangeable in term of discriminant ability since each has an 80% discriminant ability. However, diagnostic ability requires us to also consider the relative importance of false negatives and false positives.

If we regard a false negative as worse than a false positive, we would prefer Test B since it has a higher sensitivity and thus fewer false negatives. This preference for Test B would result in more false positive. However, since false negatives are considered worse than false positives, we should be willing to tolerate the increased number of false positives.[7]

When more than one index test is being compared to a reference standard, it is important to determine whether the index tests generally have the same or different false positives and false negatives. This will be important when we look at strategies for combining tests.

We have examined the results component of the M.A.A.R.I.E. framework and have found that sensitivity, specificity, and their average (discriminant ability) are the measures used to judge the information obtained from an index test. We have found that confidence intervals rather than statistical significance tests are used to report test results. We have seen that a false positive and a false negative may not be of equal importance. In addition a patient may have a false positive or false negative result on one test but not the another. Now we are ready to go on to the interpretation of the results in the next chapter.

---

[7] No attempt is made here to quantitate the relative importance of false positives and false negatives. While possible, this process is rarely seen in the research literature. The impact of different weights on false positives and false negatives usually has its impact on the cutoff point between positives and negatives. The trade-off between false negatives and false positives is also affected by the number of false negatives and the number of false negatives that will occur. This in turn is affected by the pretest probability of the disease.

17 Interpretation

Sensitivity, specificity, and discriminant ability have been chosen as measures because they are inherent characteristics of a test that should be the same when the test is applied to a group of patients in whom the disease is rare or to a group of patients in whom the disease is frequent. That is, they provide measures of a test's performance that should be the same regardless of the pretest probability of a disease—the probability of the disease before the test is performed. Ideally, this allows researchers in Boston, Bombay, or Beijing to apply the same test and interpret the results of testing despite their very different populations.

Interpretation asks us to do more than ask how much information is provided by a test or which test provides the most information. It asks us to use the information to address the following questions:

- Ruling in and ruling out disease: Interpretation asks us to compare two or more index tests to determine which performs the best for ruling in and ruling out a disease.
- Posttest chances of disease, or Bayes' theorem: Interpretation asks us to combine information from what we have called the pretest probability of disease with the information from the test to draw conclusions about the chances of disease after information from the test is included.
- Clinical performance: Interpretation also asks us to take into account safety, costs, and patient acceptance when drawing conclusions about the use of a test.

Ruling In and Ruling Out Disease

As we have seen, the ROC curve is very useful for graphing sensitivity and specificity and visualizing discriminant ability. In addition, ROC curves can be used to visualize which test does the best to rule in and rule out a disease. Figure 17.1 illustrates how we can use the ROC curve to answer these questions. Figure 17.1 indicates with a black dot the sensitivity and false positive rate (1-specificity) of a test to which other tests are being compared. The performance of a second test can be compared to this test by graphing the second test's results on the same ROC curve. The second test may be located in one of four locations labeled on Fig. 17.1. These have the following meaning:

- Superior discriminant ability—the second test is better for ruling in and also ruling out the disease
- Inferior discriminant ability—the second test is worse for ruling in and also ruling out the disease
- Superior for ruling out—the second test is better for ruling out but worse for ruling in the disease
- Superior for ruling in—the second test is better for ruling in but worse for ruling out the disease

Let us look at an example of how we can use the ROC curve.

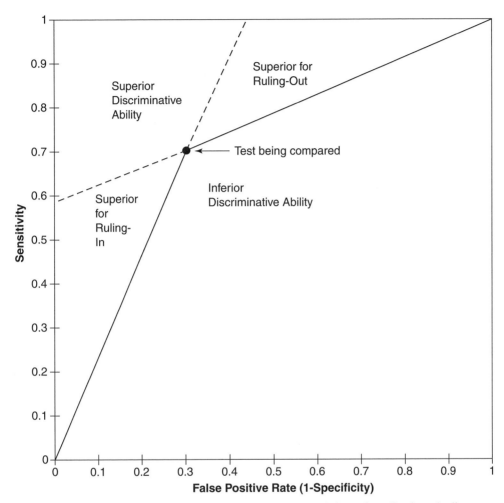

Figure 17.1. Use of ROC curve to decide which test is better for ruling in and ruling out a disease. If a test's sensitivity and false positive rate are represented by the black dot, then test results for other tests can be compared based on where they fall on the ROC curve.

Let us assume that two tests have the same discriminant ability. Test Yellow has a sensitivity of 90% and a specificity of 70%. Test Blue has a sensitivity of 85% and a specificity of 75%. Everything else being equal, which test is better to rule in the disease? Which test is better to rule out the disease?

Figure 17.2 illustrates how we can use the ROC curve. Since test Yellow is up and to the right of Test Blue, it falls within the area designated as "superior for ruling out" in Fig. 17.1. This indicates that Test Yellow is better for ruling out the disease but that Test Blue is better for ruling in the disease.

It is tempting from this example to conclude that the better test to rule in the disease is the test with the greatest specificity and the better test to rule out the disease is the test with the greatest sensitivity. While this is often true, there are exceptions, as illustrated by the following example:

Let us imagine that test Red has a sensitivity of 80% and a specificity of 70% while test Green has a sensitivity of 85% and a specificity of 50%. Everything being

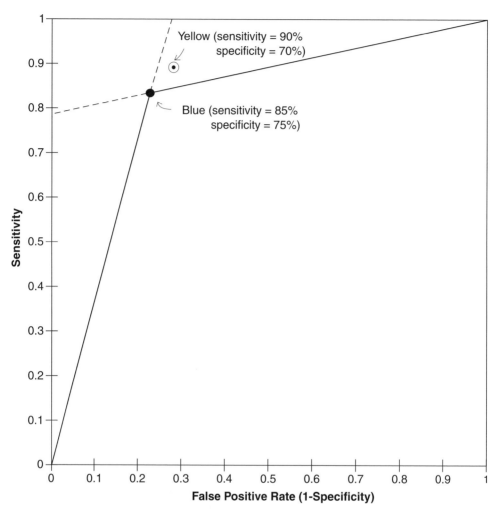

Figure 17.2. Use of ROC curve to demonstrate that Test Yellow is superior for ruling out the disease and Test Blue is superior for ruling in the disease.

equal, which test is the better test to rule in the disease? Which test is the better test to rule out the disease?

Figure 17.3 illustrates that Test Red is actually better both for ruling in and slightly better for ruling out the disease.[1] This is the solution since Test Green falls within the "inferior discriminant ability" area of Fig. 17.1.

[1] This example illustrates that likelihood ratios rather than either sensitivity or specificity alone are the best way to compare tests in order to determine which test is best for ruling in and which test is best for ruling out the disease. This may produce results that are not intuitive. Imagine for instance that Test #1 has a sensitivity of 80% and a specificity of 70%. Test #2 has a sensitivity of 85% and a specificity of 50%. Test # 1 has the largest likelihood ratio of a positive test and the smallest likelihood ratio of a negative test. Thus test #1 should be used both to rule in and rule out the disease, everything else being equal. It is important to remember, however, that this conclusion also assumes that other factors that affect our choice of test, such as cost, safety and patient acceptance, are equal. As we will see, this is rarely the situation.

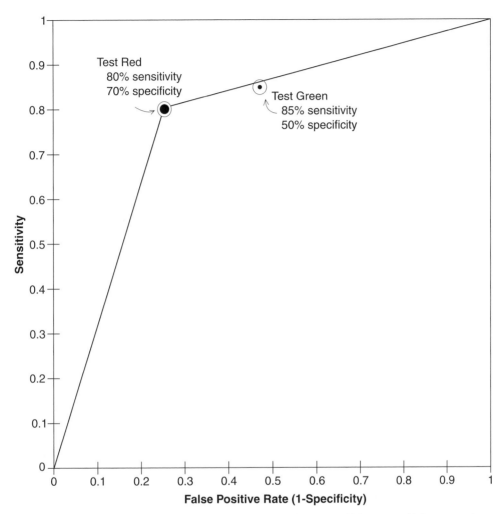

Figure 17.3. Use of ROC curve to demonstrate that a test with lower sensitivity may at times be better for ruling in a disease. Since Test Green falls within the "inferior discriminant ability" area of Fig. 17.1 Test Red is better for ruling in and also ruling out the disease compared to Test Green.

Posttest Chances of Disease: Bayes' Theorem

We have looked at how the pretest probability of a disease can be estimated based on demographic and disease factors, risk factors, and the symptom pattern. To interpret the results of a test, this pretest probability of disease need to be combined with the information that is obtained from a test using what is called *Bayes' Theorem.*

Bayes' theorem is a very useful method for combining information on the pretest chances of the disease with information from the test of interest, i.e., the index test. There are several formulae that express Bayes' theorem, but one which is particularly helpful for understanding the relationship between pretest and posttest chances of the disease is the likelihood ratio form of Bayes' Theorem. Therefore, we need to understand what we mean by *likelihood ratios.*

Likelihood ratios can be calculated from sensitivity and specificity. Likelihood ratios can be used instead of ROC curves to directly compare two or more index tests to determine which one is the best to use to rule in and to rule out a disease. In addition, we can use likelihood ratio to understand the relationship between pretest probabilities, sensitivity and specificity, and the resulting probability of the disease after obtaining a positive or negative result.

Let us use our example of a 80% sensitivity and a 90% specificity to appreciate the calculation and use of likelihood ratios. First let us define the likelihood ratios.

Likelihood ratio of a positive test (LR+) =

$$\frac{\text{Probability of a positive index test if reference standard test indicates disease}}{\text{Probability of a positive index test if reference standard test indicates free of the disease}}$$

Often it is easier to calculate LR(+) using this formulae expressed as sensitivity and specificity

$$LR(+) = \text{sensitivity}/(1 - \text{specificity}) = \text{sensitivity/false positive rate}$$

Thus for a test with a sensitivity of 80% and a specificity of 90%,

$$LR(+) = \text{sensitivity}/(1 - \text{specificity}) = 80\%/(100\% - 90\%) = 8$$

Likelihood ratio of a negative test (LR−) =

$$\frac{\text{Probability of a negative index test if reference standard test indicates disease}}{\text{Probability of a negative index test if reference standard test indicates free of the disease}}$$

Often it is easier to calculate LR (−) using this formulae expressed as sensitivity and specificity

$$LR(-) = (1 - \text{sensitivity})/\text{specificity}$$

Thus for a test with a sensitivity of 80% and a specificity of 90%,

$$LR(-) = (1 - \text{sensitivity})/\text{specificity} = (100\% - 80\%)/90\% = 0.22$$

How can we interpret these likelihood ratios? Likelihood ratio tell us the chances that an index test will be correct compared to the chances that it will be incorrect. For a likelihood ratio of a positive test (LR+), we are comparing the chances that a positive index test indicates disease to the chances that it indicates that an individual is free of the disease. A likelihood ratio of a positive test can vary from 1 to infinity, and larger is better.

A likelihood ratio of a negative test (LR−) tells us the chances that an index test will be incorrect compared to the chances it will be correct. For a likelihood ratio of a negative test, we are comparing the chances that a negative index test indicates diseases to the chances that it indicates that an individual is free of the disease. A likelihood ratio of a negative test can vary from 1 to 0, and smaller is better.

The likelihood ratios help us understand which test is best for ruling in and for ruling out disease.

- Everything else being equal, the test with the greatest likelihood ratio of a positive test is the best test to use to rule in the disease.
- Everything else being equal, the test with the smallest likelihood ratio of a negative test is the best test to use to rule out the disease.

Perhaps the most important use of likelihood ratios, however, is that they make clear the relationship between pretest probability and posttest probability. If the pretest probability of disease is known or can be estimated, Bayes' theorem allows us to calculate the posttest probabilities of a disease after obtaining the results of a test. These posttest probabilities of disease are often called the *predictive values.* The *predictive value of a positive test* indicates the probability that the disease is present after obtaining a positive result on the index test. The *predictive value of a negative test* indicates the probability that the disease is absent after obtaining a negative result on the indexed test. Thus 1 minus predictive value of a negative test tells us the probability that the disease will be *present* after obtaining a negative result on the test.

One way to appreciate this relationship is to examine the likelihood ratio form of Bayes' Theorem.[2]

Posttest odds that the disease is present if the test is positive

= (Odds that the disease is present before the test)

×(Likelihood ratio of a positive test)

Similarly,

Posttest odds that the disease is present if the test is negative

= (Odds that the disease is present before the test)

×(Likelihood ratio of a negative test)

Thus if we know or can estimate the odds that disease is present before conducting a test and we also know the likelihood ratios of the test, we can directly determine the odds of disease after the results of the test are known. We obtain the odds of disease after the results are known by multiplying the pretest odds times the likelihood ratio of either a negative or a positive test depending on the results of the test.

While this may be helpful in understanding the relationship between the chances of disease before and after knowing the results of a test, most people think in probabilities, not in odds. Fortunately, Bayes' theorem also allow us to start with pretest probabilities and, using the data we have obtained on the index test, calculate the predictive values of a positive and a negative test.

The predictive values of a positive test tell us the probability that the disease is *present* if the index test is positive. The predictive value of a negative test tells us the probability that the disease is *absent* if the index test is negative.

Table 17.1 indicates the predictive value of a positive test and the predictive value of a negative test when using a test with a sensitivity of 80% and a specificity of 90% and applying this test to populations with a range of pretest probabilities from 1% to 90%. The table shows how the pretest probabilities relate to the predictive

[2] For instance if the probability of the disease is 50%, the odds are 1:1. For our test, a likelihood ratio of a positive test is 8. Thus the posttest odds = (pretest odds) (LR+) = 1 × 8 = 8. That is, if the pretest odds are 1:1 or 1, the posttest odds are 8:1 or 8. A posttest odds of 8 is the same as a posttest probability of approximately 89% Similarly, if the probability of the disease is 50%, i.e., odds are 1, and the likelihood ratio of a negative test is 0.22, then the posttest odds are 0.22, or a probability of approximately 18%.

Table 17.1. *Relationship of pretest probability of the disease to posttest probability for a test with a sensitivity of 80% and a specificity of 90%.*

Pretest probability	Posttest probability of the disease if test positive, i.e., predictive value of a positive test	Posttest probability of being free of the disease if test negative, i.e., predictive value of a negative test
1%	7.5%	99.8%
10%	47.1%	97.6%
50%	88.9%	81.8%
90%	98.6%	33.3%

value of a positive and also the predictive value of a negative test when we use a test with a sensitivity of 80% and a specificity of 90%—that is, a test with an 85% discriminant ability. This table demonstrates the dramatic impact that the pretest probability can and often does have on the predictive values (posttest probabilities) of disease.[3]

Let us return to the examples of a 23-year-old woman and a 65-year-old man we encountered as we began the Testing a Test section. As we illustrated there, ruling in and ruling out disease requires more than the results of a test. It requires us to make our best estimates or guesses regarding the probability of disease before the test is conducted.

Now let us demonstrate with numbers the impact of pretest probability on the probability of disease after the results of a tests are known, or what we have called the posttest probability or the predictive value of the test.

Let us again look at our 65-year-old man and our 23-year-old woman. We will assume that a stress test has a sensitivity of 80% and a specificity of 90%.

- A 23-year-old female athlete with a chest pain and a family history of coronary artery disease; assume her pretest probability of coronary artery disease is 1% and her stress test is positive.
- A 65-year-old man with chest pain and multiple risk factors for coronary artery disease; assume his pretest probability of coronary artery disease is 50% and his stress test is negative.

Note that these stress test results are reversed from the test result illustrated at the beginning of Testing a Test. Let us see how these new results affect the posttest probabilities or predictive values. Looking at Table 17.1 we find that

- The 23 year old women with a pretest probability of coronary artery disease of 1% and a positive stress test has a predictive value of a positive test or a posttest probability of coronary artery disease of only 7.5%
- The 65 year old man with a pretest probability of coronary artery disease of 50% and a negative test has a predictive value of a negative test or a posttest probability of *not having* coronary artery disease of 81.8%. That is, he has approximately an 18% probability of *having* coronary artery disease.

---

[3] Note that the predictive value of a positive test and the predictive value of a negative test can be calculated from a 2×2 table if the number of individuals with and without the disease in the population are reflected in the 2×2 table. In this situation the predictive value of a positive test equals the number of true positives divided by the sum of the number of true positives plus the number of false positives. The predictive value of a negative test can be calculated as the number of true negatives divided by the sum of the number of true negatives plus the number of false negatives. The predictive value of a positive test indicates the probability that the disease is present according to the reference standard test if the index test is positive. The predictive value of a negative test indicates the probability that the disease is absent according to the reference standard test if the index test is negative.

Thus the 23 year old woman with a positive stress test actually has a lower probability of having coronary artery disease (7.5%) than the 65 year old man with a negative stress test (18%). Thus for many clinical tests, it is essential to focus not only on the test results, but on the pretest probability of the disease.

Clinical Acceptance

As we have seen, the likelihood ratios and the pretest probabilities of disease are the key issues in applying a test. However, they are not the only issues. Additional issues such as safety, cost, and patient acceptance often are important, especially when we are asked to choose between tests. Data from an investigation may be helpful in answering questions such as:

- The type and frequency of adverse effects of the test
- The frequency with which additional tests are required if the test is positive or negative, and thus some appreciation of the costs
- An estimate of the degree of patient adherence to the protocol as a measure of patient acceptance

As part of the interpretation of the test, we should be asking these types of questions. For instance, patients in the investigation may not return or complete the test, suggesting a low level of acceptance. Depending on the nature of the test, this may be due to inconvenience, discomfort, or the intrusive nature of the test.

The cost of the test is generally covered by the investigation itself and is not generally a factor in whether or not the patient participates. However, cost may affect the use of the test in clinical practice. Thus it is helpful if the investigator reports data on the resources required, including professional time to conduct and interpret the test. This provides useful information for extrapolating to the use of the test in clinical practice.

Data on safety needs to be reported, indicating side effects of the test in enough detail to enable the reader to understand the nature and timing of the adverse events.

The following example illustrates how the issues of safety, cost, and patient acceptance may influence the interpretation of which test to use.

> Two tests for gallstones were being compared. Test A has a slightly greater LR(+) and a slightly lower LR(−) indicating that Test A is slightly better for ruling in gallstones and also ruling out gallstones. However, Test A was more expensive, had more side effects, and resulted in more discomfort to the patient. The researchers recommended that Test A be used only when the patient's clinical condition suggested that the condition was life threatening.

The researchers' recommendation takes into account differences in cost, side effects and discomfort. Use of tests is often determined as much by their cost, safety, and patient acceptance as they are by small differences in their ability to rule in or rule out a disease.[4] This is especially true when the disease is not considered to be life threatening.

Now that we have gathered as much information as possible about the meaning of the test for those in the study's population, we need to go on to ask the most important question: How should the test be used for those who were not included in the investigation? This is the process of extrapolation.

---

[4] It is often not clear how to combine consideration of cost, safety, and patient acceptance, i.e., how much importance or weight to place on each one. There is no standard formulae and these factors are often considered using subjective judgments.

18 Extrapolation

Extrapolation of diagnostic test results, like extrapolation in other types of investigations, is the process of going beyond conclusions for participants in the investigation to draw conclusion about those who are not in the investigation. Extrapolation asks questions about the use of the test in other settings such as in clinical practice.

To Target Population

The aim of most investigations of tests is to draw conclusions about the use of the test in practice. That is, groups of patients in practice are the usual target population for the investigation. When asking questions about usefulness of the test in the target populations, we need to ask:

- Do the conditions for the use of the test in practice differ in ways that is likely to affect its discriminant ability—i.e., can we expect the sensitivity and specificity to be the same as under investigational conditions?
- Is a strategy proposed for combining the test with other tests?

Extrapolation of test results, like extrapolation of other types of investigations, asks us to examine the assumptions that underlie the conclusions that we have drawn for the participants in the investigation. A key assumption for tests is that their discriminant ability will remain the same when the test is applied to new populations with lesser or greater prevalence of the disease. That is, we usually assume that the sensitivity and specificity of a test is the same regardless of the setting in which it is used.

Fortunately, this assumption does generally hold up. However, when applying a test to a population with a very different severity of disease, its discriminant ability may not be the same, as illustrated in the next example.

> Urine cytology was assessed as a method for diagnosing bladder cancer by comparing those with advanced bladder cancer and those without bladder cancer. The test was shown to have very high discriminant ability. When used in practice, the test did not perform well, missing most of the patients with bladder cancer that was still in the early stages where treatment was effective.

Extrapolation requires that we step back and take a look at the assumptions that were made in investigating the test. If the test was applied to a clinical population that substantially differs from the study's population, its performance in practice may be disappointing. Thus the most cautious extrapolation is to clinical populations and clinical situations that are very similar to the ones used in the investigation.

In practice, tests often need to be combined. That is, there needs to be a testing strategy. Thus, as part of extrapolation, investigators often propose approaches to combining tests even when the combinations have not been directly studied.

Because of the importance of combining tests, we will take up this issue again in the next chapter, on screening. Combining tests, however, is not limited to screening. Often two or more tests are needed for diagnosis even in the presence of symptoms.

Often the best way to combine tests is to use one test and then use a second test only if the first test is positive. Everything else being equal, we often first use the test with the greatest likelihood ratio of a positive test. This results in fewer second tests being conducted. When using test #1 followed by test #2, Bayes' theorem may allow us to calculate the posttest probability (or odds) of the disease if both tests are positive. We do this by assuming that the posttest probability (or odds) after obtaining the results of the first test can then be used as the pretest probability (or odds) for test #2. Using the odds ratio from Bayes' theorem we can express this relationship as follows:

(Pretest Odds)(LR + of test #1)(LR + of test #2)

$$= \text{Posttest odds of disease if both tests positive}$$

Thus it is very tempting to calculate the posttest odds or probability after obtaining two positive tests.[1]

Unless this strategy for combining tests is actually examined as part of the investigation, its use is really an extrapolation. At times, the use of the posttest probability of test #1 as the pretest probability of test #2 will produce less favorable than expected results, as illustrated in the next example.

> Two tests for cervical cancer were found to each have a high discriminant ability. Test #1 was performed first and test # 2 was performed only if the first test was positive. The investigators used Bayes' theorem to calculate the probability of cervical cancer. The investigators where surprised at the large number of patients who were positive on both tests but did not turn out to have cervical cancer.

It is possible that test # 1 and test #2 produce false positives for the same types of disease. Perhaps the presence of inflammation produces false positives for both tests. When this is the situation the posttest probability of one test cannot be used as the pretest probability of the second test. If this is true, then combining them one after another will produce disappointing results.[2]

The issue of how to combine tests is an especially difficult part of the extrapolation process. In the next chapter, on screening, we will look at the advantages and disadvantages of different strategies for combining tests.

Beyond the Data

Recommendations for the use of tests in practice often require making additional assumptions. As with extrapolation of the results of other types of investigations, we often need to extrapolate beyond the data and to other settings or populations.

---

[1] Notice that this formula implies that if two tests will both be performed, it does not matter which test is performed first.

[2] Whenever we combine tests, we are making an assumption about how the information provided by one test relates to the information provided by the other test. Often we assume that the information provided by one test does not depend on the results of the other test. This is called the *independence* assumption. In order to use the posttest probability of one test as the pretest probability of the next test, the independence assumption must be fulfilled.

The timing of tests and the frequency of use are typical issues that often require extrapolation beyond the data. Issues of frequency of use are a key issue for screening programs, but also are relevant to follow-up of a diagnosis.

Conclusions about frequency of follow-up testing are often extrapolations beyond the data since they are not made on the basis of actual patient follow-up. Conclusions regarding frequency of follow-up testing are often made on the basis of current understanding of the course of a disease, as well as the available interventions. When these underlying assumptions change, it is important to be aware of the need to reconsider the frequency of follow-up, as illustrated in the next example.

> Testing for prostate cancer recurrence was advised every 6 months for 5 years based on clinical experience indicating that recurrence was generally slowly occurring and rarely if ever occurred after 5 years. A new, very successful treatment for early recurrence was developed, leading to the conclusion that more frequent follow-up was needed during year 1 and 2.

Thus the use of tests in clinical practice is subject to change over time, depending on the available treatment options. Testing always needs to be seen as a means to an end. When the options for treatment change, we often need to reconsider the use of testing.

To Other Settings or Populations

Extrapolations to other settings or populations can be obvious, such as when we apply the results obtained in one country to a country with a very different spectrum of disease. It can be more subtle as illustrated in the next example.

> A test for acute cholecystitis was recently developed and its diagnostic performance evaluated in a carefully conducted study of a spectrum of patients with symptoms compatible with cholecystitis. Patients in the investigation received the new test within 24 hours of the initial presentation with symptoms. The new test was found to improve upon the diagnosis of acute cholecystitis compared to other standard tests. To make the test practical clinically, the authors recommended using the test within 72 hours after the patient's initial onset of symptoms compatible with cholecystitis.

The investigators recommendations indicate an approach to implementation that is different than the one they investigated. The participants were tested within 24 hours of the onset of symptoms. When extrapolating to clinical practice, they have recommended that the test be performed within 72 hours of onset of symptoms. While this may be a necessary accommodation to the realities of clinical practice, it is important to recognize that the population being tested may now be very different. In making this extrapolation, the investigators are assuming that delay in testing will not affect the performance. This assumption may or may not hold true.

Extending the time period for referral beyond that in the investigation may affect both the types of patients that are referred and the performance of the test. The time extension may lead to a far more widespread use of a test, and the performance of the test may not meet expectations. With testing, as with other types of investigations, extrapolation often puts us out on a limb and leaves us in limbo.

We have now examined the application of the M.A.A.R.I.E. framework to an investigation of testing. Now let us turn our attention to an important use of testing, that of screening for disease in the absence of symptoms.

19 Screening

Criteria for Successful Screening

Screening is a special form of testing that aims to detect specific diseases in asymptomatic individuals.[1]

The goal of screening for a disease is to identify asymptomatic individuals who have the disease in order to intervene to improve outcome.

Before considering screening for a disease, the following criteria ideally should be fulfilled:

1. Substantial morbidity and mortality: The disease or condition often leads to death or disability.
2. Early detection improves outcome: Early detection is possible and improves outcome.
3. Screening is feasible: A high-risk group can be identified and tested using a testing strategy with good diagnostic performance.
4. Screening is acceptable and efficient: The testing strategy has acceptable harms, costs, and patient acceptance—i.e., one with good clinical performance.

Let us see how we can use these criteria to evaluate the use of screening tests.

Substantial Morbidity and Mortality

The importance of selecting diseases for screening which produce substantial morbidity and mortality is the key starting point for screening. Morbidity may include disabilities such as blindness or strokes, or extended period of costly health care such as kidney dialysis or treatment for coronary artery disease. Despite the importance of identifying conditions for screening that produce substantial morbidly and/or mortality, this condition may be ignored, as illustrated in the following example:

> Screening for sickle-cell trait was widely used among newborn black infants. The screening detected large numbers of infants with sickle-cell trait whose parents were informed that they carried a potentially dangerous gene.

Despite the considerable morbidity and mortality caused by sickle-cell anemia, harm from the trait has not been shown to produce substantial morbidity or

---

[1] Asymptomatic implies that the individual does not have symptoms of the disease for which the screening test is being used. They may have other diseases and/or other symptoms. The term "screening" may be used with other somewhat different meanings. Tests may be used in the presence of symptoms when the clinician wishes to test for a variety of physiological measurements or a range of possible diseases. Screening may also refer to a panel of tests designed to differentiate the cause of a clinical pattern, such as drug screening in the presence of clinical manifestations of intoxication. Screening for asymptomatic disease should also be distinguished from case finding. Case finding usually refers to identification of an individual with an infectious disease with the intention of locating and treating their contacts or cases.

mortality. A common condition that poses little short-term or long-term harm to individuals is not a good candidate for screening.

Early Detection Improves Outcome

The evidence that supports the ability to detect disease at an early stage often comes from studies that compare the stage of disease among individuals diagnosed through screening versus those whose disease was diagnosed in the usual course of health care. The probabilities of detecting disease in early stages through screening and through the usual course of health care are calculated and then compared. If there is a higher probability of detecting early disease with screening, the results suggest early detection is possible through screening.

Early detection, however, is not necessarily the same as detecting disease that will go on to cause morbidity or mortality. It is possible that the disease detected by screening may never become clinically important, as illustrated in the next example:

> A new test is able to detect thyroid cancer in 40% of all men older than 80 years. Cancers detected in these men using the new test are generally found to be microscopic foci that are at an earlier stage than thyroid cancers diagnosed during the course of health care. The investigators are enthusiastic about the possibility of early detection of thyroid cancer and argue that this test is likely to be useful in early detection.

The ability to detect cancer early is not the same as the ability to detect cancers that are likely to go on to become clinically important. Patients may die with thyroid cancer rather than die from thyroid cancer. The goal of early detection is not just to identify cancer early, but also to identify those cases that need effective therapy to prevent progression to clinically important disease.

In addition, screening should not be recommended unless an intervention is available that can alter the outcome of patients detected by screening. Thus, unless there is therapy, or other effective interventions, that are more effective when used early in the disease, there is generally no reason to conduct screening for disease.[2] Thus, the ability to detect disease at an early stage is not enough to fulfill this second criteria for screening. Treatment must be available and more be effective when used during the asymptomatic phase.

The benefit of screening is ideally demonstrated using a randomized clinical trial that randomizes patients to a screening group and a usual medical care control group.[3]

Often, however, it is not possible to perform randomized clinical trials with long-term follow-up. Thus, we often rely on studies that compare the outcome of groups that have been screened with that of groups that have not been screened by

---

[2] At times screening may be worthwhile for other reasons. It may be worthwhile to detect infectious disease in order to prevent spread even if no effective treatment is available.

[3] Even when using a randomized clinical trial, it is necessary to follow up those diagnosed with the disease. They should be monitored not just until they are diagnosed, but until they have had an opportunity to develop the adverse outcome we hope to prevent. That is because a randomized clinical trial that demonstrates improvement in early outcome is not always sufficient. The outcome in the screened group should remain better than groups undergoing the usual course of care, even years after the disease is detected.

conducting cohort studies. These studies may provide important data that suggest the ability of screening to successfully improve outcome.

Cohort studies of screening, however, are also susceptible to misleading results due to *lead-time bias*. This bias results from comparing the time from diagnosis to an outcome, such as death, between those diagnosed through screening and those diagnosed in the usual course of medical care. The potential for lead-time bias is illustrated in the next example:

> An x-ray screening program to detect lung cancer among smokers was performed among a group of smokers who were asked to participate. Their outcomes were compared with the outcomes of individuals in a control group whose lung cancer was diagnosed in the usual course of medical care. The study and control groups' individuals were matched for age and number of pack-years of cigarette smoking. The screened group had a greatly improved survival 1 year after their diagnosis of lung cancer compared with the survival 1 year after diagnosis among the unscreened control group.

Even if the treatment for lung cancer has no effect, we would expect the results for the screened group to be better. By detecting the disease earlier, screening has moved back the time of diagnosis. As illustrated in Fig. 19.1, unfortunately, it has not moved forward the time of death. The increase in time between diagnosis and death may be entirely due to lead-time bias, the early detection without improved prognosis. When using a cohort study to investigate screening, it is often necessary to make an adjustment to take into account the anticipated time between diagnosis by screening and diagnosis after the appearance of symptoms.

There is a second reason why comparing screened and unscreened populations using a cohort study to assess their outcome may not produce convincing evidence of an improved outcome among those screened. This is known as *length bias*. As illustrated in Fig. 19.2, length bias occurs when there are two or more types of disease, such as slow-growing and rapidly growing cancer. When screening is performed initially, most cases that are detected will be slow growers. This is because slow growers remain in the presymptomatic stage for a longer period of time and thus constitute the majority of cases of cancer detected by screening. Fast growers, on the other hand, remain in the presymptomatic stage for a shorter

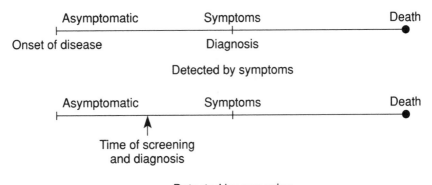

Figure 19.1. Lead-time bias in which earlier diagnosis by screening does not alter outcome.

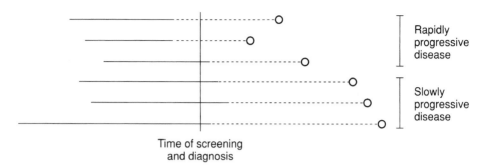

Figure 19.2. Length bias demonstrating why more slowly progressive cases of disease may be detected by screening. Solid lines indicate preclinical phase; dotted lines, clinical phase; circles, death or other endpoint.

period of time and constitute a smaller proportion of cases of cancer detected by screening.[4]

For diseases or conditions that cause substantial morbidity or mortality, and early detection improves outcome, we would ideally like to be able to provide screening to detect asymptomatic disease. However, before this can be advocated, two additional criteria should be fulfilled: Screening is feasible and screening is acceptable and efficient.

Screening Is Feasible

Need for a High-risk Group and More than One Test

As we have seen, Bayes' theorem tells us that the pretest probability of a disease usually has a very strong relationship to the probability of disease after the results of the test are obtained. Thus we need a screening strategy that allows us to identify a group at high risk of the disease and a testing approach that has good diagnostic performance.

When performing screening, we are usually testing presymptomatic individuals. Thus, we cannot rely on their symptoms to help us estimate the pretest probability of disease. Instead, we need to rely on the prevalence of the disease itself and the presence of risk factors to help us identify groups with adequately high pretest probabilities of disease.

Without being able to identify individuals who have one or more risk factors for the disease, we would often be starting with a very low pretest probability. In Chapter 17 we illustrated the posttest probabilities or predictive values when using a test with 80% sensitivity and 90% specificity on a population with 1%, 10%, 50%, and 90% probability of the disease before conducting the test. The 1% example was used to illustrate a common pretest probability when risk factors for a common disease are present in a population to be screened. In this situation, it was evident that one test alone would not be adequate for diagnosis.

---

[4] Length bias is less of an issue in randomized clinical trials if we can assume that the study and control groups have the same proportion of slow growers and rapid growers. Length bias assumes that disease that slowly progresses in the presymptomatic stage will remain slowly progressive once it enters the symptomatic phase. Length bias can be taken into account by studying groups that have previously undergone screening, thus removing from the group most of the long-standing cases of the disease.

When the pretest probability is considerably lower, screening is even more difficult. This is the situation even when a test with high sensitivity and high specificity is used, as illustrated in the next example:

> Suppose that the pretest probability of a disease is 1 per 1,000. Assume that we have available an excellent test with 99% sensitivity and 98% specificity. Using this test on a population of 100,000 with a pretest probability of disease of 1 per 1,000. This is illustrated in the following 2×2 chart.

	Disease (+)	Disease (−)	Total
Test (+)	99 = True Positive	1,998 = False Positive	2,097
Test(−)	1 = False Negative	97,902 = True Negative	97,903
Total	100	99,900	

The prevalence or pretest probability of disease is reflected by the 100 with the disease compared to the 99,900 without the disease.

The predictive value of a positive test can be calculated directly from this 2×2 table as follows:

Predictive value of a positive test = True positives/(true positives + false positives)

$$99/2,097 = .047 = 4.7\%$$

Notice that even after we have obtained a positive test, the probability of disease is still less than 5%. Thus, even when screening with an excellent test, it is usually important that we apply our tests to groups of individuals who have pretest probabilities of disease considerably greater than 1 per 1,000.

We can often identify risk factors for disease that allow us to characterize a group of individuals who have an adequately high pretest probability of disease. Age is the most common risk factor because many diseases predominantly occur among particular age groups, such as premature infants or those older than 60 years. Other risk factors may be identified by such criteria as sexual history, past illness (e.g., ulcerative colitis), occupational exposure (e.g., lead), family history (e.g., premenopausal breast cancer), and ethnicity or race (e.g., sickle cell anemia).

Even if a high-risk group can be identified with perhaps a 1% pretest probability of disease, it is still usually necessary to use at least two tests to diagnose the disease. If we apply our excellent test with 99% sensitivity and 98% specificity to a group of 10,000 with a 1% pretest probability of a disease, the predictive value of a positive test is obtained as follows:

	Disease (+)	Disease (−)	Total
Test (+)	99	198	297
Test(−)	1	9,702	9,703
Total	100	9,900	

The posttest probability of the disease after obtaining a positive test, i.e., the predictive value of a positive test, is:

$$99/297 = 0.33 = 33\%$$

The posttest probability or predictive value of a positive test is still less than 50%. This probability is certainly not adequate to make a diagnosis. Thus, in screening the use of a second test is nearly inevitable, because even with an excellent test, most of the initial positives are actually false positives. Therefore, we need to consider the implications of using more than one test or combining tests to develop a testing strategy.

Strategies for Combining Tests

There are two basic strategies for combining two tests. Using the first strategy, we label the results positive if the first test is positive and if a second test administered after the first is also positive. This strategy that we discussed in Chapter 18, may be called *positive-if-BOTH-positive*. With the second strategy for combining two tests, we label the results positive if either (or both) of the test results are positive. This strategy may be called *positive-if-ONE-positive*.

With the positive-if-both-positive strategy, we usually administer the second test only to the individuals who are positive on the first test. The advantage of this strategy is that it requires second tests on only a small percentage of individuals. Thus, when feasible, the positive-if-both-positive strategy is often the most desirable.

With this strategy, a group that has been identified with two consecutive positives generally has a very high probability of disease. This is because the posttest probability of disease after performing the first test is used as the pretest probability of disease for the second test. When we combine two tests using the positive-if-both-positive strategy, we usually make an important assumption. We usually assume that they are not prone to detect or to miss the same types of cases of disease. We call this the *independence assumption*. The independence assumption is violated when two tests are actually measuring the same phenomenon and, therefore, the tests tend to have the same types of false-negative and false-positive results. If the independence assumption does not hold true, then the posttest probability of disease after obtaining two positives will often be less impressive than expected, as illustrated in the next example:

> A testing strategy for gastric cancer included an upper gastrointestinal (GI) x-ray film performed first. A technician then performed an endoscopy without biopsy if the upper GI test result was positive. The investigators expected that those with two positive results would have a very high probability of gastric cancer and the patient could then undergo biopsy by a gastroenterologist. The results of the study, however, demonstrated that this strategy was little better than using either test alone.

These results are not surprising, because the results of upper GI x-ray examination and endoscopy provide nearly the same type of information. They both rely on the gross anatomy. Thus, the results of the two tests are not independent, and individuals with two positive results will have a less than expected probability of having gastric cancer.[5]

One of the more confusing issues in screening using the positive-if-both-positive strategy is which test to use first. A common misconception is to use the test with the greater sensitivity first. Everything else being equal, the better test to use first

---

[5] In general, tests that rely on different mechanisms of disease detection—such as exercise stress testing, thallium stress testing, and catheterization—will produce results that are more independent of each other than tests that rely on the same type of data such as gross anatomy.

is the one with the greatest likelihood ratio of a positive test. As we discussed and illustrated in Chapter 18, the test with the greatest sensitivity is not always the test with the greatest likelihood ratio of a positive test.

In practice, the issue of which test to use first is quite complicated because it also requires taking into account the relative importance of false-positive and false-negative results, safety of the tests, costs, and patient acceptance of the tests. That is, it requires consideration of diagnostic performance and clinical performance. A biopsy or angiography may be the best test to use first, for instance, but their side effects, costs, or lack of patient acceptance may limit their use to confirmation of other positive tests.

The positive-if-one-positive strategy may be implemented by having all individuals initially undergo both tests. For instance, when screening for colon cancer, testing stool for blood as well as using a flexible sigmoidoscopy is an example of a positive-if-one-positive strategy. This strategy is most useful when the two tests tend to detect different types of disease. For instance, flexible sigmoidoscopy is better for detecting left-sided colon cancers, whereas stool blood testing is better for right-sided colon cancer. The positive-if-one-positive strategy, however, is only useful when the tests detect different types of disease. If the tests detect the same type of disease, using two tests may merely increase the cost without increasing the diagnostic performance, as illustrated in the next example.

> Mammography and sonography are being studied to determine whether a strategy that uses both of these tests on all women older than 50 years will improve the outcomes of breast cancer. It was found that mammography detected 90% of the cancers, whereas sonography detected 60% of the cancers. The investigators expected to be able to detect nearly all breast cancers using both tests. They were disappointed when the results showed that performing the two tests did little better than using mammography alone.

If both mammography and sonography detect the same type of breast cancer, then administration of both tests will produce results that are no better but more costly than administration of mammography alone.[6]

Screening is Acceptable and Efficient

Before a feasible testing strategy can be put into practice for general use, it is important to consider whether it is acceptable. Issues of acceptance may relate to the patient's willingness to undergo the procedure. Colon cancer screening, for instance, faces problems with patient acceptance even though it has been shown to be fulfill other criteria. Issues of patient acceptance may be overcome as procedures become routine and as clinical skills increase. The acceptance of screening, however, also needs to take into account potential harms and costs.

The harms due to screening include side effects of the procedures that may range from colon perforation from sigmoidoscopy or colonoscopy to the anxiety produced by false positive results. The consequences of false positives need to be considered, as illustrated in the next example.

---

[6] The positive-if-both-positive strategy has been called serial *or* consecutive positive testing. The positive-if-one-positive strategy has been called parallel *or* alternative positive testing. These terms may be confusing because most screening strategies ultimately require a subsequent confirmatory test. For instance, colon cancer screening that may be called parallel screening will ultimately require biopsy.

> A screening test to identify patients with a high probability of a stroke was shown to successfully identify high-risk patients. The follow-up testing that was needed, however, produced a substantial number of side effects.

Thus the harms of screening need to be evaluated in light of the full diagnostic work-up for positive results, not merely based on the harms due to the screening procedure itself.

In addition to considerations of safety and patient acceptance, issues of cost need to be taken into account. That is, a screening program need to be efficient in terms of use of resources.

An important element in the overall cost of a screening strategy is the frequency of screening. The frequency of screening is an important issue examined in the health research literature. Screening frequency can greatly influence the cost of screening large groups of patients. The longer the interval between screenings, the more people can be screened using the same resources.

Screening a group at one time and then rescreening them a second time can be expected to produce very different results. The first time a group is screened, it is possible to detect disease that has been present for an extended period of time as well as disease that has developed recently. If there is a long presymptomatic stage, the initial screening may detect a large number of individuals with the disease. Once these individuals are treated, subsequent testing will only detect cases of the disease that have developed during the intervening period. Thus, we would generally expect subsequent screening to identify a much smaller number of individuals with the disease. Failure to appreciate this principle may result in the following error:

> An initial screening program for gonorrhea in women conducted in the only women's health clinic in one community resulted in a 5% frequency of gonorrhea. The screening was continued for every patient visiting the clinic. Over the next several years, the percentage of cultures that were positive fell dramatically. The investigators concluded that the probability of developing gonorrhea had dropped dramatically in the community.

The reduction in the frequency of positive cultures may not reflect what is really happening in the community. Rather, it may predominantly reflect the fact that repeat testing only detects the newly developed cases of a disease rather than detecting new as well as long-standing cases.[7] Most of the long-standing cases have been detected and hopefully successfully treated after the first screening.

The recommended time interval between tests must also be considered in determining the frequency of screening. Ideally, the longer the presymptomatic stage, the less frequently screening needs to be performed. However, determining the frequency of screening based exclusively on knowledge of the natural history of a disease may not be a very reliable method, as illustrated in the next example:

> One reviewer who evaluated the results of the Papanicolaou (PAP) smear concluded that PAP smears should be done every 6 months to be sure that all new cases of disease are detected at an early stage. Another reviewer recommended screening

---

[7] This is different from length bias because it occurs even if all disease had the same natural history. Notice that the first time screening is performed in a population, the number of cases of disease reflects the prevalence of the condition. If screening is repeated at a later time, the number of cases reflects the incidence of the disease since the previous screening (plus the missed cases).

patients every 5 years, arguing that cervical cancer is very slow growing and thus requires no more frequent screening.

Many screening tests depend on the adequacy of the sample obtained. In clinical practice, the PAP smear may not perform as well as in clinical studies because the sampling technique used in practice may inadequately sample the endocervical junction where cervical cancer is believed to originate. If this happens and the recommended interval is 5 years, then it can be 10 years or more before an adequate sample is obtained. Thus, in addition to the natural history of the disease, it is also important to consider the realities of testing in a clinical setting when evaluating the frequency of screening.

An additional factor affecting the frequency of screening, and thus the costs, relates to the types of individuals who seek screening tests in clinical practice. When screening depends on patients to initiate a visit, there are often two types of patients: Those who are screened repeatedly and those who rarely receive screening. This may result in *self-selection bias*. Repeating screening tests at frequent intervals leads to rapidly diminishing returns. Ensuring that those who rarely receive screening are included among those screened may produce far greater benefits. The trade-offs are illustrated in the next example:

> An organizer for a pediatric lead screening program needed to choose between testing patients every time they came in for follow-up and conducting home visits. Home visits would allow one test for every child, even those who never made an appointment. The investigators found to their surprise that they could identify far more individuals with elevated lead levels by conducting home testing in which they tested every child once.

Often those who fail to seek care are the ones who need screening the most. Factors that increase the risk of disease may be closely linked to factors that keep patients from seeking care. Social and economic factors often result in this self-selection bias.

Screening for asymptomatic disease has become an important preventive intervention in clinical practice. Its success, however, depends on being able to fulfill four key criteria: substantial morbidity and mortality, early detection improves outcome, feasible screening strategy with good diagnostic performance, and acceptable testing strategy with good clinical performance.

20 Questions to Ask and Flaw-Catching Exercises

Questions to Ask when Testing a Test

These Questions to Ask can be used as a checklist when reading research articles on diagnostic testing. For practice using the M.A.A.R.I.E. framework, please go to the Studying a Study Online Web site at **www.StudyingaStudy.com.**

The following are the Questions to Ask when Testing a Test.
Method: The investigation's purpose and population

1. **Purpose:** What is the intended purpose of the investigation?
2. **Study population:** What are the inclusion and exclusion criteria?
3. **Sample size:** What is the sample size?

Assignment: The participants and the tests

1. **Recruitment:** How are the participants recruited?
2. **Assignment process:** Does the assignment process avoid spectrum and verification bias?
3. **Conduct of tests:** How are the index test and reference standard tests conducted?

Assessment: Measurement of the outcomes for the index test(s) and reference standard test

1. **Definition of positives and negatives:** How are a positive and a negative result defined for the index test(s)?
2. **Precision:** How precise (reproducible) are the index test(s)?
3. **Completeness:** How complete and unequivocal are the test results?

Results: Performance of the index test(s) compared to the reference standard

1. **Estimates: sensitivity, specificity, and discriminant ability:** How well do the index test(s) perform among those with and without the disease as defined by the reference standard?
2. **Inference:** What are the confidence intervals around the estimate?
3. **Diagnostic ability:** How well do the test(s) perform taking into account the relative importance and characteristics of those with false positives and false negatives?

Interpretation: Conclusions for the participants in the investigation

1. **Ruling in and ruling out disease:** Which index test performs better for ruling in and for ruling out a disease?

184

2. **Posttest chances of disease (Bayes' theorem):** How well do the test(s) perform in diagnosing disease when pretest probability of the disease is taken into account?
3. **Clinical acceptance:** Is there data on patient acceptance, cost, or safety that needs to be taken into account when deciding whether or when to use the test(s)?

Extrapolation: Conclusions for those not included in the investigation

1. **To target population:** What strategy is advised for use of the index test(s), and are the test(s) expected to perform as well on groups in practice?
2. **Beyond the data:** Have the investigators gone beyond the data to draw conclusions on the timing of tests or the frequency of use, etc.?
3. **Other settings or populations:** Have the investigators indicated how the index test(s) should be implemented in other settings or populations?

Flaw-Catching Exercises

The following flaw-catching exercises are designed to illustrate the type of errors that can occur when evaluating diagnostic and screening tests. Each exercise draws conclusions. Read each exercise and see if you can identify the flaws in the conclusions as well as issues that they handled well.

Flaw-Catching Exercise No. 1: *Diagnostic Performance of Tests*

The usefulness of a new test for thrombophlebitis is being evaluated. The traditional reference standard test for thrombophlebitis has been the venogram, with which the new test is being compared. Investigators first obtained a reference interval for the new test by performing the new test on 100 laboratory technicians without a history of thrombophlebitis. They set the reference interval range to include the central 95% of the laboratory technicians' values on the new tests. Values above the reference interval were defined as positive.

To assess the precision (reproducibility) of the new test, the new test is performed on 100 consecutive patients with positive venograms. The investigators found that 98% of the patients diagnosed as having thrombophlebitis had a positive test result. The investigators then repeated the test on the same group of patients. They again found that it was positive in 98% of the 100 patients. From this, they concluded that the new test was 100% precise (reproducible).

Having demonstrated the precision of the new test, the authors proceeded to study its diagnostic performance.

The participants were carefully chosen to fulfill inclusion and exclusion criteria. The authors performed the new test and the reference standard test (venogram) on all participants. They conducted the new test and the reference standard test using the best available assessment procedures.

Next they evaluated the results. The investigation included 1,000 patients with unilateral leg pain, of whom 500 had positive venograms and 500 had negative venograms. The investigators classified individuals as positive or negative by the reference standard test and by the new test, and presented their data as follows:

New Test	Positive Venogram	Negative Venogram
Positive	450	100
Negative	50	400
	500	500

The investigators defined sensitivity as the proportion of individuals with the disease, as defined by the reference standard test, who have a positive new test. Thus,

$$Sensitivity = \frac{450}{500} = 0.90 = 90\%$$

The investigators defined specificity as the proportion of individuals without the disease, as defined by the reference standard test, who have a negative new test. Thus,

$$Specificity = \frac{400}{500} = 0.80 = 80\%$$

The investigators calculated the posttest probability of disease (the predictive value of a positive test) for their study participants. They defined this value as the proportion of persons with a positive new test that actually have the condition as measured by the reference standard test. Thus,

$$Predictive\ value\ of\ a\ positive\ test = \frac{450}{550} = 0.818 = 81.8\%$$

From these results, the investigators drew the following conclusions:

1. The reference interval used here is the only way to define a positive result and a negative result.
2. The new test is completely precise (reproducible).
3. The diagnostic ability of the test is 85% since the sensitivity is 90% and the specificity is 80%.
4. Because of the careful measurements used in this investigation, one can be confident that the sensitivity is actually 90% and the specificity is actually 80%.
5. The new test has a lower sensitivity and specificity than the venogram; thus, it is an inherently inferior test and should not be used unless the venogram is not available.
6. When applied to a new group of patients, such as a group with bilateral leg pain, a positive new test can be expected to have a predictive value of a positive test equal to 81.8%.

Critique: Exercise No. 1

Let us evaluate each of the conclusions reached by the investigators:

1. Obtaining a reference interval by utilizing a group of individuals who are believed to be free of the disease, such as laboratory technicians, is not the only or necessarily the best way to define positive and negative results. It is also possible to set the positives and the negatives by examining a series of potential

cutoff points to determine which one performs the best. This can be done by selecting the cutoff point that maximized the discriminant ability. This is the same as maximizing the area under the ROC curve.

2. If a test is performed several times on the same individuals under the same conditions, the results for each individual should be nearly identical if the test is 100% precise (reproducible). The authors stated that the total number of positive tests was identical when the test was repeated. They did not, however, indicate whether the same individuals were positive when the test was repeated. If the same individuals were not positive, the test could not be considered completely precise.

3. The investigators did a good job of performing both the index and reference standard test on all participants thus avoiding spectrum and verification bias. However, the investigators have confused the concept of discriminant ability with the concept of diagnostic performance. Diagnostic performance, in addition to taking into account sensitivity and specificity, also takes into account the relative importance of false positives and false negatives. Discriminant ability assumes that a false positive and a false negative are of equal importance. Most likely we would not regard a false negative and a false positive for thrombophlebitis to be of equal importance; thus we need to careful not to equate discriminant ability and diagnostic performance.

4. Regardless of the care and proper procedures used in an investigation, the measurements obtained from samples will never provide results that perfectly reflect the larger population from which they are obtained. The larger the investigation, the smaller the error; however, there will always be an inherent sampling error due to chance. This error should be reported as a 95% confidence interval. This investigation did not report the 95% confidence interval.

5. A reference standard test is the measure of a disease against which new or unproved tests are compared, but the reference standard test traditionally used may not be an ideal measure of the disease it is designed to diagnose. It is possible for a new test to be a more useful measure of the disease than the accepted reference standard test. When comparing the sensitivity and specificity of new tests with that of the reference standard test, we must keep in mind that disagreement between the tests may result from a reference standard test that is less than perfect rather than the inadequacy of the new test.

   When the authors concluded that the new test had lower sensitivity and specificity than the venogram, they were making the usual assumption that the venogram had 100% sensitivity and 100% specificity. When we make this assumption, there is no way for the new test to have a higher sensitivity or specificity than the reference standard test. However, it is important not to conclude that the new test is a less useful measure of thrombophlebitis. If the new test is safer, cheaper, or more convenient than the venogram, it may useful in practice. Clinical experience may eventually even demonstrate that the new test is a better predictor of the consequences of thrombophlebitis than the venogram is, allowing the new test to be used as the reference standard test. In the meantime, the best the test can do is to match the established reference standard test, assuming it has 100% sensitivity and 100% specificity and a discriminant ability of 100%.

6. The authors have used the correct definitions of the sensitivity, specificity, and predictive value of a positive test for their study participants. As they stated, the

predictive value of a positive test (the posttest probability) is the proportion of those with a positive new test who actually have the condition as measured by the reference standard test. In this study group, the chance of thrombophlebitis (pretest probability) is 50% (500 with thrombophlebitis, 500 without); thus, the predictive value of a positive test is 450 true positives divided by 550 total positives, or 81.8%.

The predictive value of a positive test, however, is different in different groups of patients, depending on the pretest probability of the disease in the group being tested. One cannot extrapolate a predictive value derived in one group of patients directly to another group with a different pretest probability of the condition. One would expect a group of patients with unilateral leg pain to have a different pretest probability of thrombophlebitis than a group of patients with bilateral leg pain.

Because the probability of thrombophlebitis in a patient who presents with bilateral leg pain is much lower than 50%, the posttest probability of disease even after a positive test would be much lower than 81.8%.

Flaw-Catching Exercise No. 2: *Screening for Disease*

Prostate cancer is known to be a disease with substantial morbidity and mortality among elderly men. A newly discovered test, known as better screening antigen (BSA), was found to distinguish between men with clear-cut prostate cancer and men without any evidence of prostate cancer.

When BSA was used as a screening test, elevated levels were followed by biopsy. Biopsy has traditionally been used as the reference standard test. It has been shown to have both a specificity and a sensitivity of nearly 100% for prostate cancer when used to follow up prostate nodules found on rectal examination. In the initial studies, among men 60 years and older, there were only a few mildly elevated BSA readings, which were identified as false positives on biopsy.

When the BSA was used in screening, the cases detected by screening were diagnosed at an earlier stage of disease compared with those diagnosed in the usual course of clinical care. The prostate cancer was almost always localized to the prostate, compared with the cases diagnosed in the usual course of clinical care in which a substantial number had spread beyond the prostate.

A systematic review of the literature on prostate cancer was conducted. The reviewers drew the following conclusions:

1. Based on the morbidity and mortality of prostate cancer and the ability of BSA to distinguish between those with and without prostate cancer, the criteria for an ideal screening test has been fulfilled.
2. Those individuals who were diagnosed through screening for prostate cancer on the basis of an elevated BSA and a positive biopsy were found to live longer from the time of diagnosis than those diagnosed in the usual course of health care. The reviewers concluded that early detection improves outcome.
3. The sensitivity and specificity obtained by comparing those with clear-cut prostate cancer to those without any evidence of prostate cancer can be expected to be the same when the test is applied in practice to patients with a full spectrum of prostate disease.

4. Because of the successful efforts at screening among men 60 years and older, BSA screening should be used among all men 50 and older since the disease may be present in the 50s.

5. Previous investigators had suggested that age and size of the prostate should be considered when determining the cut-off point for a positive test and a negative test, but reviewers concluded that it is essential to have the same cut-off point for all patients.

6. Prostate biopsy did not perform as well as expected as a reference standard test. When conducted following an elevated BSA, it did not perform as well as it had after a nodule is detected on rectal examination. The investigators could not understand this, since they argued that biopsy is the reference standard test and by definition is always correct.

7. In order to identify patients with a positive biopsy for cancer who should require aggressive treatment, investigators recommended a test known as the Grusome score. The Grusome score was advocated as a test to separate aggressive from less-aggressive cancers. However, the reviewers argued that before this test can be used, it needs to be evaluated using the same procedures as other tests.

8. After diagnosis of prostate cancer, levels above zero were found to indicate remaining disease. Progressive increases in BSA over time were strongly associated with spread of prostate cancer. The investigators rejected this use of the BSA, arguing that a test used for screening cannot also be used for another purpose.

Critique: Exercise No. 2

Let us examine each of the conclusions reached by the reviewers.

1. Substantial morbidity and mortality and the ability to detect the disease at an early stage are important when considering screening. However, they do not in and of themselves justify screening. It is key that early detection improved outcome and that screening is feasible and acceptable.

2. The fact that a group who received screening lived longer from the time of diagnosis is encouraging. However, it is possible that the earlier time of diagnosis merely extended the time between diagnosis and death rather than extending the life span. When this occurs, it is known as lead-time bias.

3. The initial efforts to evaluate a screening test were conducted comparing those with clear-cut prostate cancer to those without any evidence of prostate disease. There are a spectrum of types of patients who were not represented in these studies but who would receive the test if used in practice. This includes men with earlier stages of prostate cancer and men with other diseases of the prostate. When a full spectrum of potential patients is not used in evaluating a test, the possibility of spectrum bias exists. When spectrum bias occurs, the sensitivity and specificity observed in practice is often lower than that obtained in the investigations. Note that sensitivity and specificity can only be expected to be constant from population to population when the same spectrum of disease is present in each population.

4. Even if BSA screening has been successful among those 60 years and older, we need to be careful in applying the results to those under 60. The disease may

behave very differently among those under 60. In addition it is likely that there is lower prevalence (pretest probability) among those in their 50s. Screening may be either more or less successful among men under 60. Thus it is important that conclusions on men under 60 be drawn from data on men under 60.

5. The reference interval (range of normal) for BSA may be affected by the age of the individual and the size of their prostate. If these considerations are not taken into account, there may be a substantial increase in the false positives among older men with larger prostates. Adjusting the reference interval, especially for clear-cut factors such as age, is often a useful means of developing an improved reference interval.

6. Use of a biopsy as a reference standard test implies that the location of the disease can be clearly identified and tissue obtained for biopsy. When a prostate nodule is present and it is biopsied, these conditions are fulfilled. However, when using a blood test, the issue of identifying the location to biopsy is a problem. Thus we should not be surprised that biopsy, even multiple biopsies, is not as reliable a reference standard test after a positive BSA as it is after detection of a prostate nodule on rectal examination.

7. Tests used in preparation for treatment, such as the Grusome score, are seldom evaluated using the same criteria as those used for screening and diagnosis. While full evaluation may be desirable, it is not often practical prior to use in practice. Tests for aggressiveness of disease have often been used successfully in determining the approach to treatment. These are often based primarily on an understanding of the biology and the progression of the disease.

8. The same tests may be used for multiple purposes. Therefore, it is important to identify the purpose for which a test is used. A test may perform better for one purpose than another. A test may perform better for prognosis than it does for diagnosis. For instance, when the prostate has been fully removed, the level of the BSA may be expected to fall to zero. Subsequent increases may be a particularly good indicator of the progression of the disease.

The Testing a Test section aims to illustrate how research investigations can be used to measure the performance of tests used for diagnosis and screening. As we have seen, the M.A.A.R.I.E. framework can be used to organize a review of an investigation of a test. The use of testing relies heavily on knowledge of the rates of disease. Thus, let us turn our attention to the next section Rating a Rate.

Rating a Rate III

21 Method and Assignment

Rates of disease are often the subject of investigations. When rates are obtained and used for comparison, the investigations can be reviewed using our M.A.A.R.I.E. framework. Figure 21.1 illustrates the application of the M.A.A.R.I.E. framework to investigations that compare rates.

Method

Purpose

When examining an investigation of rates, as with the other types of investigations, the first question to ask is: What is the purpose of the investigation—i.e., what is the question being asked?

The types of investigations of rates that we will examine do more that calculate rates, they compare rates. Thus the types of questions that will be asked relate to the comparison of rates between different population or changes in rates at different times in the same population.

Specific purposes for investigating rates may include the following:

- Studies of etiology often begin with a hypothesis derived from observing a difference or change in rates of disease. For instance:

  An investigator found that countries with a high consumption of olive oil had a lower rate of death due to coronary artery disease compared to countries with a low consumption of olive oil. On the basis of this study he hypothesized an association at the individual level between consumption of olive oil and lower probability of death due to coronary artery disease.

- Testing relies on rates to estimate the pretest probability before knowing the patient's symptoms. For instance:

  An investigator found that the rate of developing coronary artery disease increases with age among men and women, with the rate among women trailing men by approximately 10 years. He used this as the starting point for estimating the risk of coronary artery disease in a 65-year-old man and a 23-year-old woman.

- Prediction of the future often rests on rates of development of disease and the subsequent rates of death or disability. For instance:

  Among those with a previous myocardial infarction, the rate of death fell steadily from 100 per 1,000 per year to 70 per 1,000 per year between 1975 and 2005. The investigators predicted that the rate would be approximately 65 per 1,000 per year by 2010.

- Efficacy may be suggested by looking at rates before and after an intervention. For instance:

  The rate of developing Reye's syndrome was 0.5 per 100,000 children under 12 years old per year during the 1960s and 1970s when aspirin was promoted for

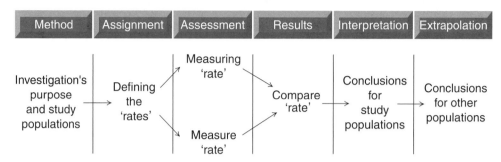

Figure 21.1. M.A.A.R.I.E. framework for investigations comparing rates.

use by children. The rate fell to 0.1 per 100,000 children under 12 years old per year after aspirin was widely considered contraindicated for young children.

Rates are often used to record the occurrence of risk factors for disease, the occurrence of disease, and the outcomes of disease, such as death or disability. When rates are used merely to record, we call the results *descriptive studies*. Descriptive statistics focus on calculating rates. Descriptive studies, unlike other types of investigations, do not aim to compare one group to another or one period of time to another. In contrast, studies that compare rates are called *analytical studies*.

The types of investigations that lead to immediately useable hypotheses or conclusions usually require comparisons. That is, when looking at studies of rates of disease, we are usually interested in the comparing rates between groups or populations, or comparing the rates from one time period to another. Thus, we will focus our attention on investigations that compare rates.

Types of Rates

In classifying rates, the most important distinction is between proportions and true rates.[1] A proportion is an expression of probability in which the numerator is derived from the denominator. That is, the numerator is a subset of the denominator, as illustrated in the following example.

> An investigator measured the number of cases of lupus erythematosus in a community and finds 100 cases. She calculated the number of cases of lupus per 100,000 people living in the community of 1 million people and concludes that there are 10 cases of lupus per 100,000 people.

This proportion is known as *prevalence*. Prevalence measures the probability that a disease is present at a particular point in time. That is, a prevalence of 10 per 100,000 represents a probability of 1 per 10,000, or 0.0001, or 0.01%.

---

[1] At times the term rate is used in this section as a generic term to indicate any fraction with a numerator and a denominator. A fraction may consist of a numerator that measures one phenomenon and a denominator that measures a different phenomenon. For example, in perinatal mortality rates, the numerator consists of the number of stillbirths in a population and the denominator is the number of live births during the same time period. This special type of fraction can be confusing because it is often referred to merely as a ratio. A better term might be *unrelated ratio*. This type of ratio does not have any predefined limits. In other words, theoretically, it can vary from 0 to infinity since the numerator and the denominator do not depend on each other.

Another important proportion that is a probability is known as a *case fatality*. Case fatality is a measure of prognosis. Case fatality indicates the probability of dying from the disease once the diagnosis is made. Thus the numerator contains the number of deaths while the denominator contains the number of cases diagnosed.

Strictly speaking, a rate, or what we might call a *true rate*, satisfies the conditions of a proportion but also includes a period of time. That is, in a true rate the numerator includes the occurrence of events over a period of time, often over a 1-year period, as illustrated in the next example.

> The lupus erythematosus investigator now identifies all new cases that develop in the community during 2005. She finds 5 cases per 100,000 people in 2005 and concludes that the rate is 5 per 100,000 per year.

This measurement is known as an *incidence rate*. It measures the probability of the occurrence of an event such as the diagnosis of lupus over the period of a year. Like prevalence, the incidence rate has a numerator that comes from the denominator and therefore measures a probability. Unlike proportions that measure the situation at one point in time, rates measure the occurrence of events over time.

Another important rate is known as the *mortality rate*. Mortality rates measure the incidence of death per 100,000 people per year. Thus, they are true rates and indicate the probability of death in a population over the course of a year.[2]

Three rates together are needed to capture a composite picture of a disease.[3] They describe the epidemiology of the disease.

- Incidence rate: the rate of development of the disease over a period of 1 year
- Prevalence: the probability of having the disease at one point in time
- Case fatality: the probability of dying once the disease has developed

These three rates aim to measure three distinct points in the progression of the disease over a period of time. Together, they aim to capture a point-in-time photograph of a moving target. We will come back to these rates in Chapter 24 on the interpretation of rates when we will ask: What is the underlying reasons for the changes or differences in rates?

Study Population

Identifying the study's population requires us to ask about characteristics of the population from which the data was obtained as well as the procedure for obtaining the data. Together, these issues can be thought of as understanding the source of the data.

---

[2] Combination measurements can be used and can cause confusion. For instance, the *proportionate mortality ratio* (PMR) which tells us the relative importance of one disease compared to another often in one particular age group. It can cause confusion if we try to use it as a probability. For instance, the fact that people older than 65 have a lower proportionate mortality ratio from trauma does not imply that the elderly have a lower probability of dying from trauma. Because many more deaths occur among people older than 65 years, even small PMR dying from trauma may represent a mortality rate from trauma among the elderly that exceeds the young.

[3] Another measurement that may be used is called *period prevalence*. Period prevalence is the number of cases that occur during a time period divided by the average size of the population. Period prevalence incorporates measures of incidence as well as prevalence. Thus, at times it may be a better reflection of the impact of a disease or condition that either one alone. Prevalence may also be referred to as *point prevalence* to distinguish it from period prevalence.

Rates may be obtained using a variety of sources of data:

- Complete data from the total population
- Incomplete data from the total population
- A representative sample of the total population
- A non-representative sample of the total population

Complete or nearly complete data in most countries is difficult to obtain. Often only a short list of types of data are available that includes births and deaths. In addition, census data from the entire population is usually obtained on a regular basis, often every 10 years. These are the basic sources of complete population data that are used to obtain rates.

Mortality rates for the entire population and infant mortality rates that measure the rate of deaths during the first year of life per 1,000 live births are usually calculated from complete population data. Many rates, however, rely on less-complete forms of data, data derived from representative samples designed to reflect the larger population or non-representative samples that do not necessarily reflect the larger population.

Most data is less complete than births and deaths. Many infectious diseases and a limited number of other conditions are collected by what is called *reportable diseases*. Reportable diseases are diseases or conditions that are expected to be reported to a governmental organization, often the local health department. This reporting is usually officially the responsibility of the clinician making the diagnosis. At times, reportable diseases may be identified on the basis of laboratory tests and reported by the laboratory itself. As we will see in chapter 22 on assessment, reporting by clinicians is often far from complete and is often non-representative. That is, it does not reflect the rates in the larger population. This has important implications for this method of data collection.

Rates may be obtained by randomly sampling the entire population to produce a subset or sample that is large enough and representative enough of the entire population to produce accurate estimates of rates in the entire population. Sampling may be done by giving each individual the same probability of being included in the sample. This is called *simple random sampling*. Alternatively, what is called *stratified random sampling* may be performed. This approach ensures that enough members of subgroups such as minority populations are included in a sample to allow accurate estimate of rates for these groups.[4]

Rates may be collected utilizing special sites sometimes called *sentinel sites*. Sentinel sites are settings such as emergency departments or ambulatory care clinics that, while not representative of the entire population, often are the sites where the first cases of a condition present for care. Sentinel sites are used for detection of influenza early in the epidemic cycle and to monitor for expected and unexpected cases compatible with bioterrorism. The use of sentinel sites implies comprehensive data collection for particular conditions at carefully selected sites.

Thus, there are a number of sources of data for rates that may be used. It is important, however, to recognize that rates can also be calculated using

---

[4] A number of national surveys are conducted using stratified random sampling. In the United States household surveys have been conducted on a regular basis and provide a wide range of data on health behaviors, risk factors, and use of health care services. In addition, these types of surveys are being used to assess the health status or degree of disability that exists at different ages and among subgroups of the total population.

easily available data that may produce misleading results, as illustrated in the next example.

> Data on myocardial infarction was readily available from 2 of 20 hospitals in a large metropolitan area. Using data on myocardial infarction from a county hospital, an investigator estimated that the community's rate of myocardial infarction was 150 per 100,000 per year. An investigator using data from a private hospital in the same community estimated that the rate was 155 per 100,000 per year. Because the rates were so similar, a reviewer concluded that the rate in the community must be between 150 and 155 per 100,000 per year.

Neither of these investigations obtain a random or representative sample of the community. The data reflect only myocardial infarctions that make it to these hospitals. The data comes from two hospitals in which the data is convenient for the investigators to obtain. It is possible that myocardial infarction patients or ambulance drivers either selectively chose one of these hospitals or selectively avoided them.

Use of this type of data is called a *convenience sample*. If data on all hospitals or a representative sample of hospitals was available, the rates might have been very different. When rates are derived from convenience samples, they usually cannot be used to represent a larger community or population.

Convenience samples may be the only available data. Though they cannot be relied on to reflect the larger population rates, repeat use of convenience samples from the same source may be useful in detecting changes, especially if the conditions for data collection remain the same. For instance, changes in rates of myocardial infarction in this community might be monitored by changes that are occurring in these two hospitals.

Thus, the first step in examining an investigation of rates is to ask, what is the purpose? what is being measured? and, where does the data come from?

Assignment

The process of assignment for rates requires us to examine the definitions of each of the components of rates. That is, the numerator, the denominator, and the period of time.

Numerator

As we have seen, rates may be measured for a variety of purposes. We can use rates to measure diseases, condition such as injuries, or administrative occurrences such as hospital admissions. Because of the wide variety of uses of rates, the term *event* is used to indicate the recognition of the condition or diagnosis that appears in the numerator of a rate.

To better understand what issues arise when defining the events that appear in the numerator, let us imagine that we are interested in comparing the rates of death and severe injury from automobiles and trucks. In order to make this comparison, we need to define exactly what we mean by death and severe injury in the numerator, as well as exactly what we mean by an automobile and a truck. While these distinctions may seem obvious, consider the following:

- Are the categories adequately distinct? What is a truck? Does it include sports utility vehicles (SUVs)?

- What is the definition of an outcome? For instance, how do we define a severe injury?
- Can an outcome be clearly attributable to one particular category? For instance, how is a death measured if a truck hits a car and kills the driver of the car? Is the death a car-or a truck-related death?

Thus, it is important to understand how the numerator of a rate is defined.

Denominator

The denominator of a rate may be defined in a number of ways as well. The choice of the denominator depends on the question being asked. For instance, imagine the following possible denominators:

- 100,000 people
- 100,000 vehicles
- 1 million miles

Each of these denominators asks us to address a different question and may produce a different answer, as illustrated in the next example.

> An investigation that used 100,000 people in the denominator concluded that automobiles had a higher death rate than commercial trucks. An investigation that used 100,000 vehicles in the denominator concluded that trucks had the higher death rate. An investigation that used 1 million miles driven in the denominator concluded that the rates for cars and trucks were similar.

The fact that there are far more automobiles than commercial trucks may in and of itself explain why there are more deaths due to automobiles. On the other hand, truck drivers may drive far more miles per vehicle than automobile drivers. This could explain the increased rate of deaths from trucks per 100,000 vehicles. The rate per 1 million miles driven may reflect both the numbers of vehicles and extent of their use.

Time

A true rate as opposed to a proportion or probability explicitly includes a unit of time as part of the measurement. The most common unit of time is a one-year calendar period, i.e., 2003, 2004, etc. At times, rates of disease may be expressed at rates per week, per month, or a variety of other time periods.

Sometimes, the people in the denominator of the rate will not be followed for the full time period. This is often the case in studies that follow individuals for varying periods of time. Thus, rates may also be expressed using what is called *person-years*. A person-year represents one individual followed for one year. However, a person-year can be made up of two persons followed for 6 months, four persons followed for 3 months, or any other combination. In addition, one person followed for 2 years would result in 2 person-years.

It is important to recognize the distinction between population-at-risk and person-years in a rate, as illustrated in the next example.

> An investigation found that the rate of developing gastroenteritis on cruise ships was 3,600/100,000 passengers. Another investigation found that the rate was 100/100,000 person-years. A reviewer examining these studies concluded that these were dramatically different results.

The results of these two studies are actually quite compatible if we assume that most passengers spend only a short period of time on board a cruise ship, perhaps 10 days. If the average of passenger spent 10 days on a cruise ship, then it would take over 36 passengers to produce one person-year. Thus, the results of these two investigations are very compatible, differing only in the unit of measurement of time.

In examining the assignment process, we have taken a look at how the numerator, the denominator, and the unit of time are defined. Understanding these definitions is key to appreciating what the rate is attempting to measure. The process of obtaining the measurement depends on how the investigator has defined the rate, as we will see in the next chapter on assessment.

22 Assessment

Assessment is the process of measurement. With rates, we are interested in how the numerator and the denominator are measured.

Measuring the Numerator and the Denominator

Let us begin examining assessment by looking at the numerator and asking how cases such as diagnosis of a disease or other events such as disability are actually measured. The identification of cases may reflect actual diagnoses made in the laboratory or by definitive criteria used in clinical practice. Alternatively, definitions of disease for purposes such as early detection of an epidemic may use definitions of disease that are less definitive, as illustrated in the following example:

> In order to monitor the rates of herpes genitalis in a community, the frequency of positive cultures obtained by all the laboratories in the community was used. A second study of patients in doctors' offices found a rate three times as high using a definition of herpes genitalis that relied on clinical findings and patient reports.

The method for measuring an event may greatly affect its rate. Often the goal is not to be completely accurate or completely precise, but rather to use a measurement that can be conveniently followed over time as a technique for identifying changes in the rate of development of a disease or in its prognosis once it occurs.

Measuring the denominator often requires the availability of data that is collected for other purposes. Census data is often the source of population data for national rates or those of smaller geographic units. Rates of disease often distinguish between the total population and what is called the *at-risk population*. For instance, what should be the denominator for the probability of becoming pregnant? All females? Females of child-bearing age? Females of child-bearing age who have not had a hysterectomy?

Regardless of the ideal denominator, investigators often need to be pragmatic and define the denominator based on the availability of reliable data. Defining a denominator that reflects women of childbearing age requires defining childbearing age and obtaining data on the female population in this age group, an achievable goal. Measuring women of childbearing age using census data may be a pragmatic choice. It is an improvement over using all women even though it does not meet the goal of using only women who have not had a hysterectomy.

Often the entire population will be substituted for those who are actually at risk of a condition, especially when it is believed to be a close approximation of those at risk, as illustrated in the next example.

> The incidence of blindness is estimated by sampling the entire population to estimate the total number of new cases of blindness per year. The total population was used as the denominator.

Use of the total population as the denominator assumes that everyone is at risk. This distinction often makes little difference when only a small percentage of the population already has the condition and thus are not at risk of experiencing it. That is, only a small percentage of the population is blind, so using the total population represents a quite good estimate of those at risk of blindness. Contrast this, however, to the following example.

> The incidence of visual impairment requiring correction for reading was estimated by sampling the population to estimate the number of new cases per year. The total population was used as the denominator.

Here, the use of the total population as the at-risk-population has a major impact on the rate since a substantial portion of the total population already has visual impairment requiring correction for reading. The use of the total population may result in underestimating the probability that those at risk will develop visual impairment.

Because the choice of denominator is often based on pragmatic considerations, it is important that the reader of the research examine not only what the investigator intended to measure in the denominator, such as the at-risk group for pregnancy, but also what they actually measured.

Derivation of Rates

At times, rates such as mortality rates can be obtained using complete population data. Complete population data may be available on births, causes of death, and the size and composition of the population.

However, the three rates that capture a composite picture of the rate of a disease—incidence rate, prevalence, and case fatality—cannot generally be obtained from complete population data. Often they need to be derived from other available data or estimated from incomplete data or samples of the population of interest.

In order to understand how these rates can at times be derived from other rates, we need to examine the approximate relationship that exist between them.

Prevalence and incidence rates are related to each other approximately as follows:

$$\text{Prevalence} = \text{Incidence rate} \times \text{Average duration of the disease}$$

Or

$$\text{Incidence} = \text{Prevalence/Average duration}$$

Thus, if prevalence is known based on an investigation conducted at one point in time and the average duration of a disease can be estimated, then it is possible to derive an estimate of the incidence rate for a disease, as illustrated in the next example.

> The prevalence of sickle cell anemia obtained using a representative sample of the population is estimated to be 300 per 100,000. The duration of the disease as estimated based on a representative sample is 30 years. From these data the incidence rate is estimated to be 10 per 100,000 per year.

Here, the estimate of the incidence of the disease is obtained by dividing the prevalence by the average duration of the disease. Alternatively, if the incidence rate and the average duration of disease can be estimated, it is possible to derive the prevalence of the disease.

At times the estimates are not really derived from data but represent the best guesses of experts, as indicated in the next example.

> The incidence of bipolar disorder is estimated by an investigation that carefully sampled the prevalence of the disease in a representative sample of the total population. They then estimated the incidence of the disease based on the clinical observations that once, present the disease is of lifelong duration.

This example illustrates that duration of disease is often estimated based on clinical impressions or knowledge of the course of a disease rather than actual measurements. Even if the prevalence can be accurately estimated using a sample, the assumption that bipolar disorder is a lifelong disease may not hold true.

The incidence rate is related to the mortality rate as follows:

$$\text{Mortality rate} = \text{Incidence rate} \times \text{case fatality}$$

Thus, if the mortality rate is known, it is possible to estimate either the incidence rate or case fatality if the other one can be estimated, as illustrated in the following example:

> The mortality rate from sickle cell anemia is found to be 4 per 100,000 per year. The previous estimate of incidence rate of 10 per 100,000 per year was used to calculate the case fatality. The case fatality as derived was 40%.

Deriving rates rather than measuring them directly can lead to problems of accuracy and precision. Estimates of incidence reflect a particular time period, while mortality rates reflect a later time period. Thus, the measures used here assume that nothing is changing, which is rarely the situation. In addition, case fatalities for conditions such as sickle cell anemia depend heavily on what is considered the cause of death. For instance if a sickle cell patient dies of a stroke, is that defined as due to sickle cell anemia or due to a stroke?

Deriving rates rather than measuring them directly may be necessary and useful in some situations. It is important to recognize, however, that derived rates are prone to problems of accuracy and precision.[1]

Completeness

As we have seen, rates may be derived from incomplete data sources. This is often the situation because our calculation of rates often relies on reported rates, which may be less than complete and less than representative of the entire population of interest. That is, they may be a biased sample of the entire population.

When rates are obtained from data on reportable diseases—a convenience sample—it is especially susceptible to be being both incomplete and non-representative, as suggested by the following example.

> Incidence rates of AIDS were obtained from physicians' reports. When these reports were reviewed, it was concluded that most of the reports occurred when requested

---

[1] Note that the relationship between incidence and prevalence is actually more complex that suggested by the simple formula prevalence = incidence × average duration. First, this formula assumes that the incidence rate and the average duration are stable over time. It also fails to recognize that duration of disease depends on the age of onset and the average life expectancy of those who develop the disease. In addition, the calculation may divide one estimate by another and thus is subject to greater error than would be the situation when only one estimate is being made.

by patients who wished to qualify for disability coverage or where the physician did not feel the disclosure would violate the patient's privacy.

The diagnosis of AIDS cannot be made exclusively on the basis of laboratory tests. It requires that the clinician put together the data. Thus, data on the frequency of AIDS may be both incomplete and unrepresentative. Whenever a judgment is required about whom to report, incomplete and biased data is likely to result. Reported data on AIDS is likely to introduce a bias that makes the types of patients reported unrepresentative of all patients with the disease.

Reporting of disease is a legal expectation protecting the clinician or laboratory that reports the disease from allegations of violations of privacy. Nonetheless, or perhaps because there are usually no consequences for not reporting, the data on reportable diseases is usually incomplete and unrepresentative of all the cases that occur.

In summary, the assessment process focuses on how rates are actually measured. It requires that we examine both the measurement of events in the numerator and measurement of the at-risk population in the denominator. It also requires that we recognize that the unit of time may be measured per year or per person-year, producing results that appear to differ. Rates may be derived by combining data collection with estimates made on the basis of expert opinion or general knowledge of the course of a disease. The relationship between incidence and prevalence and the relationship between mortality and case fatality should be used cautiously to derive rates. Finally, rates are often derived from incomplete or unrepresentative samples. It is important to recognize the potential for both inaccuracies and imprecision that can results from this approach to estimating rates.

23 Results

Estimation: Measurement of the Difference

The results component of an investigation of rates involves the comparison of rates to obtain a measurement of the differences. These comparisons may examine differences between rates for two populations such as two countries or between subgroups of the same country such as blacks vs. whites. Alternatively, the comparisons may focus on changes within the same population over time.

Thus, we need to examine how the rates measured as part of the assessment process might be combined to produce comparative measurements. Often rates are compared by subtracting one rate from another and calculating the difference between the rates, such as the difference between an incidence rate of 10/1,000 per year and an incidence rate of 5/1,000 per year. However, it is also possible to compare rates by dividing one rate by another. This combination measurement known as a *rate ratio* is illustrated in the next example.

> The investigator of lupus erythematosus noted that females have an incidence rate of 16 per 100,000 per year while males have an incidence rate of 4 per 100,000 per year. She calculated a ratio of these rates and concluded that females have four times the rate of developing lupus erythematosus.

The rate ratio is a ratio of rates, that is, one rate divided by another rate. Since the units of population and time cancel out in the ratio, we are left with a measurement without units. Rate ratios, like relative risks, tell us the relative probability of events in one population compared to another.

However, we need to distinguish rate ratio from relative risk because the rate ratio can be calculated even when it is not known whether or not those individuals with the risk factors are the ones with the increased rates of the disease. Let us review how the rate ratio is used to compare populations and their limitations using the following scenario.

> Fish consumption in the population of Italy was shown to be three times that of a population of Italians who had migrated to the United States. Coronary artery disease in Italy was one-third that among the Italian immigrants to the United States. The authors concluded that eating fish decreases the probability of developing coronary artery disease.

While this relationship may be true, it is not demonstrated using this data alone. There is no evidence that those who eat fish are the ones with a lower chance of developing coronary artery disease or that those who do not each fish are the ones at greater risk. This population comparison produces a group association but it cannot establish an association at the individual level.

In general, when we speak of a rate ratio, we do not necessarily have data on the relationships between individual risk factors and the outcomes being measures. As we discussed in the "Studying a Study" section, this is called a population comparison. When we speak of relative risk, we usually imply that we have data on the relationship at an individual level. Thus, in this example a relative risk would imply that we have established an individual association between increased fish consumption and reduced coronary artery disease.[1]

Inference: Statistical Significance Testing

When rates are obtained using data on an entire population, statistical significance testing is not needed. This is true since the aim of statistical significance testing is to draw conclusion about the larger population from the data obtained from a smaller sample of the population. When data from the total population is used, we already have the answer for the total population.[2]

Often, however, we use samples to obtain rates, and we are interested in statistical significance testing and confidence intervals.Let us take a look at what we need to know about sampling when drawing inferences.

Even when properly performed, the process of sampling is not perfect. To appreciate the process and the inherent error introduced by sampling, one must understand the basic principle that underlies sampling techniques. This principle states that if many random samples are obtained, estimates calculated from data from those samples on the average will be the same as the measurement in the original population.[3] Each sample may differ from the original population either by having a higher or a lower measurement. For example, the following figure shows an original population proportion of 10 per 1,000:

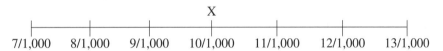

If samples of 1,000 persons were taken from this original population, the proportions might look like this:

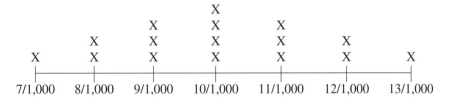

Notice that whereas some of the proportions obtained in particular samples are equal to the proportion in the original population, many of them are either higher or lower. Because samples are accurate only on the average, a single sample is said to possess an inherent sampling error. The spread of the numerical values obtained from many samples can be summarized in a measurement known as the

---

[1] At times a relative risk will be called a rate ratio since it is in fact a ratio of rates when there is a unit of time. It is possible to regard a relative risk as a special case of a rate ratio in which a risk factor can be individually related to an outcome.

[2] It has been argued that even when the entire population is used to obtain a rate, the use of statistical significance testing is important. This argument contends that even a rate based on the total population over a period of a year reflects only that particular time period rather than an average rate over an extended period of time.

[3] This is called the *central limit theorem*.

standard error. Thus, the standard error measures the size of the sampling error. Failure to appreciate the existence of sampling error can lead to the following type of misinterpretation:

> A national organization attempted to estimate the prevalence of Streptococcus carriers by culturing a random sample of 0.1% of all schoolchildren in the nation. To verify their results, the same organization used a second random sample of 0.1% of the nation's schoolchildren and conducted a second survey using an identical protocol. The first survey revealed a prevalence of 15 per 1,000 positive strep cultures; the second survey revealed a prevalence of 10 per 1,000. The authors concluded that the inconsistent results were impossible because they had used the same methodology.

The authors failed to take into account the fact that sampling has an inherent error. This sampling error may explain the differences observed in the two samples. This example merely points out that two identically obtained samples may produce different results on the basis of chance alone. Remember that large numbers of random samples, on the average, produce measurements that are identical with the true numerical value for the population, but any two samples may vary widely from one another and from the true numerical value in the larger population.

A second important principle in understanding sampling is that the more individuals who are included in a sample, the more likely a particular sample's measurement will closely approximate the numerical value in the larger population. Thus, it is the size of the sample that largely determines how close the sample's measurement is likely to be to the value in the larger population. This is not surprising because when everyone in the population is included in the sample, the sample's measurement is guaranteed to equal the population's value.

Let us look more closely at this principle. An important factor affecting the size of the sampling error is the size of the sample. Increasing the size of the sample decreases the effects of chance on the results. That is, it will reduce the random error and thus increase precision. Therefore, with a larger sample, the estimate obtained from the sample can be expected to be closer to the population's value.

The relationship between the sample size and precision is not one-to-one; it is a square root function. As the sample gets larger, diminishing returns set in, and small or moderate increases in sample size may add little to the precision of the estimate. Investigators, therefore, attempt to balance the need for precision against the financial costs of increasing the sample size. The consequence of using small sample sizes is that the sample estimates may vary widely from one sample to another and from the true numerical value in the larger population. The following example illustrates the need to take into account the effects of the sample size on the results of sampling:

> An investigator who sampled 0.01% of the nation's death certificates found that the mortality rate from pancreatic cancer was 50 per 100,000 per year. A second investigator who sampled 1% of the nation's death certificates concluded that the true mortality rate for the nation was 80 per 100,000 per year. To settle this dispute, the second investigator identified all deaths from pancreatic cancer in the country. He obtained a rate of 79 per 100,000 per year. The second investigator concluded that the first investigator had performed his study fraudulently.

The first study used a sample size only one hundredth as large as the second study; therefore, it is likely that the sampling error of the first study was much larger. The fact that the second larger sample turned out to be closer to the population's value is most likely due to its larger size rather than to fraud.

Differences in rates or changes in rates over time obtained from samples can be compared to determine if the differences are statistically significant.[4] This may be done using statistical significance testing or using confidence intervals.[5] It is important to remember, however, that the degree to which a sample represents or reflects a larger population is often a more important factor than the statistical significance of the difference.

Adjustment: Standardization

When using rates to compare the probability of developing a disease, it is important to consider whether the populations differ by a factor that is already known to affect the chance of developing the disease. This consideration is the same as adjusting for confounding variables, as discussed previously in the "Studying a Study" section. Adjustment may be needed when rates are derived using an entire population or samples of the population.

In performing an investigation comparing rates, the investigator may already know that factors such as age or gender affect the rate of developing a particular disease and is interested in other reasons for changes or differences. The investigator should then adjust for age or gender in the comparison of rates. When adjusting rates, a form of adjustment called *standardization* is often used.

Standardization for age is frequently performed. For instance, assume an investigator is interested in the incidence rate of lung cancer. Because age is a known risk factor for lung cancer, little is gained by discovering that a retirement community has a higher incidence rate of lung cancer than the rest of the community. Likewise, if one industry has a younger workforce than a second industry, it is misleading to compare the lung cancer incidence rate in the two industries directly, especially if one wishes to draw conclusions about the safety of working conditions.

To circumvent this problem, rates of disease can be standardized. Age is the most common factor used for standardization, but we can adjust for any factor that differs between groups and is known to affect the probability of developing the disease. For instance, to compare the rates of hypertension in two groups in order to study the importance of the mineral content of drinking water, one might standardize for race because blacks are known to have a higher rate of hypertension.

The principle used in standardizing rates is the same as that used to adjust for the differences in study groups discussed in the "Studying a Study" section. Investigators compare rates among individuals who are similar in age or any other factor that is being adjusted. Before illustrating the method used for adjustment, let us see how misleading results can occur if standardization is not performed.

The incidence rate of pancreatic cancer in the United States was compared with the incidence rate in Mexico. The rate in the United States was found to be three times as high as the rate in Mexico per 100,000 per year. The authors concluded that

---

[4] Statistical significance testing for comparing rates use what is called the Poisson distribution instead of the bell shaped Gaussian distribution. The Poisson distribution allows us to obtain confidence intervals directly from the number of observed events. The 95% confidence interval for a count "C" equals $C +/- 1.96\sqrt{C}$. Thus if 16 events are observed, the 95% confidence interval is approximately 8 to 24.

[5] When using confidence intervals to determine whether a difference between rates (or other differences) is statistically significant, one determines whether either of the 95% confidence intervals overlap the observed rate in the other group. If there is overlap, the differences are not statistically significant.

U.S. residents have a rate of pancreatic cancer three times as high as the rate among Mexicans, assuming that the accuracy of diagnosis was equal in the two countries.

This interpretation of this study is superficially correct; if the data are accurate, the risk of pancreatic cancer is higher in the United States. However, pancreatic cancer is known to occur more often in older persons. It may be that the younger average age of the Mexican population accounts for the difference in rates of pancreatic cancer. This may be an important issue if we are examining the cause of pancreatic cancer. If the age distribution does not explain these differences, the investigators may have detected an important unexpected difference that requires further explanation. Thus, the authors should standardize their data for age and see whether the differences persist.

Now let us see how standardization is performed. Standardization of rates is often performed by comparing a special sample that is being studied to the general population. In performing this type of standardization, we often use what is called the *indirect method*. This method compares the observed number of events, such as deaths in the sample of interest, to the number that would have been expected if the study sample had the same age distribution as the general population. When death is the outcome of interest, the indirect method produces a ratio known as the *standardized mortality ratio*.

$$\text{Standardized mortality ratio} = \frac{\text{Observed number of deaths}}{\text{Expected number of deaths}}$$

The standardized mortality ratio is a useful means of comparing a sample from a population of interest to the general population. The special population under study, however, is not expected to have the same mortality rate as the general population.

For instance, when comparing a group of employed individuals to the general population, it is important to remember that employment often requires that individuals be relatively healthy. The need to take into account this employment effect is illustrated in the next example:

A study of new workers at a chemical plant found a standardized mortality ratio of 1 for all causes of death. The investigator concluded that because the standardized mortality ratio was 1, the chemical plant was free of health risks to the workers.

When interpreting this study, it is important to remember that new workers are often healthier than persons in the general population. This phenomenon is so common that it has been called the *healthy worker effect*. Thus, we would expect them to have a somewhat lower mortality rate than the general population, or a standardized mortality ratio of less than 1. The standardized mortality ratio of 1 may actually suggest increased hazards to these generally healthy workers.[6]

When two groups from a population are under study or when changes over time in a population are being assessed, it is possible and desirable to use what is called the *direct method* of standardization. The direct method works as follows: Suppose investigators wish to compare the incidence of bladder cancer in two large industries. The bladder cancer data for the two industries are shown in

[6] Standardized morbidity ratios can also be calculated. The magnitude of the standardized morbidity ratio depends on the particular general population used. Thus, when two standardized morbidity ratios are standardized to different populations or to the same population in different years, they cannot be directly compared.

Table 23.1. *Comparison of incidence rates of bladder cancer*

Age	Number of individuals	Number of cases of bladder cancer per year	Incidence rate of bladder cancer in each age group[a]
		Industry A	
20–30	20,000	0	0 per 100,000
30–40	20,000	10	50 per 100,000
40–50	30,000	20	67 per 100,000
50–60	20,000	80	400 per 100,000
60–70	10,000	90	900 per 100,000
Total	100,000	200	200 per 100,000
		Industry B	
20–30	10,000	0	0 per 100,000
30–40	10,000	4	40 per 100,000
40–50	20,000	6	30 per 100,000
50–60	50,000	140	280 per 100,000
60–70	10,000	50	500 per 100,000
Total	100,000	200	200 per 100,000

[a]The incidence rate is obtained from the number of cases and the number of individuals in the age group. The incidence rates cannot be added down the column.

Table 23.1. Notice that the overall rates for both samples are 200 per 100,000 workers per year. Also, notice that the rates for each age group in industry A are as high or higher than in industry B.

Because of the lower rates for each age group in industry B, it may at first seem surprising that the overall incidences are the same. However, looking at the number of individuals in each age group, it becomes apparent that industry A has a much younger workforce than industry B. Industry B has 60,000 workers from ages 50 to 70 years; industry A has only 30,000 workers in these age groups. Because bladder cancer is known to increase with age, the younger age of industry A's workforce reduces the overall rates in industry A. Thus, it is misleading to look only at the overall rates because industry B's overall rate is increased by its older age structure. This is especially true if we are asking about the safety of the industry environment itself.

To avoid this problem, the authors must standardize the rates to adjust for the differences in age and thereby compare the rates more fairly. To accomplish standardization, each sample is subdivided to indicate the number of individuals, the number of cases of the disease, and the incidence rate in each age group. When data are divided into groups using a characteristic such as age, each age group is known as a *stratum*. This is also shown in Table 23.1.

The authors then must attempt to determine how many cases of bladder cancer would have occurred in industry A if the age distribution was the same as in industry B. The steps in this process are as follows:[7]

1. Starting with the 20- to 30-year-old age group, the authors take the rate of cancer for that group in industry A and multiply it by the number of individuals in the corresponding age group in industry B. This produces the number of cases that

[7] The method illustrated is not necessarily the only or best method to use for standardization. For statistical purposes, it is common to weight the strata by the inverse of the variance of the estimate in each strata as is done in the Mantel-Haenzel method.

Table 23.2. *Method of age standardization*

Age Group	Incidence rate of bladder cancer in industry A	Number of individuals in industry B	Number of cases that would occur in industry A if it had the same age distribution as industry B[a]	Number of cases of bladder cancer that actually occurred in industry B
20–30	0/100,000	10,000	0	0
30–40	50/100,000	10,000	5	4
40–50	67/100,000	20,000	13	6
50–60	400/100,000	50,000	200	140
60–70	900/100,000	10,000	90	50
Total		100,000	308	200

[a]This column is calculated by multiplying the previous two columns.

would have occurred in industry A if it had the same number of individuals in that age group as industry B.

2. The authors then perform this calculation for each age group and calculate the total number of cases from the different age groups. This produces a total number of cases that would have occurred if industry A had the same overall age distribution as industry B.

3. The authors now have standardized the rates for age and can directly compare the number of cases that occurred in industry B with the number of cases that would have occurred in industry A if industry A had the same age distribution as industry B. The authors have now age-adjusted industry A to industry B's age distribution.[8]

Let us apply these procedures to the bladder cancer data shown in Table 23.2.

If the age distribution was the same as industry B, 308 cases of bladder cancer would have occurred in industry A, but only 200 actually occurred in industry B. These figures are better measures for comparing the workers' risk of developing bladder cancer in each industry than are the unadjusted incident rates. The adjusted numbers accentuate the fact that, despite the equality of the overall rates, industry A has a rate as high or higher in each age group. Therefore, to make fair comparisons between populations that differ by age and where age is known to affect the incidence rate of developing a disease, it is necessary to age-standardize the samples. If additional factors are also known to affect the rates, the same process can be applied to standardize for these factors.[9]

---

[8] It is also possible to age-adjust the opposite way, thus age-adjusting industry B to industry A's age distribution. The general conclusion would be the same; however, the estimates would be different.

[9] Notice, however, that in performing standardization, the calculations give special emphasis to the largest strata. Thus, if there has been a substantial change in only one stratum, especially a small stratum, this effort can easily be lost in the process of standardization. In addition, progress may be made by delaying death. When death from a particular cause is moved from a younger to an older age group, this effect is not recognized by the process of standardization. As we will see, this impact of extending life without curing can be captured by measuring life expectancy.

24 Interpretation and Extrapolation

Interpretation

Real versus Artifactual

As we learned in Chapter 21 incidence rates, prevalence and case-fatality together allow us to obtain a composite picture of a disease, to describe the disease in terms of rates. When interputing rates we often wish to go beyond describing the disease to learning about changes or differences in the rates. The differences in rates may be the result of real changes in the incidence, prevalence, or prognosis of the disease itself, or they may reflect changes in the method by which the particular disease is assessed. *Artifactual differences* imply that, despite the fact that a difference exists, it does not reflect changes in the disease but merely in the way the disease is measured, sought, or defined.

Artifactual differences result from three basic sources:

1. Changes in the ability to recognize the disease. These represent changes in the measurement of the disease.
2. Changes in the efforts to recognize the disease. These may represent efforts to recognize the disease at an earlier stage, changes in reporting requirements, or new incentives to search for the disease.
3. Changes in the definition of the disease. These represent changes in the criteria used to define the disease.

The following example illustrates the first type of artifactual change, the effect of a change in the ability to recognize a disease:

> Because of an improvement in technology, a study of the prevalence of mitral valve prolapse was performed. A complete survey of the charts at a major university cardiac clinic found that in 1975 only 1 per 1,000 patients had a diagnosis of mitral valve prolapse, whereas in 2005, 80 per 1,000 patients had mitral valve prolapse included in their diagnoses. The authors concluded that the condition was increasing to an astounding prevalence.

Between 1975 and 2005, the use of echocardiography greatly increased the ability to document mitral valve prolapse. In addition, the growing recognition of the frequency of this condition led to a much better understanding of how to recognize it by physical examination. It is not surprising, then, that a much larger proportion of cardiac clinic patients were known to have mitral valve prolapse in 2005 compared with 1975. It is possible that if equal understanding and equal technology were available in 1975, the prevalence would have been nearly identical. This example demonstrates that artifactual changes may explain large differences in the prevalence of a disease even when a complete review of all cases is used.

Changes in the efforts to recognize a disease may occur when the available treatment improves, as illustrated in the next example:

> A new treatment for migraine headache is approved for use and widely advertised in the medical journals and in major newspapers. The number of patients presenting for care with migraine headaches doubles in the year after approval of the new drug. These patients meet all the criteria for a diagnosis of migraine.

This apparent doubling of the prevalence of migraine is most likely due to the increased proportion of individuals with migraine headache who present for care after becoming aware of the new treatment. A high proportion of individuals with many self-limited or nonprogressive diseases do not seek health care. Changes in the types of patients who seek care can produce dramatic but artifactual changes in the rates.

The following example illustrates how the definition of a disease may change over time and thus produce an artifactual difference in the apparent rate:

> The incidence rate of AIDS increased every year between 1981 and 1990. In one year during the early 1990s, there was a sudden, dramatic increase in the reported rate. One investigator interpreted this sudden increase as a sign that the epidemic had suddenly entered a new phase. It was later recognized that no sudden change had occurred.

The dramatic increase may have been due to a change in the Centers for Disease Control and Prevention's definition of AIDS, which meant that more individuals with HIV infection fell within the definition of AIDS. When sudden changes in the incidence rate of a disease occurs, one must suspect artifactual differences, such as changes in the definition of a disease. In this case, one suspects that an artifactual change was superimposed on long-term changes, which is called a *secular* or *temporal* trend.

Reasons for Changes or Differences

The interpretation of rates ask us to examine which rate is actually changing and why—that is, we aim to understand the underlying reasons for changes. First, we will examine how the changes in rates may reflect changes in the disease dynamics. To do this we ask how the changes may affect the rates that describe the epidemiology of the disease—i.e., the incidence rate, prevalence, and case fatality.

Artifactual differences in rates imply that the true incidence, prevalence, or case fatality has not been altered even though superficially a change appears to have occurred. Real changes, however, imply that the rates have changed. We first must ask whether any of the sources of artifactual differences are operating. If they are not operating or are not large enough to explain the differences, one can assume that real differences exist. Having concluded that real changes have occurred, we need to ask why they occured. Do they reflect a change in incidence, prevalence, or case fatality, or a combination of these measurements?

The first step in understanding the meaning of real changes in rates is to understand which of the rates is experiencing the primary change. Then we can better appreciate the effects of the primary change on the other rates of disease, as in the following cases:

1. The case fatality for Hodgkin's disease has dramatically decreased in recent years. Individuals are considered to have the disease until they demonstrate evidence of cure in long-term follow-up. Thus, the prevalence of Hodgkin's disease has increased. The incidence has remained stable; therefore, the

mortality rates, which reflect the incidence rates multiplied by the case fatality, have fallen.
2. Lung cancer incidence rates for women have increased dramatically over recent decades. The case fatality has remained very high, with most patients dying within months of diagnosis. Thus, the mortality rates have also increased dramatically. The prevalence has always been low; however, with the increased incidence rate of disease and modest improvements in treatment that increase the average duration, the prevalence has increased.

We might diagram these results as follows:

	Mortality Rates	Case Fatality	Incidence Rates	Prevalence
Hodgkin's disease	↓	↓↓↓	→	↑↑
Lung cancer for women	↑↑	→	↑↑	↑

These confusing patterns make sense when one recognizes that the primary change in Hodgkin's disease has been the decreased case fatality, whereas the primary change in lung cancer has been the increased incidence rate.

In addition to understanding the type of change in rates that is occurring, it is often helpful to examine the underlying reason for the changes. Understanding the underlying reasons for change is key to anticipating future trends.

A real change in rates may have any of the following meanings: (a) the change may herald future changes in the same direction; (b) it may reflect predictable cycles or epidemics; or (c) it may be the result of unpredictable fluctuations representing an unusual frequency of events.

In Fig. 24.1, if investigators note the increase that occurred between 1996 and 1998, they may measure the changes between 1998 and 2001 and would again find an increase. It is important, however, that investigators realize that this real change between 1996 and 2001 may be part of the natural or epidemic cycle of disease. These increases do not necessarily imply that increases can be expected in future years, as seen by the subsequent decline in rates.

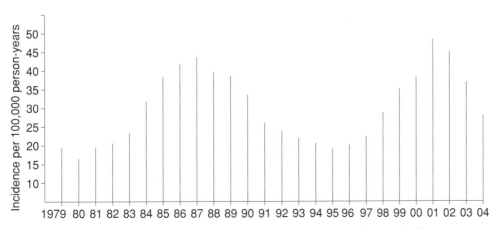

Figure 24.1. Predictable cycles or epidemics in the yearly incidence of a disease.

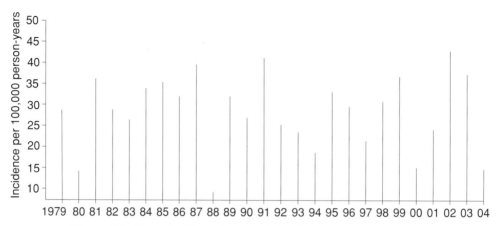

Figure 24.2. Unpredictable or chance variations in the yearly incidence of a disease.

As opposed to this predictable cycle of disease, there may be an unpredictable, random variation in the rate of disease from year to year, as illustrated in Fig. 24.2. In this situation, if investigators select a year when the rate was higher and compare it with the next year, when by chance alone the rate was lower, they may believe they are documenting important changes when, in fact, they are merely discovering the statistical principle of *regression to the mean*. Regression to the mean, or return to the average, states that unusual values are by definition rare events, and the chances are against a repetition of a rare event twice in a row. In fact, by chance alone the next measurement is likely to be nearer the mean.

Subsequent values may be less extreme because of random fluctuation of events or because of biological, social, psychological, or economic adaptive forces that react to the unusual rate. Thus, both chance and reactive forces tend to move the subsequent rate toward the mean. For instance, if one were studying how much an individual eats per meal, it is likely that the meal following a particularly indulgent one would be smaller than usual. Let us see how this principle may operate in a study of rates that produced real differences, but differences that need to be carefully interpreted.

> After a tragic accident killed several men in a factory, an accident prevention program was initiated. Investigators found that the incidence rate of accidents at the time of the tragedy was unusually high: 10 per 1,000 worker-days. The rate fell to 2 per 1,000 worker-days after the program was established. The investigators concluded that the accident prevention program was an enormous success.

The investigators have shown that a real change took place. They have not, however, shown that it was the accident prevention program that caused the change. It is possible that the 10 per 1, 000 worker-day rate was unusually high and by chance alone returned to a more usual rate of 2 per 1,000 worker-days. Even more likely, the fatal accident may have frightened the workers into taking more safety precautions.

The authors started with an unusually high accident rate, and then a tragedy occurred that may have produced adaptive changes in behavior, which resulted in the rate dropping back toward the average. It is premature to conclude that the accident prevention program would help other groups, or even this group, if it was instituted at another time. Thus, the principle of regression to the mean and adaptive changes may be the sources of real change in rates observed in this example.

It is common for an investigation or an intervention to be initiated because of a suspicion that the rate of a disease is increasing. Thus, it is important to recognize the phenomenon of regression to the mean and adaptive changes because they may start operating whenever short-term changes in rates are observed.

Another source of real differences that affects prediction of future events is known as the *cohort effect*. A cohort is a group of individuals who share a common experience or exposure. If one or several cohorts in a population have had an exposure or experience that makes them particularly susceptible to disease at a future point in time, then the possibility of a cohort effect exists. The rates for a particular age group, which include the susceptible cohort, may be temporarily increased. This temporary increase is known as the cohort effect. When a cohort effect is present, one can expect the rates for this particular age group to fall again as time passes and the susceptible cohort moves beyond this particular age group. The importance of appreciating the cohort effect is illustrated in the following example:

> An investigator was studying the incidence rate of thyroid cancer. Concern existed that past pediatric head and neck radiation, frequently used in the 1950s and into the 1960s, was a contributor to thyroid cancers. Using proper methods, the authors found that the incidence rate of thyroid cancer among 30- to 40-year-olds in 1970 was 50 per 100,000 person-years; in 1980 it was 100 per 100,000 person-years; and in 1990 it was 150 per 100,000 person-years. The authors concluded that by 2000, the rates would pass the 200 per 100,000 person-years mark. The authors were surprised to find that the incidence rate in 2000 was less than 150 per 100,000 person-years and continued to decline over the next 5 years.

The authors have established that actual changes were occurring in the incidence rates of thyroid cancer in the 30- to 40-year-old age group. The source of these changes may be a cohort effect. The cohort of individuals who were radiated carried an increased probability of thyroid cancer. By 2005, all individuals in the 30- to 40-year age group would have been born after pediatric head and neck radiation had ceased to be used. Thus, it is not surprising to observe a decline in the incidence rate of thyroid cancer in 30- to 40-year-olds rather than a continued rise. The concept of a cohort effect not only helps predict the expected future rates, but it also helps to support the theory that past radiation increased the incidence rate of thyroid cancer.

Another type of real change might be thought of as *exhausting the denominator.* Exhausting the denominator implies that the real change that is occurring relates to the size of the at-risk group. At times, the incidence rate may fall because the true population at risk that makes up the denominator has become smaller.[1]

Let us see how exhaustion of the denominator might occur and its implications in the next example.

> The incidence of HIV infection among those with hemophilia during the early years of the epidemic was extremely high due to the use of blood produced from many donors. Within a few years of after the beginning of the epidemic, the incidence of new HIV infection among hemophiliacs fell dramatically. Investigators could not explain this phenomenon because it occurred sooner than could be explained by improvements in technology.

---

[1] It can be argued that exhausting the denominator is really an artifactual change because the at-risk population has been used as the denominator. It is classified as a real change because it reflects a real decrease in the incidence of disease as experienced by the overall population, as is the situation with the other real changes discussed here.

It is possible that the occurrence of HIV infection among those with hemophilia was so rapid that the majority of those with hemophilia developed HIV infection. Once that occurred, the number at risk may have been very small, resulting in very few new cases of HIV among those with hemophilia.

What are the future implications of this fall in incidence rate? It is possible that the number of HIV-negative patients with hemophilia will increase over time. Once that occurs, there is the possibility that the incidence rate of HIV infection could again increase in the absence of measures to protect them from blood-borne infection.

Subgroups

Rates of disease are often obtained from large populations. When this is the situation, it may be possible to examine subgroups within the population. Changes in subgroups may be the same or different from the population as a whole. This information may be very useful in understanding the process that is occurring and providing insights into the underlying reasons for changes, which is the ultimate goal of examining rates.

Let us look at two examples of how changes in subgroups in the same direction and in the opposite direction can assist in the process of interpretation.

> The mortality rate from cystic fibrosis decreased among those 0 to 20 years old while it increased among those 20 to 30. The authors concluded that this may reflect the improvement in care received by younger patients. Even though they are not cured, their deaths may be delayed.

The investigators recognize that rates alone cannot definitively demonstrate the reason for these changes. Nonetheless, combining what is known about the changes that have occurred within the 0 to 20 age group and the 20 to 30 age group allows the investigators to cautiously draw a conclusion when data from subgroups changes in the opposite direction.

Let us look at changes in the same direction among subgroups in the following example.

> An investigator examined the rate of child car seat use in communities with no interventions and communities with laws requiring car seat use. Overall, the communities with laws requiring child car seat use had a higher rate of use than those with no interventions. The investigators then divided the communities into subgroups by socioeconomic level and geography. They found that the difference between car seat use was nearly the same regardless of socioeconomic level or the size of the community. The authors concluded that the consistency of the data supports the contention that the impact of car seat laws is not dependent on socioeconomic status or size of the community.

While it is important to avoid drawing cause-and-effect conclusions from rates, as illustrated here, rates for subgroups can reinforce the conclusions obtained from the population as a whole. When rates for subgroups all change in the same direction, the impact of consistency often strengthens the conclusions.

Extrapolation

The results and interpretation of rates is often designed to allow investigators to go beyond the data to draw conclusion that are useful in further research, in drawing conclusions about other populations, or in going beyond the data to predict the future. Let us look at the three basic types of extrapolation of rates that occur.

Hypothesis Generation

While comparing rates cannot establish cause-and-effect relationships, comparisons of rates in groups is often performed to generate hypotheses about the cause of disease. In these situations the investigators' interest is not limited to the population being studied. They are often trying to gain ideas or generate hypotheses that are widely applicable. Often the hypotheses generated by investigations of rates must subsequently be evaluated using the types of investigations of individuals that we examined in the "Studying a Study" section.

Investigators, as we saw previously, might note differences in rates of coronary artery disease mortality among North American Italians and Italians living in Italy. From what they know about the diets, they might hypothesize an association between fish consumption and reduced coronary artery mortality even though they do not have data on the diets of individuals.

By comparing the rates of disease and adjusting for known risk factors, it is possible to establish that a factor is increased in one group and the probability of a disease is also increased in the same group. This allows us to establish *group associations*. A group association means that in a particular group, the factor and the disease are both present at an increased rate. Note that a group association does not necessarily mean that those individuals with the factor are the same individuals as those with the disease.

Establishing the existence of a group association may lay the groundwork for subsequent studies that establish an association at the individual level and eventually a cause-and-effect relationship, such as in the case of cholesterol and coronary artery disease.

When using group data, investigators frequently have little information about the individuals who comprise the group. Thus, when comparing rates to develop a hypothesis for further study at the individual level, investigators must be careful not to imply an association among individuals when only a group association has been established. This type of error, known as an *ecological fallacy* or *population fallacy,*[2] is illustrated in the following example:

> A study demonstrated that the rate of drowning in Florida is four times higher than in Illinois. The study data also demonstrated that in Florida, ice cream is consumed at a rate four times that of Illinois. The authors concluded that eating ice cream is associated with drowning.

To establish an individual association, the authors must first demonstrate that those who eat more ice cream are the ones who are more likely to drown. Relying on group figures alone does not provide any information about the existence of an association at the individual level. It may not be people who eat more ice cream who drown. The greater consumption of ice cream may merely reflect the confounding variable known as warm weather, which increases both ice cream consumption and drowning. These authors committed a population fallacy. The

---

[2] The term population fallacy will be used because the term "ecological" is increasingly being used to indicate interaction between factors. In addition, ecological is a term that may not convey clear meaning.

establishment of an individual association between eating ice cream and drowning requires a demonstration that the relationship holds on an individual level.

When using rates in groups to develop hypotheses, it must be recognized that the use of group rates establishes group association and not individual association. Failure to appreciate the distinction between group association and individual association may lead to a population fallacy.

To Other Populations

Rates derived from one population during one particular time period may be used as the basis for decision-making in other, often quite different, populations. Thus, when extrapolating rates, as in extrapolating the conclusions of other types of investigations, we need to ask about the assumptions that are implicitly or explicitly being made.

Let us examine some of the many applications of rates to other populations. Studies of the prevalence of a disease have direct application to diagnosis and screening. As we have seen, the prevalence of a disease serves as the starting point for estimating the pretest probability. When no symptoms are present, as in screening, the prevalence of disease in particular groups or populations may be all we have to go on to establish the pretest probability.

Thus we need to be careful when extrapolating rates from one population to another, as illustrated in the next example.

> An investigation of the prevalence of breast cancer in the United States among those 50 years and older revealed a prevalence of approximately 1%. This prevalence was used to approximate the pretest probability in order to evaluate performance of a new test. The calculations proved quite accurate for women in the United States and in Europe, but when the test was applied in Japan, it did not perform well.

The prevalence of breast cancer in Japan may be lower than in the United States and Europe. We need to be careful in applying rates from one population to another. Rates may be used to draw conclusions about prognosis, effectiveness of interventions, safety of intervention, and a variety of other uses. It is important to recognize that whenever conclusions are drawn from rates obtained in one population and applied to another, we are making assumptions that may not hold true in the population to which they are applied.

Prediction

The most difficult form of extrapolation is prediction of the future. Unlike hypothesis generation and application from one population to another, with prediction of the future we cannot check up on our assumptions about the future except by waiting for the future to arrive.

As we saw in the "Studying a Study" section, many extrapolations about the future merely extend current trends, making a linear (straight-line) assumption. The linear assumption assumes that current trends will continue. This assumption is rarely true, at least over extended periods of time.

Despite the difficulties extrapolating to the future, in the interpretation component we identified three phenomenon that can help us try to extrapolate to the future: regression to the mean, cohort effects, and exhausting the denominator. Each of these can help us make educated guesses about the future rate of events.

When looking at interpretation, we asked whether any of these phenomenon are likely to be present. Each of these phenomenon suggest that changes that we have observed in the recent past may not be a good reflection of what may happen in the not-too-distant future.

A common measurement derived from mortality rates is often used to predict the future. This measurement, called *life expectancy,* is so widely used and so commonly misinterpreted that it deserved special attention. Thus, let us move on to Chapter 25 to examine life expectancy.

25 Life Expectancy

As we have seen, rates and their ratios are the fundamental tools for comparing the health of populations. They can be used to compare the health of a population in one year with that of another. In addition, they can be used to compare the health of one population, such as a nation, with the health of another population. Thus they have been called measures of *population health.*

The fundamental population health measurement tool for comparing mortality is called *life expectancy*. We can think of it as an overall summary measure of the mortality experience of a population during a single time period, usually one year.

Life expectancy, unlike the other rates we have discussed so far, has the ability to take into account prolongations in life that still result in death. Thus it has similarities to the use of life-tables we discussed in Chapter 9. This makes life expectancy very useful, since many of the improvements in health care do not cure disease but rather prolong life.

To understand what we mean by life expectancy, we need to appreciate that it is a summary measurement that combines the probabilities of death—the mortality rates—for each year of age in a population for a particular year, such as 2005. Approximations of these mortality rates are available if a nation has two forms of data: (a) adequate data from death records in a particular year indicating the age of the individuals who died; (b) data from a census or other source estimating the number of individuals at each year of age at a point in time during the year.[1]

The number of deaths at a particular age divided by the total number of individuals of the same age in the population tells us the mortality rate at each year of age. This age specific mortality rate is the key to the calculation of life expectancy. Life expectancy calculations usually also include data on gender and racial groups. Separate life expectancies can then be calculated for each gender and racial group.

Life expectancy is calculated using what are called *cross-sectional* or *current life tables*. These tables represent a snapshot view at one point in time. They are different from the life tables discussed in Chapter 9, which follow study and control groups over a period of time. Life tables that monitor patients over time are called *longitudinal* or *cohort life tables* to distinguish them from cross-sectional life tables, for which data come from the same year. Unfortunately, both types are often called life tables.[2]

The calculation of life expectancy requires us to visualize the existence of an imaginary population. This population is called a *stationary population*. It consists

---

[1] Ideally, the number of individuals is available from the beginning of the time interval because this number would indicate the total number of individuals who are at risk for death during the subsequent year. Approximations based on census data from other years are often substituted. Notice that the cause of death is not important for calculating life expectancy.

[2] Together, these two life tables can provide complementary information on life expectancy. Cross-sectional life tables provide information on life expectancy that is related to age, gender, and race, the basic demographic data. Longitudinal life tables often provide information on life expectancy associated with a specific disease. These data together may be used to estimate the life expectancy for individuals of a particular age, gender, and race with a particular disease.

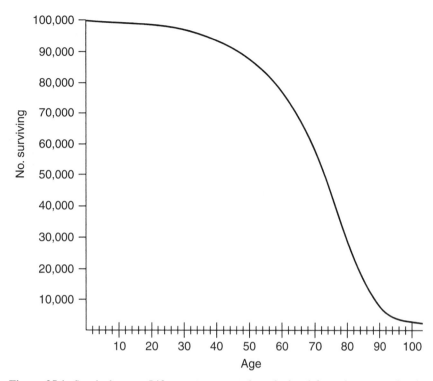

Figure 25.1. Survival curve. Life expectancy can be calculated from the area under the curve.

of 100,000 individuals born alive in the year under consideration. These individuals are assumed to live out their lives in this population, leaving only because of death. No one is allowed to move in or out of this imaginary population. These 100,000 individuals are assumed to experience the probabilities of death observed for each age group during the year in which data are obtained.

In calculating 2005 life expectancies, we are assuming that these 100,000 live births will live out their lives experiencing the probabilities of death of each of the life table's component age groups in 2005. Thus, for these people it will always be 2005 in term of their probabilities of death.

Thus, in our stationary population in 2005, the 0- to 1-year age group experience the year 2005's probability of death for the 0- to1-year age group. In 2006, the 1- to 2-year-olds will experience the probability of death of the 1- to 2-year-olds in 2005. Similarly, in 2007, the 2- to 3-year-olds will experience the probability of death of the 2- to 3-year-olds in 2005, and so on. In fact, in 2085 the life expectancy calculation assumes that the 80-year-old will still be experiencing the probability of death of 80-year-olds in 2005.

It is possible to plot a survival curve indicating the number of individuals who are alive at the beginning of each year of age, starting with our stationary population of 100,000 live births. Figure 25.1 displays such a survival plot.[3]

---

[3] Information for a survival curve can be obtained by multiplying the probability of death at each age by the number of individuals who are still alive at the beginning of the time period. Thus, if 0.01, or 1%, of individuals have died during the first year, then 99,000 enter the second year of life. If the probability of death during the second year of life is 0.001, or .1%, then 99 individuals die during the second year, leaving 98,901 individuals entering the third year of life.

The life expectancy can be calculated using the area under the survival curve. Life expectancy often refers to life expectancy at birth. However, life expectancy can be calculated at any age. These are calculated[5] using the area under the curve starting at the age of interest. Thus, if we were trying to estimate the life expectancy at age 65, we would use the area under the survival curve for ages 65 years and older.

The term "life expectancy" sounds like it should allow us to predict the future. However, the calculation of life expectancy assumes that everything in the future will remain the same; all individuals will remain in the same population; and the mortality rates will not change. This is unrealistic because the one predictable thing in life is the permanence of change. Thus, we must be careful in using life expectancy to predict the future, just as we need to recognize that all probabilities calculated on the basis of current data may not hold true in the future. The implications for prediction are illustrated in this example:

> The life expectancy at birth in a developing nation was carefully obtained and calculated to be 45 years in 1975. Over the course of the next 30 years, using life expectancy to predict survival, the probabilities of death first indicated a survival much better than expected and then indicated a subsequent decline over expected survival. The authors concluded that life expectancy measures have no value even if the data on which they are based are accurate.

Even if the data were accurately obtained, we would not expect it to predict the future perfectly. Perhaps the decline in infant mortality from diarrheal disease reduced the probabilities of death during the 1970s and 1980s. Then perhaps the AIDS epidemic took a high toll during the subsequent years. Life expectancy measures are not designed to predict the future. They are useful for comparing one population with another in one particular year, such as 2005. They are also useful for comparing the same population in different years (e.g., 2000 vs. 2005).

When life expectancy is calculated for different gender and racial groups, life expectancy measures are useful for comparing these different groups within the same population. The presence of differences in life expectancy, that is differences in population health, may be due to a variety of causes. Poorer quality of preventive or curative health services is one possible reason for these differences. They may also be due to genetics, environmental or preventive interventions at the population level.

As we have seen, when we speak of life expectancy we usually mean the life expectancy at birth. Life expectancy at birth is the average number of years of

---

[4]Notice that the median age at death, or the age at which half the population has died, can be read directly off of the survival curve. This can be done by drawing a horizontal line from 50,000 to the curve and then a vertical line down to age on the x-axis. This median age at death is not the same as life expectancy. The median age at death will generally be greater than the life expectancy because life expectancy is an average and thus is greatly affected by deaths that occur at an early age.

[5]Calculations are performed by starting with the stationary population of 100,000 and multiplying by the probability of death for the first time interval (usually the first year of life). Subtracting this number from 100,000 produces the number living at the beginning of the next age interval, that is, at age 1 year. This process is continued through each of the age intervals, producing a number living at the beginning of each age interval. Knowing the length of the age interval and the number of individuals alive at the beginning of the age interval, we can estimate the number of years of life spent in each age interval. We then add together the number of years spent in an age interval and all subsequent age intervals and divide this total by the number of individuals who enter that age interval. This allows us to calculate the life expectancy at any age we choose.

Table 25.1. *Life expectancy for males in a developed country*

Age (yr)	Life expectancy (yr)
0	75
20	57
40	38
65	15
75	10
80	6
90	4

remaining life for an individual born into our imaginary stationary population. Life expectancy at birth is not the only life expectancy that is usually available. Life expectancy at the beginning of any age can be calculated. For instance, examine Table 25.1, which might provide the life expectancies for males in a developed country.

Notice that the life expectancy at birth is 75 years. At age 65 years, the life expectancy is 15 years. If we add 15 years to the life expectancy at age 65 we get 80 years, which is greater than the 75 year life expectancy at birth This phenomenon occurs because those who reach a particular age, such as 65 years, have already survived the potential for death at an earlier age. Whether they are biologically better survivors or just lucky, they will have a longer life expectancy than at the time of their birth when they face potential mortality during each year of life. Failure to appreciate this phenomenon can lead to the following misinterpretation:

> A conference on preventive health care for 80-year-olds proposed a series of pre-ventive intervention for all 80-year-olds in a nation with a life expectancy of 78 years. The national health system refused to consider paying for these preventive procedures, arguing that the individuals had already exceeded their life expectancy.

Remember, life expectancy for groups of individuals who survive to a particular age is greater than the life expectancy at birth. The life expectancy at an ad-vanced age may be surprisingly long. For instance, note that in Table 25.1 the life expectancy at age 80 is 6 years and at 90 it is 4 years. Life expectancy is not 0 until the last person dies. Thus it is not possible to outlive your life expectancy.[6]

Using life expectancy to make recommendations for a particular individual is even more difficult than using life expectancy to make recommendations for the average member of a group, as illustrated in the next situation:

> A healthy 80-year-old man is considering elective surgery. Recognizing that the average life expectancy for 80-year-old men is 6 years, the physicians recommend against the surgery.

The ability to predict the length of survival for an individual healthy 80-year-old man has very little to do with the average life expectancy of 80-year-old men. The life expectancy at 80 years for men takes into account all 80-year-old men, whether they are healthy or have life-threatening disease. Because of the high proportion of

---

[6] Life expectancy at age 80 years may be a better predictor of the future for the average 80-year-old than life expectancy at a far younger age. This is the case because changes in the probability of death over a small number of years are usually modest compared with changes over a longer period of time.

illness among 80-year-old men, those who are healthy constitute a very different group. Averaging the healthy and the sick together produces a life expectancy that may greatly underestimate the survival of the healthy individual.

In general, life expectancy is an average that combines data from the healthy and those with disease, including life-threatening disease. The greater the proportion of those with life-threatening disease, the less useful the life expectancy will be for making recommendations for the healthy individual.

The high probability of life-threatening diseases among the elderly can lead to another misinterpretation of life expectancy data. Reduction in one important cause of death among the elderly will not necessarily have a dramatic effect on life expectancy, as illustrated in the next hypothetical example:

> A new cure for lung cancer has nearly eliminated this frequent cause of death among elderly men. The investigators had expected a dramatic increase in the life expectancy among elderly men. To their surprise, they found only a modest increase.

Unfortunately, among the elderly there are a number of competing causes of death. When one cause is reduced or eliminated, the other causes have the potential to increase in frequency. Other cancers or heart disease may become causes of replacement mortality. That is, they may increase and thus reduce the expected impact of eliminating one important cause of death. Thus, we must recognize the inherent limitation of life expectancy when dealing with the elderly.[7]

Life expectancy is an average. Using averages to summarize the health status of a population has one additional feature that needs to be recognized. Let us review how averages are calculated. For instance, imagine that we want to calculate an average for the following numbers: 2, 21, 24, 26, 27. We would first add together all the numbers and obtain 100. Then we would divide by the number of data elements, that is, by 5. Thus, the average here is 100/5, or 20.

Notice that the average is below all the numbers except 2. The inclusion of 2 has pulled the average down. This is generally the case with averages. They are heavily affected by the extreme values, especially when the extremes are far removed from the other values.

When calculating life expectancies, a parallel phenomenon occurs. The life expectancy at birth is most heavily influenced by what happens early in life. Thus, the influence on life expectancy of saving a healthy child is far greater than the influence of saving a healthy adult or a healthy 80-year-old. The implications of this phenomenon are illustrated in the next example:

> Reviewing the experience of a rapidly developing country, investigators noted that the nation rapidly gained years of life expectancy at birth when it controlled infectious diseases of the young. When it turned its attention to the diseases of the elderly and

---

[7] On the other hand, life expectancy overestimates survival for those with disease. To accurately incorporate the impact of disease on life expectancy, we need to combine life expectancy measures using data based on age, gender, and race with life expectancy data based on disease-specific survival. One such approximation is known as the *declining exponential approximation of life expectancy (DEALE)*. DEALE assumes that the life expectancy at a particular age is equal to 1 divided by the sum of the probability of survival on the basis of age, race, and gender (obtained from a cross-sectional life table) plus the probability of survival as a result of disease (obtained from a longitudinal life table). The DEALE assumes that the impact of a disease is the same regardless of a person's age. If this is not the situation, the DEALE will not be an accurate estimate of life expectancy. A new estimate called the *GAME*, independent gamma (GA) and mixed-exponential (ME) distribution, is a more accurate measurement of life expectancy. It combines survival curves based on age with those based on a specific disease.

made rapid strides in controlling these diseases, there was much less impact on the life expectancy at birth. This contradiction could not be explained by the investigators, who concluded that life expectancy was a meaningless measure.

Life expectancy at birth is strongly influenced by mortality rates among the young. This is the situation because saving a healthy child adds a large number of years to life, whereas saving a healthy adult or elderly person adds a much smaller number of years of life. Because life expectancy at birth reflects the average number of remaining years of life, it will be greatly influenced by the progress made among the young. To observe the impact on the elderly, it is necessary to calculate the life expectancy at older ages and see how they change from year to year.

Increases in life expectancy resulting from treatment of chronic disease or prevention of disease in adults may not appear to make a major impact. Increases of a few months in life expectancy from major advances in treatment may not seem very impressive. This is especially true if these months are viewed as occurring only at the end of life. In fact, a common misinterpretation of life expectancy data is to conclude that the extension of life expectancy implies that a brief period will be added on at the end of life. The impact of this misinterpretation may be seen in the following example:

> Coronary artery bypass surgery was shown to increase life expectancy by 6 months. A reviewer of this literature concluded that adding 6 months on at the end of life is not worth the other impacts of surgery.

First, the extension of life expectancy described here takes into account the fact that surgery does have immediate hazards, which may produce immediate death. In addition, the benefits of extended life do not merely get tacked on at the end of life. They are not distributed equally to everyone who undergoes bypass surgery. The benefits actually affect a modest percentage of those undergoing surgery. These patients are the ones who do not die in the months and years immediately after the surgery but who would otherwise die.

Thus, it is important when interpreting what seems like a short extension in life expectancy, for instance 6 months, to recognize that in this situation, it is actually an impressive gain in life expectancy. Its impact on some individuals may be dramatic and immediate, even though it may have little or no impact for many others. It should not be interpreted as adding 6 month on at the end of the average person's life.

There is one final limitation when interpreting life expectancy. Life expectancy has been used as the primary method for comparing the health status of one population to another, as well as to make comparisons within the same population. When used this way, it is susceptible to the misinterpretation illustrated in the next example.

> A country's life expectancy at birth was determined to be 80 years in 2005. Over the next 5 years the country experienced a major epidemic of disease that left a large segment of the population with severe disabilities. The life expectancy calculated in 2010, however, was the same as that in 2005. The reviewers of this data concluded that since the life expectancy was the same, the health status of the population had not changed.

These results are not surprising if we recognize that life expectancy only takes into account the impact of death and does not incorporate the impact of disability.

Thus, life expectancy should not be regarded as an ideal measurement of health status of a population.

Traditionally, data have not generally been available to incorporate morbidity or disabilities and their impact on the quality of health. Increasingly, population health measures are being used that incorporate the quality of health along with the length of life or longevity.

One new population health measure that takes into account the disabilities that occurs in a population and combines it with the mortality is called the Health Adjusted Life Expectancy, or HALE. HALE is increasingly being used as a substitute for life expectancy when comparing the health of populations.[8] The measurement of HALE requires knowledge of the average impact of disability in each age group. HALE can be interpreted as life expectancy that takes into account the impact of disabilities.[9]

In summary, life expectancy is a useful population health measure that summarizes the probabilities of death at different ages in a population. It is useful for comparing one population with another for the same year or for comparing how the same population changes from one year to another year. When data on gender and racial groups are available, life expectancy can be useful for comparing the mortality of these groups within a population.

It is important to remember, however, that life expectancy is not a good predictor of future survival. It combines survival for healthy and sick individuals, and it is strongly influenced by the mortality of the young. Thus, we need to be very careful when using life expectancy calculations to predict the future, to make recommendations for the healthy, and to apply these calculations to individuals. Finally, life expectancy does not take into account the impact of disabilities, New measurements such as the Health Adjusted Life Expectancy, or HALE, are beginning to be a useful measurement of a population's health status that incorporates the impact of disability as well as death.

[8] The Health Adjusted Life Expectancy has previously been referred to as the Disability Adjusted Life Expectancy, or DALE. This caused confusion with *Disability Adjusted Life Years or DALYs*. DALYs aim to address the impact of specific diseases or conditions by comparing one population to the current best-performing population in terms of mortality and morbidity.

[9] Life expectancy is increasingly being combined with measures of the quality of health for decision-making investigations as well as for comparing populations. As we will see, the measurement most commonly used in decision-making aims to include both the impact of mortality as reflected in life expectancy as well as disability. This measurement is known as Quality Adjusted Life Years or QALYs.

26 Questions to Ask and Flaw-Catching Exercises

Questions to Ask: Rating a Rate

The following Questions to Ask can serve as a checklist when reading a journal article that compares rates. To see how these questions can be applied see the Studying a Study Online Web site at **www.StudyingaStudy.com.**

Method: Investigation's purpose and study population

1. **Purpose:** What is the purpose for investigating rates?
2. **Types of rates:** What rates does the investigation intend to measure?
3. **Study population:** What is the study's population?

Assignment: Defining the rates

1. **Numerator:** How are the events in the numerator defined?
2. **Denominator:** How is the population in the denominator defined?
3. **Time:** Is a unit of time being incorporated to produce a true rate?

Assessment: Measuring the rates

1. **Numerator and denominator:** How are the numerator and the denominator measured?
2. **Derivation:** Are rates derived from other measurements instead of being directly measured?
3. **Completeness:** Is the measurement complete, and if not, are the data representative of the larger population?

Results: Comparing rates

1. **Estimation:** What measurements are used to compare rates?
2. **Inference:** Are statistical significance testing and/or confidence intervals used?
3. **Adjustment:** Is adjustment for confounding variables performed?

Interpretation: Conclusions for populations included in the investigation

1. **Real vs. artifactual:** Are the changes or differences artifactual or real?
2. **Reasons for changes or differences:** Are conclusion drawn about underlying reasons for the changes or differences?
3. **Subgroups:** Are subgroups examined?

Extrapolation: Conclusions for populations not included in the investigation

1. **Hypothesis generation:** Are rates used to generate a hypothesis for populations similar to those in the investigation?
2. **To other populations:** Are rates obtained in one population applied to another?
3. **Prediction:** Is prediction of future rates attempted?

Flaw-Catching Exercises

The following flaw-catching exercises are designed to give you practice in applying the principles of Rating a Rate to hypothetical research articles. The flaw-catching exercises include a variety of errors. Read each exercise. Then write a critique pointing out the types of errors committed by the investigators. A sample critique is provided for each exercise.

Flaw-Catching Exercise No. 1: Rates of Cancer—Is It Progress?

A study of progress in survival after diagnosis of cancer in the United States compared the rates in 1975 with the rates in 2005 to assess changes. Data on incidence rates and mortality rates of cancer were collected. Incidence data were obtained from an intensive search of hospital records on a random sample of 1% of the nation's hospitals. Data on mortality rates were obtained from a complete review of all the death certificates in the nation. Case fatality was derived from the following formula for long-term changes:

$$\text{Mortality rate} = \text{Incidence rate of disease} \times \text{Case fatality}$$

The data from these studies are summarized in Table 26.1. The investigators found that the overall age-adjusted mortality rates had not change very much. Looking more closely at the data, the researchers reviewed randomized clinical trials on cancers that caused nearly all of the cancer deaths among people 20 years and older. They found that among people with incurable cancers, the trials showed a 3-year increase in life expectancy should be obtainable when applying new therapies developed since 1975.

Finally, the researchers calculated the proportion of all deaths that are due to cancer—that is, the *proportionate mortality ratio*. They found that the proportionate mortality ratio for cancer overall had increased from 22% to 24%.

The researchers confessed complete confusion, saying that it was possible to make any of the following arguments:

1. There has been substantial progress on the basis of the decreased mortality rates for people younger than 20 years, decreased case fatality for all age groups, and the increased survival rates in randomized clinical trials among those 20 years and older.
2. The situation is getting worse on the basis of the increased incidence rates among people older than 20 years. The increased cancer mortality rates among those older than 65 years and the increased proportionate mortality ratio support a worsening of the situation.
3. No change has occurred on the basis of the nearly constant overall age-adjusted mortality rates.

Table 26.1. *Changes in cancer rates from 1975 to 2005*

Age (yr)	Incidence rate	Case fatality	Mortality rate
0–19	No change	20% decrease	20% decrease
20–65	1% increase	1% decrease	No change
65+	15% increase	10% decrease	5% increase

The investigators throw up their hands and ask you, the readers, to explain how the data could support such inconsistent results.

Critique: Exercise No. 1

These rates are all compatible. They reflect different ways to look at and to argue about rates. Incidence rates reflect the rate at which new cases of the disease develop over a period of time. Case fatality reflects the probability of dying over a period of time if the disease develops. Thus, incidence rates and case fatality measure two very different phenomena. Incidence rates primarily reflect the underlying causes of disease. They may be artifactually changed by interventions that alter the effort to detect disease, the ability to detect disease, or the definition of disease. Primary prevention efforts, such as smoking cessation, may alter the underlying incidence. In general, however, incidence rates do not reflect the usual therapeutic efforts that are part of clinical care. Case fatality, on the other hand, is a measure of how successful therapy is at curing disease.

When an intervention successfully prolongs life but does not cure a disease, this intervention has little or no effect on the long-term mortality or the case fatality. Thus, the 3-year increase in life expectancy among people with incurable cancers is compatible with the more modest decrease in case fatality. The increased proportionate mortality ratio tells us very little about the progress in survival after diagnosis of cancer over those years. It does suggest, however, that mortality from other diseases is becoming less frequent compared with cancers. Proportionate mortality ratios are useful measures of the relative frequency of various causes of death. The increase in the proportionate mortality ratio suggests that deaths from cancer are becoming more common relative to deaths from other causes.

This exercise demonstrates how it is possible to argue for quite different conclusions from the same data. The argument presented by the researchers reflects different concepts about what is meant by progress. Is progress a reduced incidence of new disease? Is progress an increased cure rate for diagnosed disease? Alternatively, is progress a prolongation of life for people with disease?

Flaw-Catching Exercise No. 2: Life Expectancy in Econotiger and Developed Country

A developing country known as Econotiger compared its life expectancy with its own previous life expectancy and those of Developed Country. It found the following years of life expectancy:

	At birth	At 65 years	At 80 years
Econotiger			
1985	50	15	5
2005	72	15	5
Developed Country			
1985	72	15	5
2005	75	18	5

The investigator drew the following conclusions:

1. A child born in Econotiger in 1985 will, on average, live until 2035 because the life expectancy in Econotiger in 1985 was 50 years.

2. The dramatic improvement in life expectancy at birth experienced in Econotiger will result in a longer life expectancy at birth in Econotiger than in Developed Country sometime during the twenty-first century.
3. The 1985 Econotiger life expectancy of 15 years at age 65 cannot be accurate because the life expectancy at birth is only 50 in 1985.
4. The increase from 15 to 18 years in life expectancy at age 65 years in Developed Country represents a very modest improvement.
5. The identical life expectancies at age 80 in both countries in both years suggest that once an individual has lived to 80 years, life expectancy is 5 years regardless of whether their health is good or poor.
6. Life expectancy is the only way to measure and compare the improvement in population health because it is a measure that incorporates prolongations of life, even in the absence of cure.

Critique: Exercise No. 2

Life expectancy calculations require only accurate measurement of the number of individuals in each age group in a population and the number of individuals who die in that age group in the year being considered. Thus, life expectancy is a useful measure for comparing the same country over time and making comparisons between countries. However, life expectancy has a number of limitations and potential misinterpretations, some of which are illustrated in the six conclusions that were drawn from the previous data.

1. Life expectancy is not usually a useful measure for predicting the future. Life expectancy provides a snapshot view of the experience of each age group in a particular year. To use life expectancy to predict the future, we need to assume that nothing will change in the future. It is clear that many things are changing in Econotiger. Individuals born there in 1985 will not actually experience the probabilities of death at each age that were present in Econotiger in 1985. Rather, they will experience the reduced probabilities of death that are present in the subsequent years. Thus, the life expectancy at birth in 1985 of 50 years is a particularly poor predictor of how long the average person born in Econotiger in 1985 will actually live.
2. In general, extensions in life expectancy at birth are most dramatically achieved by controlling infectious diseases of infants and children. By saving the life of an otherwise healthy infant or child, a large number of years of life expectancy is gained. Once these gains are obtained, further progress, as measured by life expectancy at birth, is often more difficult to achieve. Improvement in longevity for the elderly may represent important progress, but it has only a modest effect on the life expectancy at birth. This progress is better reflected in the life expectancy at age 65 years. The data suggest that Developed Country has experienced this type of progress between 1985 and 2005. If Econotiger experiences this same progress in subsequent years, it would cause the life expectancy at birth to change very little.
3. The life expectancy at 65 in Econotiger is 15 years in both 1985 and 2005. This might be surprising because the life expectancy at birth is only 50 years in 1985 and 72 years in 2005. Once individuals have survived to a particular age, such as 65 years, they have managed to avoided a number of potential causes of death.

Thus, upon reaching an age such as 65, their expected life span will be greater than the life span expected at birth. Remember, individuals never outlive their life expectancy because life expectancy increases with age. Even in a country where the life expectancy is only 50 years, some individuals will live to age 65 years and beyond. Their life expectancy is dependent on the probabilities of death at more advanced ages. These probabilities of death in a developed and a developing country may be quite similar even if the life expectancies at birth are dramatically different.

4. In Developed Country, an improvement in life expectancy at age 65 of 3 years between 1985 and 2005 represents an impressive increase of 20%. The data suggest that the entire increase in life expectancy at birth that occurred in Developed Country is the result of the improved probabilities of death in people older than 65 years.

5. Life expectancy at advanced ages, such as 80 years, must be interpreted carefully. Life expectancy at all ages comprises the life expectancy of both the healthy and the diseased. At advanced ages, however, the proportion of people with potential life-threatening disease is much greater than at younger ages. The smaller group of healthy individuals at an advanced age may have a much better prognosis than the larger number with potential life threatening disease. Thus, life expectancy should not be used to predict longevity for the healthy elderly.

6. Life expectancy does have the advantage of reflecting advances that prolong life rather than cure disease. Despite the usefulness of life expectancy in comparing a country's progress over time and making comparisons between countries, it also has important limitations. Life expectancy does not take into account improvements in the quality of life that are not also reflected in the length of life. Many of the benefits of health care are improvements only in the quality of life. Efforts to improve vision, mental health, and mobility, for instance, are not often reflected in increased life expectancy. Newer measures such as the Health Adjusted Life Expectancy (HALE) aim to incorporate the quality of health as well as the length of life. That is, they aim to include the impact of disability as well as death.

Summary

Rates are the basic measurement for describing disease. They can also help us generate hypotheses about causation, help us establish the pretest probability of disease, and with great caution, predict the short term future. Changes or differences in rates may be real or artifactual. Real changes or differences may be the result of a cohort effect, regression to mean, or depletion of the denominator. As we will see in the next section, rates are also central to the process of quantitative decision making.

IV
Considering Costs and Evaluating Effectiveness

27 Introduction and Method

Introduction: Considering Costs and Evaluating Effectiveness

Decision-making in medicine and public health has traditionally relied on subjective judgments, expert opinions, and non-quantitative decision-making. Today, we increasingly rely on quantitative methods. Potential interventions, from prevention to palliation, are subjected to measurements of outcome that take into account the desirable outcomes (benefits), the undesirable outcomes (harms) and the financial costs. Thus, decision-making has become the art and science of balancing the benefits and harms, and considering the costs. Benefits, harms, and costs have become the measures of medicine.

Why has this change occurred? In balancing benefits and harms and considering costs, it has become increasingly clear that qualitative and subjective decision-making is affected by inherent limitations in how our brains process information.[1]

Not being computers, we have limited ability to store and manipulate information, and can be biased in how we structure our decision-making processes. These might be classified as limitations in data handling and limitations in data framing.

Data-handling limitations relate to our limited ability to simultaneously consider and utilize large quantities of information. To address these limitations, we often use simplified approaches or rules of thumb called *heuristics* to assist in our decision-making. For many activities, including such complicated activities as diagnosis, these rules of thumb work remarkably well. However, when simultaneously examining and selecting between the available options for intervention that incorporate data on benefits, harms, and costs, our simplifying rules of thumb often reveal their limitations.[2]

---

[1] Our current understanding of the subjective process of decision-making is due in large part to the work of Amos Tversky and Daniel Kahneman, as reflected in their *prospect theory* of decision-making. For a useful overview of this theory and the relationship of quantitative and subjective decision-making, see H. Hastie and R.M. Dawes, *Rational Choice in an Uncertain World: The Psychology of Judgment and Decision Making* (Thousand Oaks, Calif.: Sage Publications), 2001.

[2] Our limitations in data handling include at least three elements: (a) limited ability to handle more than two options at a time; (b) limited ability to objectively judge the probability of rare events such as death or side effects; (c) limited ability to combine data such as two or more probabilities. Our limited ability to handle data thus often leads us to overly simplify the complexities of decision-making. For instance, when faced with three or more options, we often reduce them to two-at-a-time comparisons, leaving out options or giving an advantage to an option that does not need to compete in the early rounds. When a side effect is rare but serious, such as death, we often either dismiss it as too unlikely to matter or focus on it as an especially important outcome. One-step procedures such as surgery may be viewed as more desirable than multiple-step procedures that may have multiple complications and side effects.

Limitations in data framing imply that we can be influenced in our selection of the preferred option by the way the question is posed or the alternatives presented.[3] The impacts of framing often result from the fact that there are many versions of the truth, and we are remarkably prone to being influenced by the way the truth is told.

Quantitative decision-making aims to overcome these limitations by using quantitative measurements rather than qualitative conclusions and by objectively combining these measurements rather than subjectively drawing conclusions. There are a number of potential advantages of quantitative decision-making over subjective, non-quantitative decision making, including:

- The ability to simultaneously compare three or more options
- The potential to objectively consider events with low probability
- The ability to explicitly state which factors are being taken into account in making a decision
- The ability to identify the reasons for disagreements
- The ability to identify the factors which have the most influence on the preferred option

For these and other reasons, quantitative decision-making is growing in importance in medicine and public health. As we will see, quantitative decision-making often has advantages in objectively structuring decision-making and identifying areas that are critical to selecting between options. We will also see, however, that quantitative decision-making also has inherent limitations that we need to recognize when reading the rapidly growing decision-making research literature.

Decision-making investigations may be used as the basis for making recommendations. However, as we will see in Section V, "A Guide to the Guidelines," recommendation or guidelines usually require additional considerations beyond those that can be quantitatively considered in a decision-making investigation.

The process of quantitative decision-making research can be quite complex. Nonetheless, the investigations that quantitatively examine decision-making can be reviewed using the M.A.A.R.I.E. framework. Figure 27.1 illustrates the application of the M.A.A.R.I.E. framework to decision-making investigations.

A decision-making investigation often requires the investigator to do the following:

1. **Model the decision:** This requires defining the alternatives that are being considered and the paths that eventually lead to potential outcomes. Decision-making investigations require the researcher to identify which options are being compared and what outcomes are being considered.
2. **Incorporate probabilities:** The investigator must determine which probabilities to use for measuring the favorable and unfavorable outcomes. These probabilities may come from the research literature, but they may need to be "guesstimated" based on expert opinion.

---

[3] Framing effects our tendency to (a) compare new options to a "reference point" which may reflect past or envisioned states of health rather than an objective assessment of the status quo; (b) favor alternatives that are framed optimistically such as percent survival rather than pessimistically such as percent mortality; (c) favor options expressed with certainty as opposed to those expressed with ambivalence. Thus, options for intervention that are presented optimistically as percent survival and that may return patients to their past state of good health may be especially valued by clinicians and patients. When uncertainty is minimized by expressions such as "in my hands" or "in my experience," the bias toward action may be especially strong.

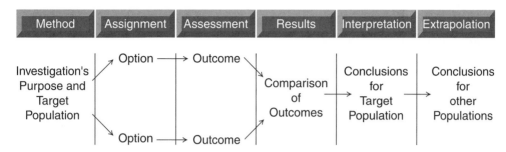

Figure 27.1. Application of M.A.A.R.I.E. framework to decision-making investigations.

3. **Incorporate utilities:** A measurement of the degree of preferences for each of the favorable and unfavorable outcomes is required. As we will see, these preferences are measured using what are called *utilities*.

4. **Incorporate costs:** As the cost of health care has increased along with the number of available options, researchers are also increasingly expected to measure and compare the financial consequences of each option being considered.

Thus, the health research literature now includes more than investigations that measure the probability of good outcomes or benefits and bad side effects or harms. Increasingly, decision-making investigations aim to measure or quantify the entire process of decision-making. These decision-making investigations aim to model the decision-making process, to measure each of the components, and at times to offer recommendations or guidelines based on the research. Decision-making investigations now appear in most major medical, management, and public health journals.

In examining decision-making investigations, we will focus on two hypothetical examples.

The first example examines three alternatives for treating single-vessel coronary artery disease. Conventional treatment is a combination of medications, angioplasty, and surgery. There are also two new treatments. One treatment is called transthoracic laser coronaryplasty (TLC). The other is a new drug called Cardiomagic. We will be looking at how we can compare these alternatives to decide which is the most effective for treatment and which is the most cost-effective.

The second example examines options for approaching a disease that we will call Paresis A. We will examine the following situation:

> Paresis A is a common contagious disease of childhood that is usually self-limited. However, a small percentage of children who experience the illness develop paralysis, and a few develop life-threatening complications. Long-term paralysis and late complications can occur. The conventional treatment for Paresis A has been only supportive treatment which we will call a do-nothing approach. Recently, an expensive vaccination has become available to prevent Paresis A. We will discuss how we can compare the results of the vaccine to the do-nothing approach.

These types of decision-making investigations require a wide variety of information drawn from multiple sources. Thus, they can be very confusing to read and understand. However, decision-making investigations, like the other types of studies that we have examined, can be understood by using the M.A.A.R.I.E. framework.

Method

Study Question and Study Type

Decision-making investigations differ from other types of investigations that we have examined because they generally do not begin by stating a study hypothesis. Rather, they begin by defining a study question and then identifying the options that will be considered to address the study question. Thus, the investigator does not begin by hypothesizing which option is best. Rather, the investigator's study question should be to fairly identify and compare the options using predefined criteria.

A variety of study questions can be addressed by decision-making investigations. The specific type of decision-making investigation used should depend on the question being addressed.

Let us begin by outlining the common types of decision-making investigations. Then it should be possible for you to determine whether the study type is appropriate to the study question.

Decision-making investigations can be divided into two general types. The first type includes efforts to consider benefits and harms—that is, favorable and unfavorable health effects. This type of investigation is often called a *decision analysis*.[4]

The second type of decision-making investigation is called *cost-effectiveness analysis*. Cost-effectiveness analysis will be used as a general term that includes all types of decision-making investigations that consider costs and relate them to a measure of favorable and adverse outcomes.[5]

Both decision analysis and cost-effectiveness analyses can be subdivided into several different types of investigations, depending on the factors that are considered.

DECISION ANALYSIS

One type of decision analysis in the literature is an *outcomes profile*.[6]

Table 27.1 shows the favorable and unfavorable outcomes with TLC and Cardiomagic. This profile provides considerable data that may be helpful in making decisions. However, it does not in and of itself lead to preference for one option over another. The outcome profile actually raises a series of questions that need to be considered in making decisions that can be incorporated into more complex investigations.

---

[4] The term "decision analysis" is often used even more generically to refer to all decision-making investigations that use a quantitative approach to decision-making under conditions of uncertainty. In this context, all investigation types discussed here, including those that incorporate costs, can be considered decision analyses. In addition, the term "decision analysis" has been used more narrowly than we use it here to imply the use of a decision tree as the method for modeling the options being considered.

[5] As we discuss later in this chapter, the term "cost-effectiveness" is also used to describe one particular type of decision-making investigation in which the investigator is interested in comparing different alternatives for obtaining the same outcome. In this special type of investigation, the results are stated as additional costs per additional outcome. The term "effectiveness" as used in cost-effectiveness has a somewhat different meaning than when used in the "Studying a Study" section of this book. Effectiveness in the context of cost-effectiveness combines the favorable and adverse outcomes. When we viewed outcomes previously, we regarded effectiveness as including only favorable outcomes. Considerations of adverse outcomes or safety were discussed separately. Thus, in decision-making investigations, we should regard the term "effectiveness" as implying net effectiveness.

[6] The term "balance sheet" has been used to describe this type of investigation; however, this term may be misleading. This is an accounting term that refers to assets and liabilities measured in monetary terms such as dollars. The type of analysis being considered here does not imply the use of costs, and it is often not possible to directly compare the favorable outcomes with the adverse outcomes.

Table 27.1. *Favorable and unfavorable outcomes with TLC and Cardiomagic*

TLC outcomes:	Cardiomagic outcomes:
Successful 96%	Successful 80%
Unsuccessful 3.9%	Unsuccessful 19.8%
Death 0.1%	Blindness 0.2%

Let us examine Table 27.1 to see what information is provided and what is left out. First, note that the outcomes profile provides estimates of the probability of favorable and adverse outcomes. In an outcomes profile, however, the timing of the events are not necessarily made explicit. In addition, in an outcomes profile there is no attempt to combine or summarize the impact of favorable and adverse outcomes or long-term and short-term impacts. This process is left to the reader. An outcomes profile does not really provide a conclusion and may not allow us to determine which is the best alternative. Therefore, we may consider an outcomes profile to be a preliminary, partial, or incomplete decision-making investigation.

An outcomes profile may provide enough information to make a decision if it is clear that both the harms and the benefits of a therapy such as TLC are more favorable than the harms and benefits of Cardiomagic. It is important to recognize, however, that the outcomes of TLC and Cardiomagic are not directly comparable. Looking at the adverse effects of these two treatments requires us to compare two outcomes: death and blindness. These have very different implications. We may need to quantitate the importance of outcomes such as death and blindness and incorporate these measurements into a decision-making investigation if we wish to compare TLC and Cardiomagic. In decision-making investigations, incorporating the relative importance of an event is accomplished by measuring utility.[7]

A utility is designed to measure the preference of a decision-maker for a particular health outcome or state of health. As we will see in Chapter 29 on assessment, there are a variety of methods for measuring utilities and considerable controversy about which is best. Regardless of the method chosen, the aim is to measure utilities on the same scale as probabilities. By doing so, it is possible to combine probabilities and utilities.

Thus, our goal is to measure the utilities of blindness and death on the same numerical scale. In addition, our goal is to combine the measurements of utilities that we obtain for blindness and death with the probabilities that they will occur.

Remember that probabilities are measured using a scale of 0 to 1, which is often converted to percentages from 0% to 100%. On this scale, there are no measurements greater than 1 or less than 0. The utility scale generally defines 0 as death and 1 as full health or an individual's state of health in the absence of manifestations of disease or other health-related conditions.

Once utility and probability are measured on the same scale, the probability can be multiplied by the utility to produce what is called an *expected utility*. We can consider expected utility to be the probability of an outcome that takes into account its value or utility. The calculation of expected utilities is an essential step in performing a decision-making investigation that attempts to compare options

---

[7] At times, outcomes profiles may be adequate for decision-making when one option is clearly better than the other, regardless of the utility that is placed on each outcome. In decision-making investigations, when one alternative is clearly more favorable than another, the alternative with the better outcomes is said to be *dominant*.

and draw conclusions. Thus, an investigation that measures utilities and combines them with probabilities is called an *expected utility decision analysis*.

The possibility that death may occur raises an additional factor to consider in a decision-making investigation. At times, we may want to consider the expected life span lost as the result of death. We have already encountered the measurement of life expectancy, which despite its limitation is our standard measurement of average life-span. For cases in which we hope to return an individual to his or her state of full health, we can use life expectancy measures, as derived from the age or average age of the individuals being treated, to estimate average remaining life span.[8]

Life expectancy can be incorporated into decision-making investigations along with utilities. When this is done, the investigation usually produces a measurement called *Quality Adjusted Life Years* (QALYs).[9]

Decision analyses that use QALYs to take into account life expectancy as well as utilities represent what many experts consider a fully developed decision analysis. We will call this form of decision analysis a *Quality Adjusted Life Years decision analysis* (QALY decision analysis).

We have now defined three types of decision analyses:

1. Outcomes profiles: This type of investigation merely states the probabilities of the known favorable and adverse outcomes from each of the alternatives being considered.
2. Expected utility decision analyses: This type of investigation combines the probabilities and utilities of each favorable and each adverse outcome and summarizes the results as overall expected utilities. Thus, expected utility decision analyses, as opposed to outcomes profiles, summarize the outcomes of each alternative and allow them to be directly compared.
3. QALY decision analyses: Like expected utility decision analyses, these allow direct comparison of alternatives, taking into account the favorable and adverse outcomes. However, QALY decision analyses go beyond expected utility in that they incorporate life expectancy.

COST-EFFECTIVENESS ANALYSIS

Cost-effectiveness analyses, in contrast to decision analyses, incorporate costs as well as considerations of favorable and adverse outcomes. Cost-effectiveness analyses, like decision analyses, can be divided into several types.

---

[8] If the investigator is dealing with a women's disease, then life expectancy by age and gender should be used. Similarly, if the author is dealing with a disease generally limited to blacks, such as sickle cell anemia, use of life expectancy by age and race would be appropriate. As discussed in the next chapter, the relevant life expectancy is not always the life expectancy derived from population data. For diseases that substantially reduce life expectancy, the appropriate life-expectancy measures take into account life expectancy for a particular disease as well as life expectancy defined by age and possibly gender and race.

[9] QALY is the standard but not the only method for incorporating utilities and life expectancy. A method known as *Health Adjusted Life Expectancy* or HALE is gaining recognition for combine life expectancy and quality of life measures at the population level. HALE is gaining acceptance for cost-effectiveness analysis in public health, for instance when comparing population-wide investments. However, HALE cannot be used when examining the impact of a particular disease or condition. Another measure known as Disability Adjusted Life Years or DALY is useful when comparing different reasons for mortality and morbidity, but does not provide the basis for comparing the impact of different interventions for the same disease or condition. Thus QALY is the routine measure used in a fully developed decision analysis or cost-effectiveness analysis.

Table 27.2. *Possible data from a cost-consequence analysis for Paresis A*

Paresis A vaccine	
Outcomes:	Successful immunization 97%
	Unsuccessful immunization 2.9%
	Complications 0.1%
Costs:	$50 per use

As with outcomes profiles, cost-effectiveness analysis may simply measure or describe the various costs as well as the probabilities of the potential outcomes. The reader then needs to combine these outcomes to reach conclusions. This type of investigation is called a *cost-consequence analysis.* The data from a cost-consequence analysis might look like that in Table 27.2.

Cost-consequence analyses are really partial analyses because they do not generally allow us to directly compare two or more alternatives. To compare alternatives, the investigators need to bring in outside data or judgments.

A second type of cost-effectiveness analysis has unfortunately been called a *cost-effectiveness analysis.* Using this term to describe a specific type of cost-effectiveness analysis can be very confusing. To minimize confusion, we will call this type of analysis a *cost-and-effectiveness study.*

A cost-and-effectiveness study looks at the costs required to produce an additional unit of desired outcome. For instance, imagine the following situation with Paresis A:

> The cost of the new Paresis A vaccine including the total costs of providing the vaccine and treating any complications is $15,000 per case of Paresis A prevented.

This type of investigation compares the cost per additional desired outcome. It does not ask about the importance of the outcome or the life expectancy of the people treated. That is, cost-and-effectiveness studies do not consider utility or life expectancy. This type of cost-effectiveness analysis can be used to compare any outcomes, such as disease prevented or correct diagnosis, as well as lives saved. However, most comparisons of intervention options produce more than one outcome, most of which require consideration of utilities and life expectancy.[10]

Thus, a full cost-effectiveness analysis incorporates considerations of utility and life expectancy as well as cost. This type of cost-effectiveness analysis is called a *cost-utility analysis* or a *cost-effectiveness analysis using QALY* as the measure of effectiveness. Let us see what we mean by a cost-utility analysis:

> Paresis A vaccine was found to reduce the cost by $2,000 per quality-adjusted life year saved when it was compared with the conventional approach. The investigation took into account the utility of the outcomes as well as the life expectancy of people who experienced favorable and adverse outcomes.

This form of cost-effectiveness analysis represents a fully developed analysis. It allows us to compare any alternative, taking into account all the relevant costs and health outcomes including the probability and utility of favorable and adverse

---

[10] At times, the key issue for an analysis is the relative costs. The effectiveness of two options may be comparable and the investigation is directed only at considering costs. This type of cost-and-effectiveness study is called a *cost analysis.*

outcomes as well as the life expectancy. Cost-utility analyses are increasingly considered the method of choice for most decision-making in health care. They allow us to directly compare alternatives and determine the costs relative to the health consequences.

COST-BENEFIT ANALYSIS

At times, however, the question posed in an analysis does not relate to comparing the costs and health consequences of an intervention. Decision-making may at times require looking at trade-offs between money spent on health and money spent on other important outcomes such as environmental protection, economic growth, or education. To make these types of comparisons, it is necessary to translate effectiveness as well as costs into monetary terms.

The form of analysis that converts effectiveness as well as costs into monetary terms is known as a *cost-benefit analysis.*[11] Let us examine how a cost-benefit analysis of might look:

> An analysis was conducted to compare the economic costs and consequences of providing insurance coverage for paralysis vaccine compared with the alternative of providing college scholarships. The analysis assumes that one QALY could be converted to $50,000. The investigation found that coverage of paralysis provided $2 in benefits for every $1 in cost. The alternative of paying for college tuition provided $3 of benefit for every $1 of costs. Thus, paying for college tuition was considered the better alternative.

Note that cost-benefit analyses must make the conversion of QALY into dollars. This is a big step, and there is no agreement on the value of a year of life. Thus, this type of analysis remains controversial. Fortunately, it is not often necessary to directly compare health expenditures with other uses of money. Therefore, cost-benefit analyses are not frequently seen in the health research literature.

We will not examine cost-benefit analyses. However, the conversion from a cost-utility study to a cost-benefit study is mechanically simple even though it represents a major intellectual leap. The key is determining the proper monetary value to place on a year of life. Once the monetary conversion of QALYs to dollars or other currency is agreed upon, that monetary figure merely replaces each QALY.

Thus, decision-making investigations can be classified as follows:

Decision Analysis
Outcomes profile: Probabilities of favorable and unfavorable outcomes
Expected utility decision analysis: Probabilities and utilities of favorable and unfavorable outcomes
Quality adjusted life year (QALY) decision analysis : Probabilities, life expectancy, and utilities of each outcome

Cost Effectiveness
Cost-consequence analysis: Costs and probability of favorable and unfavorable outcomes

---

[11] The term "benefit" is also used to imply a favorable outcome. In the context of cost-benefit analysis, benefit means net effectiveness measured in monetary units. Net effectiveness implies favorable outcomes minus unfavorable outcomes.

Cost-and-effectiveness study: Costs to produce an additional unit of desired outcome such as lives saved

Cost-utility analysis: Costs compared to a unit of outcome that incorporates utilities and life expectancy

Cost-Benefit Analysis

Costs compared with health outcomes that are converted to a monetary value

Target Population

As with all investigations, it is important to define the target population, the population to which the results will be applied. This is important because it tells us three things:

1. What type of individuals are being included and excluded
2. What type of sources can be used to provide the necessary data
3. What types of extrapolations to similar populations will be possible if the results favor one of the alternatives

The population that is the target of the decision-making study ideally should guide the investigator to the type of data to use. Unfortunately, data may not be available from the target population. To understand the implications of the choice of data, let us return to our coronary artery disease example and ask which population's data should be used to address the following study question:

> We are evaluating the costs and effectiveness of three types of treatments for single-vessel coronary artery disease: conventional treatment, i.e., a combination of medications, angioplasty, and surgery.

When obtaining data to address the effectiveness or cost-effectiveness of the three alternative treatments, it is important that the data come from individuals with single-vessel coronary artery disease. These treatments may also be used on patients with more extensive disease. Such individuals are likely to be older and have other related arterial disease. Thus, data derived from a population of patients with severe coronary artery disease would not be the type of data that should be used in addressing the study question. Now let us look at our other hypothetical situation:

> We are evaluating the costs and effectiveness of a new vaccine for Paresis A, a common contagious disease of childhood that is usually self-limited but can produce short- and long-term complications.

When obtaining data to address the costs and effectiveness of this vaccine, the data should be obtained from a population like the one on which it will be used. It would not be useful to obtain data from a population of severely ill children, especially if they had a high frequency of complications and required large expenditures if they did develop complications. Likewise, it would not be useful to obtain data from a population in which a high level of natural immunity already existed and therefore the fully developed disease was rarely experienced.

Thus, when examining a decision-making investigation, the reader must ask, "From what population (or populations) was the data obtained?" and "Is the population appropriate to the study question?"

Perspective

To evaluate whether appropriate data were included in an investigation, it is important to consider the study *perspective*. Perspective asks about how broadly we should look when measuring the effectiveness and the costs of an alternative. Let us examine some of the possible perspectives by returning to the use of Paresis A vaccine. We could view the costs and effectiveness of the vaccine from at least the following perspectives:

- The patient who receives the vaccine and pays out of pocket
- The insurance company that pays for the vaccine as well as the short-term costs of treating Paresis A
- The government insurance system that pays for the care for individuals who develop Paresis A
- The society that, through one payment mechanism or another, receives the effectiveness and pays the costs of the administration of the vaccine and of the disease

The first three perspectives can be viewed as *user perspectives*. They reflect different ways for recipients or payers to view the costs and effectiveness of the vaccine. In theory, an investigation could be conducted from the perspective of the user of the investigation.

The fourth perspective is a *social perspective*. A social perspective implies that we are interested in the impact of the effectiveness and the costs regardless of who obtains the benefits, who suffers the harms, or who pays the costs. The choice of perspective guides the investigator in determining what should be included or excluded in the measurement of benefits, harms, and costs. Therefore, we can look at perspective as parallel to the inclusion and exclusion criteria used in other types of investigations.[12]

In general, decision-making investigations should use the social perspective. Other perspectives may also be used for additional analyses. There are two basic reasons for using the social perspective. First, it is the only perspective that never counts an adverse outcome for one individual as a favorable outcome for another individual. Similarly, the social perspective is the only perspective that never counts a financial lose to one individual as a financial gain for another individual. Thus, social perspective is the only perspective that considers all the favorable and adverse outcomes and all the costs regardless of where they fall in society.

The perspective chosen should apply equally to the benefits, the harms, and the costs. If different perspectives are used for each, we cannot fairly compare or summarize the relationship between net effectiveness and costs. Use of the social perspective thus considers all the favorable and adverse outcomes regardless of who they affect and all the costs regardless of who pays the bills. Using the social perspective allows us to compare net effectiveness and costs in a consistent manner and to compare the results of one investigation with another.

As is often the case in study design, we do allow investigators to have it both ways. It is legitimate to conduct a decision-making investigation from the perspective of a potential user. If this is done, however, it is recommended that the

---

[12] The perspective of the decision-making investigation should be distinguished from the identity of the decision-maker. For instance, a clinician may make a recommendation by attempting to view the situation from the perspective of an individual patient, an institution, or even society as a whole.

investigation begin with a presentation from the social perspective. The social perspective is usually considered the ideal perspective for conducting a cost-effectiveness analysis. When a cost-effectiveness analysis is conducted from other perspectives, the results are often compared with the results obtained using the social perspective. The use of the social perspective in cost-effectiveness analysis has been called the *reference case*.[13]

It is also important to recognize that many readers of a cost-effectiveness analysis do not look at the issue from a social perspective but rather from one or more user perspectives. Ideally, the data is presented in such a way that it is possible for readers who want to take a user perspective to selectively use the data to reach their own conclusions. Recognizing the perspective used in an investigation is especially important when we try to extrapolate the results to individuals or situations not included in the study.

In summary, when reading a decision-making investigation, we first need to address the three basic questions of study design[14]:

- What is the study question, and is an appropriate study type being used to address the study question?
- What is the target population?
- What is the study perspective?

Having addressed these questions, we can turn our attention to assignment and see what we mean by a decision-making model. In the next chapters in this section, we examine net effectiveness using probabilities, utilities, and life expectancy, and we consider costs as well as net effectiveness from the social perspective.

---

[13] Throughout Section IV the basic principles addressed are derived from M. Gold et al., *Cost-Effectiveness in Health and Medicine* (New York: Oxford University Press), 1996.

[14] In decision-making investigations we do not need to consider sample size since we are not collecting original data.

28 Assignment

Options

The process of assignment in a decision-making investigation involves modeling, diagramming, or otherwise structuring the decision options. The selection of the options to consider is under the investigator's control. As the reader, it is very important to review which options have been selected and, conversely, which potential options have not been included.

First, let us examine what we mean by modeling the decision-making process. To conduct a decision-making investigation, the investigator needs to propose what is called a *decision-making model*. A decision-making model outlines the steps the investigator will follow in the decision-making and the *final outcomes* that occur. By final outcomes, we mean the outcomes that may occur at the completion of the decision option.[1] With TLC and Cardiomagic, the decision-making model may be described as follows:

> TLC and Cardiomagic will be compared. TLC or Cardiomagic may be chosen, but not both. The outcomes of TLC are successful, unsuccessful, and death. No other therapy may be used if TLC is unsuccessful. Alternatively, Cardiomagic may be chosen. The outcomes of Cardiomagic are successful, unsuccessful, and blindness. If Cardiomagic is unsuccessful, surgery will be performed. The outcomes of surgery are successful, unsuccessful, and death. No other intervention will occur.

A common method for diagramming the decision-making process is a *decision tree*. A decision tree graphically depicts the decision options and the choices that must be made to implement each option. The decision tree also depicts the events that occur through a chance process, outside the control of the decision-maker.[2]

Let us use our example of TLC and Cardiomagic to demonstrate the essential components of a decision tree.

Figure 28.1 represents a decision tree outlining the choice between TLC and Cardiomagic for patients with symptomatic single-vessel coronary artery disease. Note the following: First, there are two and only two options to choose from, TLC and Cardiomagic. The choices of TLC and Cardiomagic are the decision options. Second, note that there is a square connecting the two decision options. This square is called a *decision node*. A decision node is connected with each of the decision options using a vertical line. The decision-maker must choose one of the available

---

[1] The term "final outcome" is not in common usage. It is being used here to distinguish the outcomes at the right end of the decision tree from intermediate outcomes. In decision analysis the outcomes at the right-hand side of the decision tree are the outcomes of interest. Thus, death is death and full health is full health regardless of the process of getting there. Decision analysis focuses on final outcomes not the process of getting there.

[2] The term *decision-maker* intentionally evades the question of who is making the decision. Thus, at times the decision-maker may be a clinician, a patient, an administrator, etc.

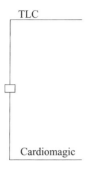

TLC

Cardiomagic

Figure 28.1. A decision tree outlining the choice between TLC and Cardiomagic for patients with symptomatic single-vessel coronary artery disease.

decision options. Once the choice of option is made, the decision tree depicts the subsequent course of events.[3]

In the decision tree for TLC depicted in Fig. 28.2, we see only events that subsequently occur by chance.

For TLC, one of three final outcomes occur: successful, unsuccessful, or death. Any individual can experience only one of these outcomes; that is, the outcomes are considered mutually exclusive.[4]

These three final outcomes are connected by a *chance node*. Chance nodes are represented by a darkened dot or circle. The "successful" and "death" final outcomes each brings us to the end of the TLC portion of the decision tree.

Figure 28.3 displays the option to use TLC and also the option to use Cardiomagic. Cardiomagic, unlike TLC, may be followed by surgery if it is unsuccessful. Thus, in the Cardiomagic alternative, there are two chance nodes. The first reflects the fact that the outcome can be successful, unsuccessful, or blindness. The

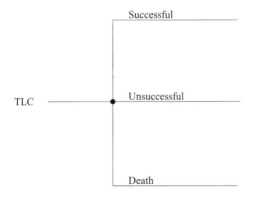

Successful

TLC

Unsuccessful

Death

Figure 28.2. Decision tree for TLC depicting three branches of the decision tree indicating events that occur by chance.

[3] Choice nodes may again appear later in a decision tree, implying that the decision-maker will need to make a subsequent decision as part of implementing a specific option.

[4] The mutually exclusive assumption may at times make the decision tree less than a true reflection of reality. In reality, any individual can experience both an unsuccessful procedure and an adverse effect. An outcome in which more than one outcome occurs can be included as an additional potential outcome. Often, combined outcomes are not included. Fortunately, at least from the social perspective, the unusual occurrence of more than one outcome often has little overall effect on the recommendations derived from the analysis. However, for the individual experiencing both an unsuccessful procedure and an adverse event, this is a particularly poor outcome.

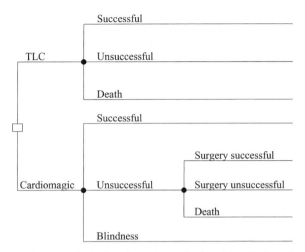

Figure 28.3. Decision tree displaying the options of using either TLC or Cardiomagic.

second chance node shows that the surgery following unsuccessful Cardiomagic will be successful, unsuccessful, or will result in death.

Relevant Options and Realistic Outcomes

Now let us see what our decision tree has and has not achieved. When looking at a decision tree, we need to ask whether the options being considered are relevant to the study question. We also need to ask whether the outcomes are realistic—that is, do they include the final outcomes that are important in practice.

When looking at a decision tree, the first question to ask is: "Were the relevant options considered?" Notice that there is no option to use conventional treatment such as surgery, angioplasty, or medications. Furthermore, observing the natural course of events without intervening is not included as an option. Whether or not these options should be included in a decision tree depends on the question being asked and the current state of knowledge. The choice between TLC and Cardiomagic may be appropriate if one of these must be selected for a particular group of individuals or both of these have been clearly shown to be superior to the other available options. When another option is considered, it should generally be included in a decision tree.

The other key question to ask in examining a decision tree is: "Does the decision process include the final outcomes that are important in practice. That is, do they reflect realistic decision-making?" This question is more complicated than it first appears since all decision trees simplify the real decision-making process. Decision trees generally leave out unusual events, especially if they are not directly related to the therapy. For instance, a procedure that requires hospitalization may result in side effects unrelated to the therapy itself. Hospitalization may increase the chances of developing hospital-acquired pneumonia or experiencing a medication error, yet a decision tree is not generally expected to incorporate these types of events.

In addition, as we have already seen, a decision tree often skips potential options. For instance in the decision tree for our example, it was not permitted to stop after unsuccessful Cardiomagic treatment results. The greater the number of chance nodes, the more data that are needed to complete the decision tree. Thus, these types of simplification are usually necessary and acceptable to make the decision-making model manageable.

The ideal way to construct a decision tree is to think of all possible final outcomes of the options being considered and to display a decision tree that reflects all of these possible outcomes. This process will usually produce a large number of unusual outcomes and a number of similar outcomes. The researcher then combines outcomes that are similar and decides whether certain outcomes are so unusual or so inconsequential that they can be deleted from the decision tree. This very common practice is referred to as *pruning the decision tree*.[5]

Timing of Events

The timing of occurrence of potential outcomes is an important consideration in structuring the options in a decision-making investigation.[6] Some events occur immediately, and others may take years to occur. Some events may occur only once, while others may recur in the near or distant future. Whether or not to include events that occur in the future depends on the study's *time horizon*.[7]

The time horizon is the follow-up period that determines which outcomes are included in the model. The time horizon tells us how far into the future to look for favorable or unfavorable outcomes. The investigation may be interested only in short-term outcomes, such as hospital mortality, long-term outcomes such as late recurrences, or even consequences for the next generation. Notice that the TLC decision tree that we used only considers the immediate outcomes. However, what if TLC could damage the coronary arteries and increase the probability of late complications? If this is the case, a decision tree for TLC with a longer time horizon would need additional chance nodes displaying additional outcomes.

Ideally, the time horizon should extend throughout the life of the individuals who receive the intervention option. When shorter time horizons are used, the reader should ask: "Was the time horizon long enough to include all important favorable or adverse outcomes?"

The choice of appropriate time horizon may itself be quite complex. With genetic interventions, the appropriate time horizon may extend to future generations. The time horizon may also be important in determining the proper structure of a decision tree, including which complications to consider. For instance, if the time horizon is extended long enough, the disease may recur; that is, the treated coronary artery may experience restenosis or disease may develop in additional

---

[5] In addition, the reader must ask the bigger questions of whether the approach used in outlining the decision tree is a realistic reflection of clinical or public health decision-making. Remember that the decision tree used here implied that the choice was between TLC and Cardiomagic. However, if there is an alternative to use Cardiomagic first, and if it is not successful to use TLC, then the decision tree does not reflect realistic decision-making.

[6] When examining a decision tree and considering the options it is also important to identify the *time frame* of the analysis. The time frame is the period during the course of the disease when it is possible to use the intervention. Here, TLC and Cardiomagic are being used at the time when single-vessel coronary artery disease has become symptomatic. If the time frame of the analysis had extended to an earlier period in the course of the disease before symptoms had developed, it may have been possible to select preventive interventions. Thus, the choice of time frame can be very important in selecting decision options.

[7] The time horizon is also called the *analysis horizon*. "Time horizon" is used here because the issue is the time period that is considered in structuring the decision model.

arteries. It is possible to construct more complicated decision trees incorporating recurrences and applying techniques known as *Markov analysis* to incorporate recurrent events into decision trees. Markov analysis allows the development of complex models in which one individual can potentially move back and forth through stages of disease over extended periods of time.

The assignment process in decision-making investigations can be thought of as structuring the decision-making model. An important technique for displaying or diagramming a decision model is a decision tree.[8] Having created the decision-making model, the next step in the process is to look at how the data in the model were obtained. This issue is addressed in the assessment process, which is discussed in the next chapter.

[8] Decision trees are not the only technique that can be used to diagram a decision-making investigations. *Influence diagrams* can be used. These display the relationships between events and the factors believed to be relevant to decisions. Influence diagrams may be combined with decision trees, which may make complex decision trees, easier to display and understand.

29 Assessment

The assessment process in decision-making investigations requires the investigator to obtain information from a variety of sources and to plug these pieces of information into a decision-making model that adequately describes the decision-making process. To better understand this process, let us see what need to be done to complete our decision tree on TLC and Cardiomagic.

A decision tree is a particularly attractive technique for diagramming decision-making because it allows the investigator to incorporate not only probabilities, but also utilities, life expectancies, and even costs. We will look at how we incorporate these measurements, beginning with probabilities.

Probabilities

So far we have looked at the components of method and assignment. In our coronary artery disease example, we have described the choices to be considered (TLC and Cardiomagic) and the meaning of decision nodes and chance nodes. Assume that TLC and Cardiomagic are the appropriate choices to consider and that TLC and Cardiomagic cannot be used together. Let us refer again to our decision tree before we proceed to look at what is needed to complete the decision tree. Figure 29.1 includes the probabilities of each potential outcome of TLC and Cardiomagic. Notice that the three potential outcomes of TLC are successful (0.96), unsuccessful (0.039), and death (0.001). The probabilities total 1 for each option. Figure 29.1 also outlines the potential outcomes and probabilities for Cardiomagic: successful (0.80), unsuccessful (0.198), and blindness (0.002). Calculating the probabilities of the final outcome for Cardiomagic requires us to combine probabilities. We will see how to do this a little later in this chapter.

If possible, probabilities should be obtained from studies found in the research literature. Often, however, these estimates are not available and educated guesses must be used instead. When educated guesses are used to obtain probabilities, they may be referred to as *subjective probabilities*.[1]

When using subjective probabilities, it is important to recognize that it is very difficult to accurately estimate probabilities, especially when the probability is very high (99% or more) or very low (1% or less). Thus, this problem often arises with estimates of the probability of adverse effects. In these situations, it is a common practice to either overestimate the probability, magnifying the chances of death for instance, or to underestimate the probability and therefore ignore the possibility of a rare side effect such as blindness or death.

The reader of decision-making literature needs to closely examine how the probabilities of rare but serious events were measured. When they are based on

---

[1] Underestimating and overestimating the probability of events are even greater problems in the types of nonquantitative decision-making that is used for most decisions. One advantage of quantitative techniques, such as decision trees, is that they force the investigator to be explicit about which outcomes are being included and the probabilities that are attached to each outcome.

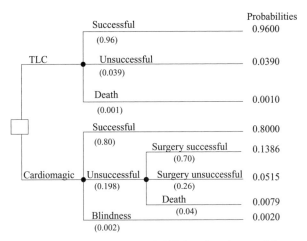

Figure 29.1. Decision tree including the probabilities of each potential outcome.

educated guesses or subjective judgments, these probabilities are especially prone to errors that need to be taken into account in the analysis.[2]

Utilities

It is possible to directly compare the successful and unsuccessful outcomes of TLC and Cardiomagic using probabilities alone. However, it is not possible to directly compare the consequences of death and blindness using only probabilities. Thus, to complete the decision tree, it is also necessary to include a measure of the relative value or importance of death and blindness. This is performed using utilities.

Figure 29.2 includes utilities for all the final outcomes. Success is given a utility of 1, which implies that the individual returns to full health. Death is given a utility of 0, which represents the lowest possible utility. Blindness is given a utility of 0.5, which implies that it is considered to be halfway between full health and death. We will examine methods for measuring these utilities and their implications in greater detail later in this chapter. For now, we examine how utilities are incorporated into the decision tree.

When utilities are used in a decision-making investigation, they must be measured on the same 0-to-1 scale as probabilities.[3] Using the same scale allows us to combine probabilities with utilities. This is performed by multiplying probabilities and utilities to obtain *expected utilities*. Expected utility can be viewed as a

[2] Overall probabilities are calculated based on the *independence assumption*. This assumption implies that the probability of success at surgery is not influenced by whether or not Cardiomagic was successful. At times, the independence assumption may not hold in decision-making situations. It is possible that a factor that led to failure of Cardiomagic also influences the probability of unsuccessful surgery.

[3] The question often arises as to who should be asked to assess utility. Should the investigator ask people who are already blind and have thus gained experience with blindness, or should we ask those who may become blind as a result of choosing the alternative to use Cardiomagic? The literature tells us that people who have already experienced a condition tend to score it with a slightly higher utility than those who have not experienced the condition. That is, people who have experienced blindness tend to adapt to its limitation and don't find it quite as bad as those confronted with potential blindness. The difference, however is not great and studies of utilities may use either people who have experienced or those who have not experienced the condition to obtain measures of utility.

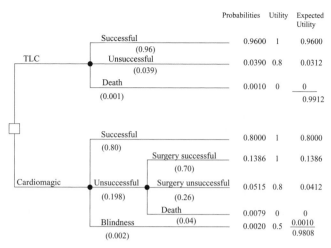

Figure 29.2. Decision tree displaying utilities for all outcomes.

probability that takes into account the utility of the outcome. In expected-utility decision analysis, the expected utilities are compared. Let us see how the expected utilities would be calculated for TLC and Cardiomagic by looking at Fig. 29.2.

The expected utilities of each outcome are obtained by a process known as *folding back the decision tree*. With this process, we calculate the probability of each of the final outcomes that may occur in the decision process. Once the probability of each final outcome is calculated, we multiply the probability by the utility of that outcome. For the Cardiomagic option in our example, the following outcomes may occur: (1) successful; (2) unsuccessful then successful surgery; (3) unsuccessful then unsuccessful surgery; (4) unsuccessful then death from surgery; (5) blindness.

Outcomes 2, 3, and 4 require combining two probabilities to obtain the probability of the final outcome. For instance, the probability for unsuccessful Cardiomagic followed by successful surgery is obtained by multiplying the probability of being unsuccessful with Cardiomagic (0.198) by the probability of experiencing successful surgery (0.70). This equals 0.1386, which is the probability of the final outcome.

Figure 29.2 displays the probabilities and utilities of the final outcome. These probabilities are multiplied times their utility to produce the expected utilities for each potential final outcome of TLC and Cardiomagic, the two decision options.

One more step must be completed before we can directly compare the final outcomes of the TLC and Cardiomagic options. This step summarizes each of the options by adding together the expected utilities relevant to each option. This process is known as *averaging out the expected utilities*. In averaging out the expected utilities for TLC and Cardiomagic, we would perform the following calculations:

$$\text{TLC expected utilities} = 0.9600 + 0.0312 + 0 = 0.9912$$

$$\text{Cardiomagic expected utilities} = 0.8000 + 0.1386 + 0.0412 + 0 + 0.0010$$
$$= 0.9808$$

Now we have folded back and averaged out to calculate overall expected utilities. For an expected-utility decision analysis, these numbers represent the last step. They reflect a completed decision tree. This decision tree leads us to the conclusion that TLC is a better choice than Cardiomagic since it has a greater overall expected utility.

As we have already discussed, utilities need to be measured on a scale of 0 to 1, the same scale used to assess probabilities. Utilities, unlike probabilities, are inherently subjective; they depend on how they are viewed by each individual. Each individual measures utilities differently. Thus, there is no right utility.

What, then, are we measuring when we attempt to measure utilities? When decision-making investigations are conducted from the social perspective, the investigator is attempting to measure the average utility for individuals who are potentially affected by the outcome. Let us see what we mean in the case of blindness.

There are several techniques used to measure utilities, each of which measures a slightly different phenomenon. Currently, there is no consensus on which is best.[4] The most straightforward method for measuring utilities is called the *rating scale* method. Using the rating scale method, individuals indicate their own utility for blindness using a linear scale from 0 to 1, as seen in the following example:

Imagine your quality of life if you became permanently and completely blind. Indicate on the following scale the relative worth of blindness. Notice that the scale extends from 0, which stands for immediate death, to 1, which stands for your state of full health.

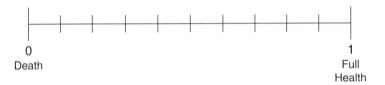

0
Death
1
Full
Health

How did you score the utility for blindness?

When the scores of individuals are averaged, the utility of blindness is usually approximately 0.50. However, there is great variability from individual to individual. Perhaps you scored permanent and complete blindness as carrying a utility as high as 0.80 or as low as 0.20. This type of variability is not unusual. In addition, it is not always obvious why one individual perceives a condition as carrying a high utility and another perceives it as carrying a low utility. At times, an individual's profession, age, or current state of activity may explain how they rate a condition's utility. More often, however, a large difference exists between similar individuals

---

[4] The technique demonstrated for directly scoring utilities on a scale of 0 to 1 is known as the *rating scale* approach. There are a growing number of other methods for scoring utilities. The *time trade-off* and *reference gamble methods* are commonly used. There is considerable controversy over the best method to use. None of the currently available methods is ideal. The time trade-off method asks the decision-maker to determine the percentage of their remaining life span that they would trade off for a return to full health (a utility of 1). It incorporates considerations of life expectancy and discounting. The reference gamble methods ask the rater to choose between a secure outcome at a specific utility and a gamble that will bring them to either full health (a utility of 1) or alternately will produce death (a utility of 0). Reference gamble methods thus incorporate risk-taking into the measurement. The rating scale measurement has the advantages that it can be used to measure the quality of health at one point in time without incorporating issues of life-expectancy, discounting for time, or risk-taking attitude.

without obvious explanation. Usually the best way to estimate a condition's utility is to ask the individual.

Estimates of average utility are often quite similar from population to population but greatly differ from individual to individual within a population. Thus, it is important to recognize that wide and unpredictable variation in utilities from person to person often exists and must be taken into account if the decision analysis is used for individual decision making.

The 0 to 1 scale used to measure utility creates issues at both ends of the scale. At the upper end, 1 is considered full health for the individual. For many medical conditions, it is impossible to bring an individual to full health. This is especially so for those with severe disabilities. Thus, when comparing an intervention designed for disabled people with one designed for people who can potentially be brought to full health, the disabled are at a disadvantage in terms of the extent of improvement that is possible as measured by utilities. An intervention may have a greater potential for improving the utility score among the potentially healthy compared with the disabled. To understand why this may be the case, consider the use of Cardiomagic in the following situation:

> Cardiomagic is being evaluated for use in otherwise healthy middle-aged men compared with its use in middle-aged men on dialysis. Despite its comparable probabilities of success, no success, and blindness, the procedure was found to produce greater expected utility when used on otherwise healthy individuals.

When dialysis patients return to their previous state of health, they do not return to a utility of 1. Rather, they return to the state of health for a dialysis patient who is doing well. This explains the greater expected utility when Cardiomagic is used on otherwise healthy individuals. When dialysis patients return to their previous state of health, their utility may only increase to approximately 0.6 compared to a previously healthy individual whose health may return to a utility of 1. As suggested by this example, decision-making investigations have been criticized as having a bias against the disabled.

There are also problems at the other end of the scale. In most decision-making investigations, 0 is defined as death. Considerable research and everyday experience tell us that, for many individuals, there are conditions worse than death. Prolonged vegetative states, severe mental incapacity, and intractable pain are typically viewed as having a utility worse than death. To use a scale that is the same as the one used for probabilities, it is not possible to incorporate negative utilities. It is possible to set immediate death as greater than 0 and to set 0 as a state worse than death. Despite the possibility of using this scale, it is rarely seen in the decision-making literature.[5]

Life Expectancy

The questions addressed so far may be the only issues addressed in a decision-making investigation. If so, the investigation is an expected-utility decision

---

[5] There is an additional problem inherent in the utility scale. The utility scale is linear—that is, the difference between 0.00 and 0.01 is the same as the difference between 0.50 and 0.51 or between 0.80 and 0.81. However, 0.00 is death and 0.01 implies continued life. Life and death are not measured on a continuous scale; they are discrete either/or conditions. Thus, it is important to recognize that the scale used to measure utilities cannot truly reflect the true situation, especially at the lower end of the scale.

Table 29.1. *Quality adjusted life years (QALYs) for TLC and Cardiomagic*

	Probability	Utility	Life expectancy	QALYs
TLC				
Successful	0.9600	1	18	17.28
Unsuccessful	0.0390	0.8	5	0.16
Death	0.0010	0	0	0
Total QALYs				17.44
Cardiomagic				
Successful	0.8000	1	18	14.40
Successful after surgery	0.1386	1	18	2.49
Unsuccessful after surgery	0.0515	0.8	5	0.21
Death after surgery	0.0079	0	0	0
Blindness	0.0020	0.5	18	0.02
Total QALYs				17.12

analysis. That is, it considers only the probability of favorable and unfavorable outcomes and the utilities attached to these final outcomes.

When a decision analysis incorporates life expectancy measures, the results are usually presented using quality adjusted life years (QALYs) as the measurement of effectiveness. Let us see how we can incorporate life expectancy into the decision-making process using the following data:[6]

> In examining the options, assume that the average individual being considered for treatment is 62 years old. Further assume that if the treatment is successful, they will return to having an average life expectancy of 18 years. If unsuccessful, assume that they will have a life expectancy of 5 years. Death produces a life expectancy of 0.

To see how these life-expectancy measures can be incorporated into the decision analysis process let us take a look at Table 29.1

The QALYs for each final outcome are obtained by multiplying the probability of each final outcome, the utility of each final outcome, and the life expectancy of the average individual who experiences the final outcome. Adding the QALYs together, we can average out and obtain the following results:

$$TLC = 17.44 \, QALYs$$

$$Cardiomagic = 17.12 \, QALYs$$

Once again, we can conclude that TLC is a better choice.

The measurements used to obtain life expectancy for a decision analysis can be very complex. The life-expectancy measurements derived from cross-sectional life table that we examined previously are designed as an average for all individuals of the same age and, sometimes, of the same gender or race. This type of life expectancy is not designed to take into account the consequences on life span of a specific disease that is being treated. Life expectancy derived from cross-sectional

---

[6] This approach to lining up life-expectancy measures along with utilities and probabilities as the outcomes of a decision tree is rarely used in the literature. It does, however, illustrate key issues. It also points out the need to define what is included in a utility. If life expectancy is included as a separate measure, utilities should not incorporate consideration of longevity. Unfortunately, this distinction is not always made in the literature.

or population data overestimates survival for those with disease. To accurately incorporate the impact of disease on life-expectancy, we need to combine life-expectancy measures using data based on age, gender, and race with data based on disease-specific survival.[7]

The implications of reduced life expectancy for those with disease is illustrated in the following example:

> A decision-making investigation is being conducted to determine whether use of TLC or Cardiomagic is better for dialysis patients with coronary artery disease whose average age is 50. The average 50-year-old is assumed to have a life expectancy of 30 years.

The average 50-year-old may have a life expectancy of 30 years based on a population's life-table data, but those on dialysis may have a much shorter life expectancy regardless of the success or failure of treatment of their coronary artery disease. Thus, the life expectancy that must be incorporated into each outcome of a decision tree is the life expectancy of the average individual on dialysis. That is, if we are dealing with dialysis patients, the relevant life expectancy may be 10 years instead of 30.

The impact of life expectancy is even more dramatic when the goal is to compare two very different treatments—one aimed at young people and the other aimed at an older population. For instance, consider the following:

> QALY decision analysis examined the favorable and unfavorable outcomes of treating single-vessel coronary artery disease with TLC or Cardiomagic in individuals with an average age of 62. It compared these results with the prevention of Paresis A by using a vaccine in children. The prevention of Paresis A was shown to produce considerably more QALYs than the treatment of single-vessel coronary artery disease.

When comparing a treatment or a preventive intervention that is applied to very different age groups, it is important to recognize that a successful intervention among children results in a far greater improvement in life expectancy than an equally successful intervention among 62-year-olds. Thus, many more QALYs result from successful efforts to prevent Paresis A in children compared with treatment of coronary artery disease among 62-year-olds. Decision-making investigations that incorporate life expectancy, i.e., when using QALYs, tend to favor the young. This tendency may or may not be justifiable, but the reader must recognize this tendency, especially when comparing different types of treatments aimed at different age groups.

---

[7] One such approximation is known as the *Declining Exponential Approximation of Life Expectancy* (DEALE). DEALE assumes that the life expectancy at a particular age is equal to 1 divided by the sum of the probability of survival on the basis of age, race, and gender (obtained from a cross-sectional life table) plus the probability of survival as a result of disease (obtained from a longitudinal life table). The use of DEALE would imply that the reduction in life expectancy due to the need for dialysis is the same regardless of whether the patient is 65 or 35 years old. That is, the need for dialysis might shorten average life span by 10 years. A recent, more accurate approximation is known as GAME (Gama Mixed-Exponential Estimate). GAME takes into account the often observed declining motality from a disease over time. DEALE assume that the impact of the disease continues without decline over time, thus resulting in an underestimation of life expectancy. (W.B. van den Hout, "The GAME Estimate of Reduced Life Expectancy," *Medical Decision Making* 24(2004):80–88.)

Costs

Costs are not generally incorporated directly into a decision tree. Rather the decision tree is used to calculate the effectiveness, and costs are then compared to effectiveness.[8]

To appreciate the costs that must be considered in a cost-effectiveness analysis, let us return to our example of Paresis A:

> Paresis A is a common contagious disease of childhood that is usually self-limited. However, a small percentage of children who experience the illness develop the complication of permanent paralysis, and a few develop life-threatening complications. Long-term paralysis and late complications can occur. The conventional treatment for Paresis A has been only supportive treatment, which we will call a do-nothing approach. Recently, an expensive vaccination designed to prevent Paresis A became available. A rare complication of the vaccine is development of a form of paralysis that is similar but usually less severe than the disease itself.

We will see how we can compare the costs of the vaccine with the do-nothing approach. When assessing the costs of an intervention, it is necessary to consider the types of cost discussed in the next three sections.[9]

Short-Term Health Care Costs

Health care costs include the cost of delivering the service and treating the short-term complications. For the conventional treatment of symptoms and complications, the costs include visits for health care and the cost of providing hospitalization and treatment. For Paresis A vaccine, this would include the costs of the vaccine and the associated costs of delivering the vaccine, as well as costs of treating the short-term complications that develop as a result of administering the vaccine. It would also include the costs of care and complications for those who developed paralysis despite use of the vaccine.

In general, short term can be thought of as costs that occur within a year of treatment.

Short-Term Nonhealth Care Cost

Nonhealth care costs include the time and expense to access care by the patient, as well as for anyone else who must provide paid or unpaid services. These especially include the costs of providing care outside the medical system, even when this care is provided by family members without charge.

---

[8] Occasionally, costs are directly incorporated into a decision tree as an outcome measure. When this is done, the outcome is called *expected value* rather than expected utility.

[9] These categories attempt to present the concepts incorporated into the recommendations of Gold, et al. The separation of short-term and future health care costs is presented to clarify an important distinction for the reader. The use of one year for short term implies that no discounting for harms, benefits, or costs is needed. The omission of the use of the term "direct" is an attempt to avoid confusion with other uses of this term, such as the use of "direct" and "indirect" to indicate program cost and institutional costs respectively. Both of these costs are included in the concept of direct as used in cost-effectiveness analysis. Note that this section does not attempt to define the methods used for actually measuring costs. The accuracy of the measurement of costs is an important issue, but one that is beyond the scope of this section. However, it is important to distinguish between costs and prices. Costs aim to measure resource use, as opposed to prices that are affected by additional factors, especially in health care.

For the conventional approach, there are no costs of obtaining the vaccine, but there will be considerable costs of taking care of the illness and the short-term complications.

For Paresis A vaccine, these costs include the time required from the parent or other caregiver to obtain the vaccine and time required to care for short-term complications of the vaccine or the disease if the vaccine is not successful.

Long-Term Health Care Costs

Long-term health care costs can theoretically be separated into costs that are and are not related to the disease or the treatment. The related costs of caring for long-term consequences of the disease or its treatment should be included in a cost-effectiveness analysis. In general, unrelated long-term health care and nonhealth care costs are not included.[10]

For conventional treatment, the long-term health care costs include the long-term cost of caring for those who experience the disease and survive the short-term life-threatening effects.

For Paresis A vaccine, related long-term health care costs include the costs of providing ongoing care for all those who experience the complications of the vaccine and the costs of long-term treatment of those who experience the disease despite receiving the vaccine. Long term can be thought of as beginning 1 year after the treatment and continuing for the lifetime of the individual.

In this chapter, we have looked at what each of the variables needed to complete a decision-making investigation attempts to measure. Probabilities, utilities, life expectancy, and costs are included in the assessment. Depending on the question being addressed and the type of investigation being conducted, the investigator may need to obtain the best available measurements of probabilities, utilities, life expectancies, and costs. These are called *base-case estimates*. When doubt exists about the accuracy of the base-case estimates, the investigator may need to make educated guesses of what are called *realistic high* and *realistic low values*. These provide a means of quantitatively incorporating uncertainty into the decision-making process.

In the next chapter on results, we examine how the results are presented and look at how the realistic high and realistic low estimates can used to incorporate uncertainty into the decision-making investigation.

---

[10] Unrelated costs include the cost of treating other diseases that occur unrelated to the disease being treated. For a condition like Paresis A, these costs should be approximately the same for the vaccine and the conventional treatment. At the discretion of the investigator, these may be included for any added years of life. Gold recommends that the costs of treating unrelated disease be included during the years of life that would have been lived without the intervention and either included or excluded for the additional years of life. In addition, Gold's recommendations allow either inclusion or exclusion of nonmedical future costs, such as food and shelter. We will assume that these are excluded, as is increasingly the practice in most cost-effectiveness analyses. If long-term nonhealth care costs are included, an otherwise successful intervention may be viewed as very expensive because it requires society to provide support for the additional years of life. The exclusion of these costs implies a social decision to consider the value of a year outside the work force to be just as valuable as a year in the work force.

30 Results

The results component of the M.A.A.R.I.E. framework for decision-making investigations asks us to address the issues of estimation, inference, and adjustment. The aim of estimation is to provide the best possible estimation of the strength of the relationship. Inference produces what we will call a sensitivity analysis that is parallel to confidence intervals in other types of investigations. Adjustment aims to take into account the key differences between the timing of events using a process called discounting.

Let us look more closely at what we mean by estimation, inference, and adjustment in a decision-making investigation.

Estimation

Estimation is a summary measurement that results from an investigation. Each type of decision-making investigation produces one or more summary measurements. The measurement is different, however, if we are dealing with an expected-utility decision analysis, a QALY decision analysis, a cost-and-effectiveness analysis, or a cost-utility analysis.

The differences between the summary measurements used in different decision-making investigations depend largely on the factors that are used to measure the outcomes. Probabilities alone may be used, or life expectancy may be incorporated. Cost may be used, or the investigation may focus exclusively on effectiveness.

To see what we mean by these different estimates, let us return to our TLC and Cardiomagic example.

Figure 30.1 reproduces the previous decision tree for TLC and Cardiomagic incorporating probabilities and utilities of each final outcome. The summary measurement for this decision-making investigation is the difference in expected utility:

$$0.9912 - 0.9808 = 0.0104$$

This measurement may have little intuitive meaning in and of itself. However, what we will call a quality-adjusted number needed to treat can be calculated as 1 divided by this difference between the expected utilities. Here, the quality-adjusted number needed to treat equals the following:

$$1 \div 0.0104 \approx 96$$

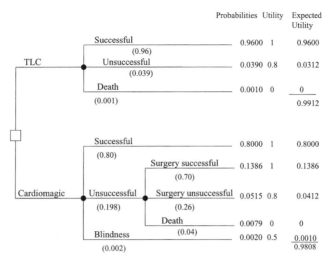

Figure 30.1. A decision tree incorporating probabilities and utilities for each outcome of TLC and Cardiomagic.

This quality-adjusted number needed to treat tells us that on average, 96 individuals need to be treated with TLC instead of Cardiomagic to produce one additional life at full health.[1]

Now let us look at the summary measurement that can be used when a decision-making investigation produces results measured in QALYs. The data from the QALY decision analysis we discussed in chapter 29 is presented in Table 30.1.

Table 30.1. *Quality adjusted life years (QALYs) for TLC and Cardiomagic*

	Probability	Utility	Life expectancy	QALYs
TLC				
Successful	0.9600	1	18	17.28
Unsuccessful	0.0390	0.8	5	0.16
Death	0.0010	0	0	0
Total QALYs				17.44
Cardiomagic				
Successful	0.8000	1	18	14.40
Successful after surgery	0.1386	1	18	2.49
Unsuccessful after surgery	0.5150	0.8	5	0.21
Death after surgery	0.0079	0	0	0
Blindness	0.0020	0.5	18	0.02
Total QALYs				17.12

[1] The quality-adjusted number needed to treat is being interpreted as the number of individuals who need to be treated with TLC as opposed to Cardiomagic to obtain one additional life at full health that would otherwise have resulted in an outcome with a utility of 0 (death) if treated with Cardiomagic. That is how many individuals, who would have otherwise died, need to be treated to obtain the equivalent of one life saved at full health. As with all uses of expected utility, the meaning of the results assumes that we are willing to add together changes in utility from different individuals. Thus, we are assuming that preventing two cases of blindness, which provide two individuals an increase in utility from 0.5 to 1, is worth the same as providing full health at a utility of 1 compared with death at a utility of 0 for one individual.

This data allows us to easily present the difference in QALYs per use by subtracting the 17.12 QALYs for Cardiomagic from the 17.44 QALYs for TLC:

$$17.44 - 17.12 = 0.32$$

Again, this may not have very much meaning in and of itself. In parallel to the measurement of expected utilities, we can calculate a quality-adjusted number needed to treat as follows:

$$1 \div 0.32 \approx 3$$

Thus, on average, an additional QALY results from treating approximately three patients with TLC instead of Cardiomagic. The quality-adjusted number needed to treat to produce an additional life or alternatively an addition QALY are thus useful summary measures for effectiveness. They tell us the number of individuals who need to receive the intervention of interest, as compared to the alternative, to produce one additional life or alternatively one additional life year at full health.

Cost-Effectiveness Measures

In contrast to the measures of effectiveness, the estimates for cost-utility analyses are presented in two ways that need to be understood and distinguished. Table 30.2 shows us the QALYs produced by TLC and Cardiomagic and also the costs of TLC and Cardiomagic. The table also shows this data for conventional treatment. These data allow us to calculate two types of summary measures. One is the *cost-effectiveness ratio*. The other is known as the *incremental cost-effectiveness ratio*.[2]

Let us examine the data for the decision using the three alternatives for single-vessel coronary artery disease (Table 30.2).

The cost-effectiveness ratios for the decision alternatives for single-vessel coronary artery disease would be calculated as follows:

Cost-effectiveness ratio of TLC $= \$116,600 \div 17.44 \,\text{QALYs} = \$6,686/\text{QALY}$

Cost-effectiveness ratio of Cardiomagic $= \$50,000 \div 17.12 \,\text{QALYs} = \$2,920/\text{QALY}$

Cost-effectiveness ratios measure the average cost of an option divided by the average health outcome if that option is used. The comparison being used in a cost-effectiveness ratio is sometimes called the *do-nothing option*. The do-nothing option implies that there is an option that has no cost and produces no benefit. Thus it might be called a zero-cost zero-effectiveness option. Cost-effectiveness ratios allow us to compare options for intervention for different diseases or conditions because all options are compared to the same do-nothing or zero-cost zero-effectiveness option.[3]

Incremental cost-effectiveness ratios, as opposed to cost-effectiveness ratios, make what is often a more relevant comparison between two options. That is, they ask about the additional cost to obtain additional effectiveness. Incremental

---

[2] The special type of cost-effectiveness analysis called a cost-and-effectiveness study can also use cost-effectiveness and incremental cost-effectiveness ratios. However, for these studies, the cost-effectiveness ratio is cost per outcome, such as cost per life saved or cost per diagnosis made. The incremental cost-effectiveness ratio then measures the additional cost required to achieve an additional outcome such as a life saved or diagnosis made.

[3] The costs are compared with the do-nothing or zero-cost zero-effectiveness option which is assumed to have zero cost and zero effectiveness even when that is not a realistic possibility. For instance, even when there is no intervention, there may be costs such as custodial care.

Table 30.2. *Cost and QALYs of the TLC, Cardiomagic, and conventional treatment*

	Cost	QALYs
TLC	$116,600	17.44
Cardiomagic	$50,000	17.12
Conventional treatment	$20,000	15

Cost-effectiveness Ratios
TLC, $116,600/17.44 = $6,686/QALY

Cardiomagic, $50,000/17.12 = $2,920/QALY

Conventional treatment, $20,000/15 = $1,333/QALY

cost-effectiveness ratios compare the option of interest with the conventional treatment, that is, the current standard treatment. Thus, incremental cost-effectiveness ratios are the preferred comparison when we are asking about the best option to address one particular disease or condition.

Using the data from Table 30.2, let us look at the incremental cost-effectiveness ratios comparing TLC to conventional treatment and Cardiomagic compared to conventional treatment.

TLC vs. Conventional treatment

$$= \frac{\$116,600 - \$20,000}{17.44\,\text{QALYs} - 15\,\text{QALYs}} = \frac{\$96,600}{2.44\,\text{QALYs}} = \$39,590/\text{QALY}$$

Cardiomagic vs. Conventional treatment

$$= \frac{\$50,000 - \$20,000}{17.12\,\text{QALYs} - 15\,\text{QALYs}} = \frac{\$30,000}{2.12\,\text{QALYs}} = \$14,151/\text{QALY}$$

Notice that the incremental cost-effectiveness ratios are much greater than the cost-effectiveness ratios. This is the usual situation and reflects the different questions addressed by these two types of ratios. The cost-effectiveness ratio asks about the average cost of obtaining an outcome such as a QALY. This cost is really being compared with the do-nothing option that is assume to have zero costs and zero effectiveness.

Incremental cost-effectiveness ratios, on the other hand, are usually comparing a new intervention with the existing conventional intervention. To the extent that the conventional intervention already has a reasonable degree of effectiveness, it should not be surprising that there are substantial costs per additional unit of effectiveness (i.e., per QALY). Thus, it is important to recognize that the incremental cost-effectiveness ratio is asking about the additional cost per additional unit of effectiveness measured as QALYs.[4]

Which ratio to use depends on the question being asked. Usually the question has to do with a choice between alternative treatments. In this situation the incremental cost-effectiveness ratio is the most informative. In fact, incremental cost-effectiveness ratios are now expected as part of a cost-effectiveness analysis. In general, comparing each new treatment to conventional treatment is the most helpful means of comparing different interventions for the same condition.

---

[4] Incremental cost-effectiveness ratios may at times also be used to compare two new treatments, such as TLC versus Cardiomagic. When this form of comparison is made, however, we need to be aware of what is being compared; otherwise, considerable confusion can result.

Inference: Sensitivity Analysis

In Section I, "Studying a Study," we showed how confidence intervals can be used to perform inference. A similar approach, called *sensitivity analysis,* is used in decision-making investigations. Sensitivity analysis is a general term used to describe a series of methods for isolating factors in a decision-making investigation and determining the influence each factor has on the results of the investigation. The analyses we have looked at so far use measures that are called base-case estimates. Base-case estimates represent the best available data or the investigators' best guess at the true value for the factor. Sensitivity analyses are an effort to examine the consequences if the base-case estimate does not turn out to be accurate. Thus, investigators often try to define a realistic high value and a realistic low value that reflect the potential range of values. Together we can think of these as parallel to the 95% confidence interval. This interval has been referred to as the *credibility interval.*

Sensitivity analyses are often classified as *one-way* or *multiple-way sensitivity analysis.* In one-way sensitivity analysis, one factor at a time is examined to determine whether varying its level within the credibility interval alters the conclusions of the investigation.

Let us look at how a one-way sensitivity analysis might be performed:[5]

Table 30.3 summarizes the results of a one-way sensitivity analysis that varys measures of the utility of blindness for the comparison of TLC and Cardiomagic. For this one-way sensitivity analysis, a high and a low estimate are used in addition to the base-case estimate that was used in the original analysis. The high estimate is designed to reflect the upper end of what is felt to be a realistic range of possible values, while the low estimate is designed to reflect the lower end of this realistic range.

When looking at the results of a one-way sensitivity analysis, we are interested in determining whether the relationships between the decision options change when the high or the low estimate is substituted for the base-case estimate. If using the realistic high or realistic low estimate for a factor such as cost, probability, or utility alters our preference for one option over another, then we say that the recommendation is sensitive to a particular factor. For instance, in constructing the decision tree for Cardiomagic, we used a base-case utility for blindness of 0.5. Now look at what happens in Table 30.3 if we alter the utility of blindness from a high of 0.8 to a low of 0.2. This change has very little impact on the expected utility,

Table 30.3. *Cardiomagic vs. conventional therapy: one-way sensitivity analysis for utility of blindness*

	Incremental cost (base-line)	Incremental QALYs	Incremental cost-effectiveness ratio
Blindness utility 0.8 (high)	$30,000	2.13	$14,085
Blindness utility 0.5 (base-case)	$30,000	2.12	$14,151
Blindness utility 0.2 (low)	$30,000	2.11	$14,218

[5] Other one-way sensitivity techniques are used for special purposes. One is *threshold analysis*, which varies key factors to determine the level of these factors that would alter the conclusions obtained from a particular decision-making investigation. Threshold analyses aim to determine the toss-up points or thresholds at which a different recommendation would be made.

Table 30.4. *Cardiomagic vs. conventional therapy: one-way sensitivity analysis for costs*

	Incremental cost	Incremental QALYs (base-line)	Incremental cost-effectiveness ratio
Cardiomagic cost high	$60,000	2.12	$28,302/QALY
Cardiomagic cost base-case	$30,000	2.12	$14,151/QALY
Cardiomagic cost low	$20,000	2.12	$9,434/QALY

and the recommendation to use Cardiomagic is not affected. When a decision is not affected by changes in a factor within its realistic range, we say that the decision is not sensitive to the factor.

Table 30.4 shows a one-way sensitivity analysis for Cardiomagic and cost. Notice that the impact of the realistic high and realistic low cost estimates on the incremental cost-effectiveness ratio is substantial. However, even the use of the high estimate produces an incremental cost-effectiveness ratio of $28,302/QALY, which is well below the $39,590/QALY incremental cost-effectiveness ratio for TLC. Thus, despite the substantial change in cost per QALY, the conclusion that Cardiomagic is more cost effective than TLC is not sensitive to the estimates of cost.

It is important to look at key factors one at time and examine how their realistic high and low values may influence a recommendation. However, these one-way sensitivity analyses underestimate the uncertainty that exists, because in practice, variation in more than one factor is at work at the same time. Thus, it is often important for the investigators to perform a multiple-way sensitivity analysis, altering two or more factors simultaneously.

An extreme but commonly used and easy to understand form of multiple-way sensitivity analysis is called the *best case/worst case analysis*. Best case/worst case analysis reflects the investigators' attempt to create scenarios in which two or more key factors are favorable within a realistic range (best case) or unfavorable within a realistic range (worst case). These scenarios are not designed to reflect the very worst or very best possible outcomes, but rather the extremes of the realistic range.[6]

Table 30.5 shows how a best case/worst case analysis might look for the incremental cost-effectiveness ratios of TLC compared with conventional treatment. Two important factors, the probability of success and the cost, are initially set at the most favorable realistic estimates and then both are set at the least favorable realistic estimates.

When the probability of success and the cost for TLC are set at their most favorable realistic level (best case), the incremental cost-effectiveness ratio is $31,202/QALY. This best-case situation for TLC can then be compared to the base-case estimate for Cardiomagic. This best-case situation for TLC is still far

---

[6] The best case/worst case sensitivity analysis is often considered too demanding an approach because it is unlikely that uncertainties in multiple key variables will act in the same direction. Other forms of multiple-way sensitivity analyses are increasingly being used to calculate the confidence intervals or credibility intervals. A number of complicated mathematical approaches are used to obtain these estimates. The best known is the *Monte Carlo Simulation* which aims to establish credibility intervals by randomly selecting levels of each of the key variables using computer simulations. By performing a large number of these simulations, a distribution of results can be obtained and used to calculate a credibility interval.

Table 30.5. *Cost effectiveness of TLC vs. conventional treatment:*
best case/worse case analysis

	Incremental cost	Incremental cost-effectiveness ratio
TLC best case success = 98%	$85,000	$31,202/QALY
TLC base case success = 96%	$96,600	$40,000/QALY
TLC worst case success = 90%	$120,000	−$500,000/QALY

greater than the $14,151/QALY base-case estimate for Cardiomagic. This provides convincing evidence that Cardiomagic is more cost effective than TLC, and this conclusion is not sensitive to the cost of TLC or its effectiveness within the realistic ranges.[7]

When the probability of success and the cost of TLC are set at their least favorable realistic level (worst case), the incremental cost-effectiveness ratio is −$500,000. This negative number implies that, given these unfavorable assumptions, TLC is now less cost effective than conventional treatment. If these unfavorable assumptions are true, then by spending $500,000 on TLC, we are reducing the effectiveness by 1 QALY compared with using conventional treatment. Thus, our multiple-way sensitivity analysis has raised some degree of uncertainty as to whether TLC is actually a better treatment than conventional therapy.

Adjustment and Discounting

In general, adjustment is performed to take into account differences in alternatives that can affect the results. In decision-making investigations the timing of events is a very important factor that needs to be taken into account as part of the adjustment. Timing of events is important for both decision analysis and cost-effectiveness analysis.

To understand the impact of the timing of events, let us take another look at TLC. Recall that using the base-case estimate, TLC has been found to be more effective in treating single-vessel coronary artery disease compared with conventional treatment. It produces a substantially greater probability of favorable short-term outcomes despite its slight increase in adverse outcomes.

Short-term net effectiveness in comparison with conventional treatment still leaves open questions regarding TLC's impact on favorable outcomes in the long term, as well as possible long-term adverse outcomes. Assume that the following information is now available:

> More than a decade after the widespread use of TLC began, it was recognized that late effects on the coronary artery made it more likely to close, producing a higher incidence of late myocardial infarction.

In most decision-making situations, not all events occur at the same time. The impacts of treatment may be immediate or delayed for many years. Even in the absence of an intervention, a disease may not have an impact until many years later.

---

[7] The comparison should generally be made between the credibility limit and the base-case estimate of the other option in parallel to the way that confidence intervals are used to determine statistical significance. Overlap of credibility intervals, like overlap of confidence intervals, often occurs and is not the criteria used to determine either statistical significance or sensitivity to a factor.

Note that people who experience the late effect on the coronary artery have still received the advantage of the favorable short-term outcome. That is, on average, they have lived longer.

The most common and accepted method for taking into account the consequences of the timing of events is *discounting*.[8] Discounting considers the fact that the benefits, harms, and costs that occur in the future are given less importance than those that occur immediately. The concept of discounting comes from economics and is most easily understood in terms of costs. However, it is important to recognize that discounting or taking into account the timing of events needs to be conducted for costs, benefits, and harms. An adverse outcome in the distant future is not as bad as an adverse outcome that occurs in the immediate future. Similarly, a favorable outcome in the distant future is not valued as highly as a favorable outcome that occurs in the immediate future. For instance, with Paresis A vaccine, the favorable outcome of prevention of paralysis does not necessarily occur immediately. A case of Paresis A prevented may occur a number of years in the future.

The concept of discounting can be understood by recognizing that most people prefer to receive $100 today rather than $100 a year from now. This is the situation even if the payoff a year from now takes inflation into account. That is, most people prefer $100 now to receiving $100 plus a guaranteed adjustment for inflation a year from now. As economists see it, if you receive $100 today, you generally can invest the money and, on average, receive a *real rate of return*. The real rate of return means that 1 year from now, you will have more than $100 even after the adjustment for inflation.

Looked at the other way, most people would prefer to pay $100 a year from now rather than today. A dollar paid in the future is not as costly as a dollar paid today. In fact, when performing discounting, the investigator is really calculating the amount of money that needs to be invested today to pay bills that are not due until a future time. The amount of money that needs to be invested today is called the *discounted present value* or *present value*. To calculate the discounted present value, the investigator needs to choose what is called a *discount rate*. Choosing a 3% annual discount rate implies that approximately $97 need to be put aside and invested today to ensure the availability of an inflation-adjusted $100 a year from now. If the discount rate is 5%, only about $95 needs to be put aside today to ensure the availability of an inflation-adjusted $100 a year from now.[9]

What is the proper discount rate? Economists generally agree that costs should be discounted to reflect the real rate of return, which is the rate that can be expected on average from investing money after taking into account the impact of inflation. There the agreement ceases because the real rate of return is neither constant nor

---

[8] The two basic approaches to taking into account the effects of timing are discounting and incorporating the timing of events into utilities. Most experts consider discounting of costs, favorable outcomes, and adverse outcomes to be the proper approach for decision analysis and also for cost-effectiveness analysis. In decision analysis, however, timing of events may at times be incorporated into utilities. Note that decision trees are structured to reflect the sequence of events, but they do not tell much about the time intervals between events. Long-term consequences are not necessarily distinguished from short-term consequences in a decision tree. Unless explicit discounting occurs, outcomes are usually dealt with as if they occur simultaneously. That is, a discount rate of 0% is used or the impact of timing is incorporated into the measurement of utilities.

[9] Note that if the discount rate is 0%, then $100 needs to be put aside to ensure the availability of $100 a year from now. Thus, if discounting is not performed, the investigator is really assuming a discount rate of 0%.

predictable. However, the accepted range of discount rates is between 3% and 5%. A 3% discount rate is recommended when performing a sensitivity analysis. A second analysis to determine the consequences of using a 5% realistically high and a 1% realistically low discount rate can also be performed.

The discount rate for favorable and adverse effects should generally be the same as the discount rate used for costs. If different rates are used, the following situation can occur:

> In discounting costs, favorable outcomes, and adverse outcomes for Paresis A vaccine, costs were discounted at 5% but favorable outcomes were discounted at 3%. The authors concluded that since interventions that could be implemented in the future were much less expensive, it is desirable to wait to implement a Paresis A vaccine campaign.

Discounting costs at a greater discount rate than favorable outcomes always encourages delay. If costs are discounted at a greater rate than favorable outcomes, then every year, it looks desirable to wait until the next year because in future years it will cost less to produce a favorable outcome. Thus, regardless of the discount rate that is used, it is important to discount cost, favorable outcomes, and adverse outcomes at the same discount rate. It is not enough just to discount costs. It is generally accepted that favorable and adverse outcomes also need to be discounted, and at the same discount rate as costs.

We have now examined the results that are produced through a decision-making investigation. Let us now turn our attention to the interpretation component of the M.A.A.R.I.E. framework.

31 Interpretation

Cost-Effectiveness Ratios

As with other types of investigations, interpretation is designed to evaluate the implications of the results for the types of individuals who are included in the investigation. With decision-making investigations, no individual or group is actually included in the investigations. Rather, the investigator usually creates a model designed to simulate the situation facing particular types of individuals. Thus, the interpretation of a decision-making investigation should address the investigation's implications for the types of individuals for which the investigation was designed.

Often, the most important and confusing interpretation in a decision-making investigation is the meaning of the cost-effectiveness ratios. Let us take a close look at how we interpret these ratios for the types of studies on single-vessel coronary artery disease and Paresis A vaccine that we have already examined. Since we are comparing interventions directed against two different conditions, we need to use the cost-effectiveness ratios when making comparisons. That is, we need to compare each of our options to the do-nothing or the zero cost-zero effectiveness option.

As we have seen, the cost-effective ratios of the three options for treating single-vessel coronary artery disease are obtained as follows:

$$\text{TLC: } \$116,600 \div 17.44 \, \text{QALYs}$$
$$\text{Cardiomagic: } \$50,000 \div 17.12 \, \text{QALYs}$$
$$\text{Conventional treatment: } \$20,000 \div 15 \, \text{QALYs}$$

In Chapter 27 we found that Paresis A vaccine reduced the cost by $2,000 per QALY compared to the do-nothing option—the only available alternative. Thus

$$\text{Paresis A vaccine: } -\$2,000 \div 1 \, \text{QALY}$$

To compare the Paresis A cost-effectiveness ratio to the TLC cost-effectiveness ratio, we need to calculate the cost of 17.44 QALYs as follows:

$$\text{Paresis A vaccine: } -\$34,888 \text{ to produce } 17.44 \, \text{QALYs}$$

To examine the implications of these cost-effectiveness ratios, their components can be plotted on a cost-QALYs graph. Figure 31.1 is a cost-QALYs graph. Notice that it contains four areas, or quadrants, labeled A, B, C, and D. The zero point for the graph is the do-nothing or zero cost-zero effectiveness option with which all other options are compared. Figure 31.2 plots the cost-effectiveness ratios for the options to treat single vessel coronary artery disease and to prevent Paresis A.

Use of a cost-QALYs graph allows visual comparison between options for the same condition and/or different conditions using cost-effectiveness ratios. Each of the four quadrants has a different implication. Quadrant D, where Paresis A vaccine is located, is the ideal quadrant. Here, there is increased effectiveness as measured

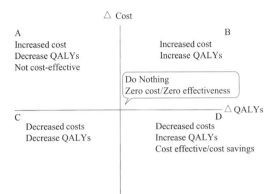

Figure 31.1. A cost–QALYs graph.

by QALYs and reduced cost as measured in dollars. The cost-effectiveness ratio in quadrant D is thus negative. When an option is located in quadrant D, it is cost-saving/effectiveness-increasing. This is a special situation where we can unequivocally say that the results are cost-effective.

At times, this situation is called *cost savings*. Use of this term results in considerable confusion because, as we shall see, cost savings can also result when the number of QALYs are reduced. This is the situation when the results are in quadrant C, in which there is a cost reduction accompanied by an effectiveness reduction as measured by reduced QALYs. Quadrant C is more accurately labeled cost-reducing/effectiveness-reducing.

When interpreting decision options that fall into quadrant C, it is important to recognize that they may be labeled cost-effective if the decision-maker concludes that a relatively small reduction in QALYs is worth the substantial reduction in cost. At times, it may be reasonable to substantially reduce costs even though effectiveness is also reduced. However, calling this approach cost-effective obscures what is happening. It is better to label this cost-reducing/effectiveness-reducing and

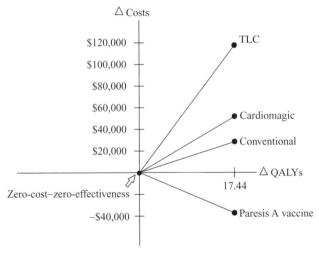

Figure 31.2. Cost-QALYs graph depicting cost effectiveness ratios. This graphs allows comparison between options for the same condition or for different conditions. Note that cost-effectiveness rather than incremental cost-effectiveness ratio are used.

then to separately determine whether the reduction in cost justifies the reduction in effectiveness.

Quadrant A is also a clear-cut result. In this quadrant, the costs are increased and the effectiveness is decreased. Therefore, neither costs nor effectiveness support a decision option that falls in quadrant A, and such options should be labeled as not cost-effective.

Most alternatives being considered by QALY cost-effectiveness studies end up in quadrant B. These decision alternatives increase both cost and effectiveness. When an alternative is located in quadrant B, it is very important to determine the magnitude of the cost-effectiveness ratio and to be sure their meaning is clear.

When treatments are located in quadrant B, where both costs and effectiveness are increased, we are faced with the difficult questions of where to draw the line. When determining where to draw the line, it is important that we compare the options to conventional treatment, not to the do-nothing option. Thus incremental cost-effectiveness ratios rather than cost-effective ratios should be used.

Let us review the data we have obtained on incremental cost-effectiveness ratios for TLC and Cardiomagic:

> The incremental cost-effectiveness ratios for TLC compared with conventional treatment is approximately $40,000 per QALY and the incremental cost-effectiveness ratio for Cardiomagic compared with conventional treatment is approximately $14,000 per QALY. Should either or both of these options be considered cost-effective?

The answer depends on how cost-effectiveness is defined. Considerable controversy exists regarding the methods for interpreting these results and deciding which treatments should be labeled cost-effective. A variety of methods have been used to try to categorize the results of incremental cost-effectiveness ratios to be able to establish a level which is considered cost-effective. This has been very controversial because determining what dollar figure to use to draw a line requires placing a monetary value on a QALY.[1]

Today, there is a general consensus that the question really is what can a society afford, not what is a QALY worth. Often the per capita gross domestic product (GDP) is used as an approximation of what a society can afford to pay for a QALY.[2]

---

[1] One method used to place a monetary value on a QALY is the *human capital approach,* which attempts to convert a QALY into a dollar value based on recipient's ability to contribute economically. This approach has been criticized because it only includes activities that result in financial payments and thus undervalues those who work without monetary payments, the retired, and low-wage groups. Efforts have been made to use what economists call a *willingness-to-pay approach*. These approaches are attractive to economists but have been very difficult to implement, and special situations such as legal cases may distort the data. Two other approaches with less theoretical foundations are also used. Past practice with drawing lines and refusing to pay may be used as evidence of where a society is willing to draw the line. A simple approach that takes into account the ability to pay is to use the per capita income, or the per capita gross domestic product of the nation in which the investigation is conducted or to which the results will be applied.

[2] Acceptable and unacceptable ranges depend heavily on a society's ability to pay. The per capita gross domestic product is one method for helping to define this range. The $14,000 figure is clearly within the per capita income for North America and most of Europe and Japan. However, the $40,000/ QALY may not be considered cost-effective even in many developed countries. In addition, neither of these options would be considered cost-effective in a developing country with a per capita income of $3,000. However, in nations with low per capita incomes, the costs may also be substantially lower. When a definitive value is set on a QALY, the investigation is really a cost-benefit analysis because equating a QALY with a set monetary figure allows all outcomes to be converted to dollars. Remember that the essential difference between cost-effectiveness analysis and cost-benefit analysis is that in cost-benefit analysis, outcomes and costs are both measured in monetary units.

In the United States the following general approach is often used.

1. Incremental cost-effectiveness ratios of less than $50,000/QALY are generally considered cost-effective.
2. Incremental cost-effectiveness ratios of $50,000 to $100,000 are considered borderline cost-effective.
3. Incremental cost-effectiveness ratios of $100,000 or greater are generally considered not cost-effective.

This approach makes it clear that the approximately $14,000 incremental cost per QALY for Cardiomagic is considered cost-effective in the United States. The incremental cost of approximately $40,000 per QALY for TLC would also be considered cost-effective in the United States as long as conventional therapy is used as the comparison option.

However, if Cardiomagic becomes accepted as standard or conventional treatment the use of TLC looks very different.

Let us calculate the incremental cost-effectiveness ratio comparing TLC with Cardiomagic:

$$\text{TLC vs. Cardiomagic} = (\$116{,}600 - \$50{,}000)/(17.44 - 17.12 \text{ QALYs})$$
$$= \$66{,}600/0.32 \text{ QALYs} \approx \$208{,}000/\text{QALY}$$

This large incremental cost-effectiveness ratio tells us that to produce an additional QALY using TLC instead of Cardiomagic costs over $200,000 per QALY.

What are the implications when an intervention falls clearly outside the range of cost-effectiveness from the social perspective? First, it is important to note that when an intervention is clearly outside the cost-effectiveness range, it may still be more effective than the alternatives. In fact, TLC has been found to be slightly more effective than Cardiomagic, producing 17.44 QALYs per use compared with 17.12 QALYs for Cardiomagic. These additional QALYs, however, are very expensive to achieve.[3]

It is important to recognize that an intervention that has been declared not cost-effective from a social perspective may look quite different from an individual perspective. An individual who has the personal resources or adequate insurance coverage may well favor the use of TLC rather than Cardiomagic despite the extremely high cost per extra QALY.

Subgroups: Distributional Effects

We have already seen that cost-effectiveness analysis may be viewed as being biased in favor of the young over the old. In addition, we have seen that a bias exists in cost-effectiveness analysis towards the healthy as opposed to the permanently and severely disabled. In particular situations, there may be additional tendencies to favor one group over another. To understand these impacts, it is important to

---

[3] The fact that a country cannot afford to generally provide everyone in need with an expensive service does not preclude a society from paying for its use under specific circumstances or for unique group(s) of patients. Ideally these are justified as being subgroups who obtain substantial benefit. A number of political, economic, and even research rationales may be made for heavily subsidizing a limited number of expensive services.

examine the results of a decision-making investigation to determine what types of individuals receive the favorable outcomes and what types experience the adverse outcomes. In addition, it is important to focus on the types of individuals who bear the financial costs. This is parallel to looking at subgroups.

The process of interpreting the results of a decision-making investigation is not limited to interpreting the summary measures such as incremental cost-effectiveness ratios. Summary measures, by definition, are averages. They are designed to summarize the average results. Average results do not tell the whole story for two fundamental reasons. First, the average does not in and of itself say much about what types of individuals experience the favorable outcomes and what types experience the adverse outcomes or must pay the additional costs. Examining the types of individuals who experience the favorable and adverse outcomes in decision-making investigations is known as examining the *distributional effects* of the intervention.

To illustrate the distributional effects, let us return to the Paresis A example and consider an aspect of the vaccine that we have not focused on previously. That is, which type of individual experienced the favorable and the adverse outcomes of the vaccine.

The favorable outcome of the Paresis A vaccine is the prevention of paralysis. The adverse outcome is the rare occurrence of a Paresis A like illness among children of parents who have voluntarily had their children vaccinated.

It is unfortunate whenever anyone experiences the adverse outcomes of an intervention. However, when children (or their parents) voluntarily agree to accept the treatment after they are made aware of known adverse effects, they are accepting the adverse outcomes as part of the treatment. However, that is not the situation if the treatment is not accepted voluntarily. Imagine that the following new information is available on the impact of the Paresis A vaccine:

> It has been found that the virus contained in the vaccine can spread to other children. Children exposed to their vaccinated peers are often protected, while a few children unknowingly exposed to vaccinated children may experience the Paresis A-like illness.

Thus, the impact of the adverse effects of the vaccine may fall on persons who never voluntarily agreed to receive the vaccine. Some may argue that submitting individuals to harm without their (or their parents') agreement is not an acceptable approach even if it results, on average, in improved outcomes at reduced costs. Regardless of how you view this controversy, it is important to recognize the distributional effects.[4]

Meaning from Other Perspectives

As we have seen, the initial analysis in a decision-making investigation should be performed from the social perspective. That is, we need to consider the harms,

---

[4] Distributional effects often raise issues of social justice related to the impact on groups in society who have a lower socioeconomic status or are otherwise disadvantaged. Disproportionate negative impacts on groups who are already at a social disadvantage are often seen as violating principles of social justice.

benefits, and costs regardless of who experiences the benefits or harms and regardless of who pays for the costs.

However, in addition to conducting a decision-making investigation from a social perspective, it may also be presented from the perspective of particular users of the investigation. These users may be insurance companies who pay the bills over the short run; government insurance systems that pay the bills over the longer run; or hospitals, health systems, or groups of professionals that receive payment for providing services.

When an analysis is conducted from a user perspective, it may not include all of the benefits, harms, and costs that should be considered from the social perspective. This can lead to potentially conflicting interpretations, as illustrated in the next example:

> A decision-making investigation conducted from the social perspective found that TLC cost approximately $40,000/QALY and Cardiomagic cost approximately $14,000/QALY. The data was then examined from the perspective of a hospital system and an insurance company. The hospital system received payment for the TLC procedure and favored use of TLC. The insurance company was not responsible for the cost of medications and its findings strongly favored use of the medication Cardiomagic.

In addition to the focus on reimbursement, providers of care are also concerned with their costs of providing services. Costs from the social perspective are very different from costs from a provider's perspective, as illustrated in the next example:

> A reviewer of TLC, Cardiomagic, and the Paresis A vaccine literature looked at the relative costs and effectiveness from the social perspective. He concluded that for the same expenditure of funds, more QALYs could be obtained by providing all children with Paresis A vaccine and reducing the use of TLC. A hospital administrator whose hospital performed large number of TLC procedures argued in response that from the hospital's perspective, if TLC procedures were reduced in half, it would only serve to substantially increase the cost of performing the remaining TLC procedures.

The provider or institutional perspective is reflected in the approach of the hospital administrator. From his perspective, costs are seen quite differently than from the social perspective. For instance, institutions have fixed costs, such as equipment, that remain regardless of how many TLC procedures they perform. The social and institutional perspectives may both be true as seen from different points of view.[5]

These examples indicate the limitations of cost-effectiveness analysis when conducted from specific user perspectives. Decision-making investigations are designed for the social perspective and should be interpreted primarily from the social perspective. That is, cost-effectiveness analysis is most useful for setting policies that apply to large numbers of institutions or a large population. Most users are interested primarily in their own reimbursements or costs. Thus,

---

[5] In addition, institutions may have personnel costs that can't be reduced for lower volume because they need the equipment to be staffed regardless of volume of services. In addition, change itself involves economic (and psychological) costs. Institutions may have special concerns regarding the effect that the change will have on its reputation, cash flow, or other local effects. The social perspective views all costs and outcomes as averages for the future and does not take any of these factors into account. Thus, any one institution looking at a cost-effectiveness study will not necessarily agree that the conclusions drawn from the social perspective apply to them.

cost-effectiveness analysis may be presented from user perspectives, but the results should be interpreted with great caution.[6]

In this chapter, we have examined how the results of a decision-making investigation can be applied to the type of individual included in the decision-making model. Finally, as with other types of investigations, we turn our attention to efforts to extrapolate the data.

---

[6] Note that the government perspective and the social perspective are not the same. If a government provides insurance coverage, it may have a payer perspective. When comprehensive lifetime benefits are provided, including Social Security, that provide living expenses for the elderly, the tendency is even to go beyond the social perspective to try to include the additional living expenses for the additional years of life. Inclusion of these costs has been controversial, but they are not generally included from the social perspective. Payer perspectives may also be influenced by the special characteristics of the subgroup of individuals for whom they are responsible. Insurance companies that cover generally healthy individuals may look at recommendations quite differently than an insurance plan that covers the general population or individuals who have advanced disease.

32 Extrapolation

In decision-making investigations, as in other types of studies, we need to consider the impact of extrapolation to similar populations, beyond the data, and to other populations. We first need to consider the impact of extrapolating the results to all individuals who are similar to those included in the investigation.

To Similar Populations

Decision-making investigation may form the basis for the development of recommendations for practice. The development and use of practice guidelines is the focus of the next section, "A Guide to the Guidelines." Before decision-making investigations can serve as the basis for practice recommendations or guidelines, we need to examine their implications for those who are similar to the populations in the investigations.

Let us assume that a decision-making investigation has indicated that additional QALYs can be obtained at a cost that is considered cost-effective. If we want to extrapolate these results to a similar population in a practice setting, we need to consider the impact that will occur in practice.

First, it is important to address the meaning of effectiveness. The QALYs gained are not gained equally by all individuals who undergo the treatment. Some will experience a major positive outcome, some will experience no change, and some will experience only an adverse effect.

An appreciation of the impact of QALYs gained helps to avoid the following common but incorrect extrapolation of the results of a cost-effectiveness study:

> A reviewer of the cost-effectiveness literature noted that the effectiveness of Cardiomagic was 17.12 QALYs per use compared with 15 QALYs per use for conventional therapy. The reviewer concluded that this was a quite small difference, especially because the impact occurs by adding years at the end of life.

The additional 2.1 QALYs gained per use are actually quite impressive. Few interventions provide this large an increase in QALYs. Cardiomagic is being used to treat single-vessel coronary artery disease, a condition that can be immediately fatal in middle-aged patients. For those who experience the benefit, the impact is immediate and substantial. That is, when it is effective, it can be expected to prolong the life of younger individuals, as well as extend the longevity of the elderly. Thus QALYs gained should not be viewed as added on only at the end of life.

In addition, to understand the impact of a decision-making study on a target population similar to the one included in the investigation, it is also important to appreciate the overall or *aggregate effects*. When extrapolating to a target population that has similar characteristics to the population used to construct the decision tree, the investigators are interested in the aggregate effect. The aggregate effect will often depend on the size of the target population.

In decision analysis using QALYs, for instance, aggregate effectiveness may be reported as the total number of QALYs that would result if the intervention was applied to all individuals in a particular population who are similar to those included in the investigation.

Let us see the potential aggregate population impact by comparing the results of TLC and Paresis A vaccine in the next example:

> A reviewer of the Cardiomagic and Paresis A vaccine cost-effectiveness literature noted that Cardiomagic provides on average 2.5 additional QALYs per use, while Paresis A vaccine provides far less than 1 QALY per use. Nevertheless, he noted that in the United States, using Cardiomagic for all patients with single-vessel coronary artery disease will provide 1.5 million QALYs compared with conventional treatment. Because of the large number of children who are susceptible to Paresis A and the large number of QALYs gained per case prevented, using the Paresis A vaccine for all children will provide 4 million QALYs. Therefore, he concluded that Paresis A vaccine is more effective than Cardiomagic.

Care must be taken when using measures of aggregate effectiveness to compare different types of interventions such as Paresis A vaccine and treatment of single-vessel coronary artery disease, that are applied to two very different target populations. In parallel to attributable risk percentage, cost-effectiveness ratios address the impact on a group with the condition. Aggregate population impact addresses a different question than the cost-effectiveness ratios. Aggregate population impact like population attributable risk, asks questions that depend on the particular composition and size of a target population. Aggregate population impact does not compare one procedure or approach with another. Rather, it compares the impact of the procedure plus the characteristics and size of the target population. This approach may be useful at times for making population-based decisions, but it requires additional data and additional assumptions that are not part of the results of cost-effectiveness analysis. Thus, as with other types of investigations, we need to distinguish between the impacts at the individual, at-risk group, and population levels.

Beyond the Data

Extrapolation often requires that we extend the results to situations for which we do not have data. We have called this extrapolation beyond the data. An investigator may conduct this form of extrapolation using *linear extrapolation*. That is, the investigator may assume that more effort to implement an intervention will produce additional QALYs in direct proportion to the increased effort. This linear assumption may not hold true, especially when extending beyond the range of the data.

Cost, for instance, may not increase in a linear fashion as volume increases. The costs of increasing the scale or volume of services provided are referred to as *marginal costs*. Let us see what we mean by marginal costs in the following example:[1]

---

[1] The term *marginal costs* is sometimes equated with incremental costs. The two terms are not consistently used in the literature. However, it is important to distinguish between two very different concepts. Incremental cost addresses the question of the additional costs that occur when comparing one option to another under the conditions being modeled. Marginal cost relates to the changes in cost that occur when the conditions of practice are used rather than the conditions modeled in the investigation. Specifically, the conditions of practice often include a larger scale of operation that the one assumed in the decision-making investigation.

As Paresis A vaccine programs were implemented, it was found that the cost per vaccine delivered fell initially as the program grew and could more efficiently use personnel and publicize the program using mass media. However, as the program continued to expand, costs per vaccine delivered began to rise again as extra efforts were needed to identify and to obtain access to the most difficult-to-reach individuals.

Economists refer to *economies and diseconomies of scale*. The initial reduced cost per vaccine delivered is an example of an economy of scale, whereas the eventual increase in cost per vaccine delivered is an example of a diseconomy of scale.

To Other Populations

Extrapolation to populations with different characteristics can lead to very misleading results. Let us first look at the potential for problems when we extrapolate the results of a decision-making investigation to a new population, nation, or culture.

Paresis A vaccine was introduced into the rural areas of a developing country where a dependable source of electricity for refrigerating the vaccine could not always be assured. In this setting, the results of the intervention were very different in that the cost was considerably reduced, but so was the effectiveness. Once the problems with handling the vaccine were addressed, the intervention was found to cost only $1,500 per QALY. Unfortunately, this was considered more than the developing nation could afford to pay.

This example illustrates many of the problems with extrapolating from one population to another. The costs of labor and of delivering services may be much less in a developing country. However, if special training or equipment is needed for effectiveness, then effectiveness may also be reduced. Even if the cost-effectiveness ratios are substantially lower in a developing nation, the nation may not be able to afford the treatment. Thus, it is a very difficult task to extrapolate cost-effectiveness data and results from one society to another.

Extrapolation to groups with different characteristics can also produce misleading conclusions. For instance, imagine the following extrapolation of the TLC and Cardiomagic results:

The successful use of Cardiomagic for single-vessel coronary artery disease was so convincing that the results were widely extrapolated to recommend use of Cardiomagic for patients with severe coronary artery disease in two or more vessels. The favorable outcomes were not as great and the adverse outcomes were greatly increased when Cardiomagic was applied to this new group of individuals.

It is not surprising that the outcomes will be different when an intervention is applied to groups with more severe or different types of disease. Therefore, just as in other types of investigations, it is very important in decision-making investigations to carefully examine the types of individuals who are included in the options being compared. Extrapolation to other groups carries assumptions that may not hold true among the new group of individuals to whom the results are extrapolated.

Finally, it is important to remember that cost-effectiveness investigations, like all studies, are conducted assuming a set of current alternatives and data. The alternatives may change rapidly, and unfortunately, cost-effectiveness analyses may sometimes be considered out-of-date by the time they are completed.

Despite the potential problems and difficulties in conducting decision-making investigations, it is important to recognize the contributions that these types of investigations make to clinical care and public health. The requirements to measure and express results quantitatively can improve communication. Decision-making investigations require the investigator to apply numbers to vague terms such as "rare" and "common," and "likely" and "unlikely." The need to explicitly define the decision-making process means that consequences must be defined and uncertainties recognized. Uncertainty always exists in decision-making. Formal decision-making investigations help us to measure and to determine the impact of uncertainty.

The decision-making literature is an important part of the movement toward evidence-based decision-making in health care and public health. Decision-making investigations require the investigator to spell out in great detail the available evidence and the assumptions that have been made in filling the holes where evidence is not available. In decision-making investigations, the investigator must be able to respond to demands to show the evidence and justify the assumptions.

The forms of decision-making investigations that incorporate costs have added an entire new dimension to the health research literature. Previously, clinical and public health decision-making relied almost exclusively on issues of benefits and harm, i.e., favorable and adverse outcomes. Technological advances in recent years have opened up so many therapeutic and preventive alternatives that no society can afford to do everything. Cost-effectiveness studies, despite their many limitations, often present the best available method for systematically choosing between the available options. For this reason, cost-effectiveness studies are now widely published in the health research literature.

33 Questions to Ask and Flaw-Catching Exercises

Questions to Ask: Considering Costs and Evaluating Effectiveness

The following Questions to Ask can serve as a checklist when reading a decision-making investigation. To see how these questions can be applied see the Studying a Study Online Web site at **www.StudyingaStudy.com.**

Method: Investigation's purpose and target population

1. **Study question and study type:** What is the study question and the type of decision-making investigation?
2. **Target population:** What is the target population to which the investigator wishes to apply the results?
3. **Perspective:** From what perspective is the investigation being conducted?

Assignment: Options and outcomes being investigated

1. **Options:** What options are being evaluated?
2. **Relevant options and realistic outcomes:** How are the options modeled? Are the options relevant to the study questions and do they include realistic outcomes?
3. **Timing of events:** Is the timing of events properly incorporated into the decision process?

Assessment: Measurement of outcomes

1. **Probabilities and utilities:** How are the probabilities and the utilities obtained, and are they accurate and precise?
2. **Life expectancy:** Are life expectancies used and if so, were they appropriate to the study question?
3. **Costs:** How are the costs obtained, and do they accurately and precisely reflect the social perspective?

Results: Comparison of outcomes

1. **Estimation:** Is the summary measurement appropriately expressed, e.g., QALYs, incremental cost-effectiveness, etc?
2. **Inference:** Is an appropriate sensitivity analysis conducted?
3. **Adjustment:** Is an appropriate method of discounting for present value used?

Interpretation: Conclusions for the target population

1. **Cost-effectiveness ratios:** Are the estimates such as cost-effectiveness ratios correctly interpreted?
2. **Subgroups:** Are the distributional effects on subgroups examined?

3. **Meaning from other perspectives:** What are the implications from perspectives other than the social perspective?

Extrapolation: Conclusions for other populations

1. **To similar populations:** Is the meaning for the average individual as well as the aggregate population impact addressed?
2. **Beyond the data:** If extrapolation beyond the data was conducted, is only a linear extrapolation used and are marginal effects of the scale of operation considered?
3. **To other populations:** If extrapolation to other populations is conducted, are differences from the target population of the investigation considered?

Flaw-Catching Exercises

The following Flaw-Catching Exercises are designed to give you practice using the M.A.A.R.I.E. framework for decision-making investigations. Read the exercise then take a look at critique that follows. See if you can answer each question before reading the answer that follows.

Flaw-Catching Exercise No. 1: Pulverizer—Evaluating Its Costs and Effectiveness as a Treatment for Kidney Stones

An evaluation of the costs and effectiveness of Pulverizer, a newly approved method for treatment of calcium-containing kidney stones for otherwise healthy individuals, was investigated. Pulverizer has been shown to have a high probability of breaking apart first kidney stones of 2 cm or less and allowing them to pass down the ureter. Immediate side effects are minimal, but there is a concern that the use of Pulverizer increases the probability of recurrence of kidney stones over the following decade.

An investigator decided to compare the use of Pulverizer with the conventional method in a decision-making investigation. The standard or conventional method consists of treating symptoms and observing the natural course of kidney stones and intervening only if the stone does not pass. Surgery, which includes an average of 4 days in the hospital, is performed only if the stones do not pass after a week.

In the decision option to use Pulverizer, this treatment was assumed to have a 95% chance of success and a 5% chance of failure. If Pulverizer fails, it is immediately followed by surgery, which is assumed to have a 99.5% success rate and a 0.5% chance of death. Pulverizer is assumed to be used at the time of diagnosis, thus avoiding hospitalization and returning the patient to work an average of a week earlier.

The alternative to use, standard treatment, is assumed to require an average of 4 days in the hospital, during which 80% of the stones pass. Surgery is performed on individuals whose stones do not pass in a week or who develop complications. Surgery is assumed to have a 99.5% success rate but to result in death in 0.5% of the patients. Under the above assumptions and assuming that successful treatment with either option returns the patients to full health, the two treatments were found to be equally effective.

The costs considered for Pulverizer are the cost of treatment, surgery, and subsequent hospitalization. The costs considered for conventional treatment are the

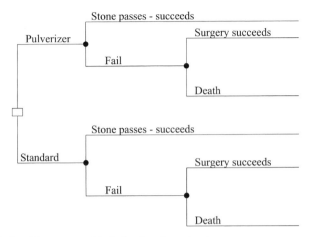

Figure 33.1. Decision tree used in Pulverizer investigation.

costs of hospitalization, surgery, and subsequent hospitalization. Costs are included regardless of who pays the bills.

The conventional treatment was found to cost $15,000 per successful outcome, whereas Pulverizer was found to cost $10,000 per successful outcome. A sensitivity analysis taking into account the length of hospitalization required for the conventional treatment found that if hospitalization could be shortened from an average of 4 days to an average of 2 days, the cost per successful outcome would be identical.

The investigators concluded that since both methods cost less than $50,000 per use, they were both cost-effective based on the current criteria in the United States. However, Pulverizer was more cost-effective. They concluded that Pulverizer was the best treatment available and should be tried on all stones at the time of diagnosis.

Figure 33.1 displays the decision tree used in this investigation. Figure 33.2 includes the probabilities and utilities, and calculates the expected utilities.

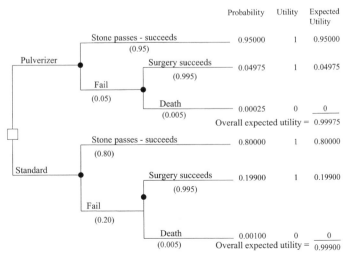

Figure 33.2. Decision tree for Pulverizer investigation including probabilities, utilities, and expected utilities.

Critique: Exercise No. 1

METHOD

- What type of decision-making investigation is being conducted?

The results of this investigation are measured in costs per successful outcome. This approach makes the assumption that the two treatments are equally effective. When the results are expressed as cost per successful outcome, it is called a cost-and-effectiveness study, as opposed to a cost-consequence study or a cost-utility study. In a cost-consequence study, the outcomes are merely described rather than combined. A cost-utility investigation expresses the outcomes incorporating utilities and often incorporating life-expectancy measures, and therefore expressing the results as QALYs.

- What is the study question and what target population does it address?

The investigators were trying to evaluate the relative cost and effectiveness of Pulverizer versus conventional therapy for treatment of initial, calcium-containing kidney stones of 2 cm or less in otherwise healthy individuals. Pulverizer is used at the time of diagnosis. Recognition of the study question directs the investigator to the type of population that should be used to collect the necessary data for the decision-making investigation. In this case, the data should reflect effectiveness and costs for healthy individuals with initial kidney stones of moderate size and should not consider stones not containing calcium.

- From what perspective is the investigation being conducted?

The investigators do not explicitly state the perspective being used in this investigation. However, the fact that costs are calculated regardless of who pays the bills implies that the investigation is appropriately conducted from the social perspective.

ASSIGNMENT

- What options are being considered? Are any options for using Pulverizer omitted?

The decision options chosen include only use of Pulverizer or the conventional combination of treatment of symptom relief and surgery for stones that do not pass. Other options are not considered. For instance, there is no mention of the alternative to use Pulverizer as a substitute for surgery after stones fail to pass.

- Is the time horizon appropriate?

The investigation only considers effectiveness and costs during the duration of the initial stone episode. The investigators do not consider the possibility of recurrences. Analysis of recurrence could be handled in a number of ways, including use of a Markov process that allows the investigators to vary the probability, timing, and cost of recurrences.

ASSESSMENT

- What utilities are being used in calculating effectiveness?

The investigators explicitly state the utilities they are using, with successful outcome equal to 1 and death equal to 0. As is often the situation, the investigators do not distinguish utilities for different routes to the favorable or the unfavorable outcomes. Thus, decision-making investigators are accused of considering only outcomes not the process of getting there.

- Is the assessment of costs complete?

The measurement of costs is incomplete. To include all the appropriate costs from the social perspective requires consideration of nonmedical expenses, such as the cost of accessing care, as well as the future costs, such as treatment of recurrences.

RESULTS

- What is the quality-adjusted number needed to treat for this investigation?

The overall expected utility for Pulverizer is 0.99975 compared with 0.99900 for the conventional treatment, as shown in Fig. 33.2. The quality-adjusted number needed to treat is equal to:

$$1/(0.99975 - 0.99900) = 1/0.00075 = 1,333$$

This quality-adjusted number needed to treat tells us that, on average, over 1,000 individuals need to be treated using Pulverizer rather than conventional therapy to produce one additional favorable outcome—that is, full recovery rather than death. This represents a large number needed to treat, but it indicates that the investigators should not have assumed the two treatments were equally effective.

- What type of sensitivity analysis is being conducted?

The investigators conducted a sensitivity analysis for cost by varying the number of days of hospitalization needed for the conventional treatment. This sensitivity analysis varied one factor at a time and thus is an example of a one-way sensitivity analysis. The investigators used this analysis to conclude that if the hospitalization could be shortened to 2 days, the cost per successful outcome would be identical. When an investigator uses a sensitivity analysis to determine the toss-up point, the sensitivity analysis is called a threshold analysis. The fact that decreasing hospital days to less than 2 could reduce the costs of conventional treatment below that of Pulverizer implies that the recommendations are sensitive to the length of hospitalization.

- Is discounting performed to take into account the timing of events?

The investigators act as if all the outcomes of interest occur in the immediate future. The investigators do not consider future events such as recurrence. Here, as with many decision-making investigations, it is important to consider the occurrence and timing of future events. If recurrences were included in the decision-making investigation, it would be important to discount the costs as well as the harms and benefits of the treatment of the recurrence.

INTERPRETATION

- Does this investigation establish that Pulverizer is cost-effective for treatment of first kidney stones of 2 cm or less in otherwise healthy individuals?

Whenever the results of a one-way sensitivity analysis suggest that the recommended option is sensitive to a modest change in a variable, such as length of hospitalization, the investigators need to be especially careful in interpreting the results. In addition, the results of this investigation are expressed as cost per successful treatment. By indicating that the costs per case were less than $50,000, the investigators are interpreting the results the same way they would if the results were expressed as incremental cost per QALY. Incremental cost per QALY would have required the results to explicitly incorporate life expectancies as well as utilities and compare Pulverizer with conventional treatment.

EXTRAPOLATION

- What assumptions need to be made to conclude that Pulverizer should be tried on all stones?

This extrapolation would require the investigators to extrapolate from otherwise healthy individuals with kidney stones of 2 cm or less to all patients with kidney stones. This extrapolation assumes that Pulverizer has the same probability of favorable outcomes, probability of adverse outcomes, and costs when applied to patients with larger stones, noncalcium stones, and to those additional conditions that may complicate treatment. Since Pulverizer is being investigated for patients with stones of 2 cm or less, it may already be known that Pulverizer's effect on larger stones is different than its effect on these smaller stones.

Flaw-Catching Exercise No. 2: GREAT Dialysis versus Hemodialysis

A new dialysis method known as GREAT dialysis (Gradient Re-Entry Abdominal Thoracic dialysis) is being evaluated to compare its cost and effectiveness with hemodialysis, which is the conventional treatment for adult patients. The cost and effectiveness are being evaluated based on use of the treatments for the lifetime of the average adult dialysis patient who requires dialysis beginning at an age of 60 years.

Both methods of dialysis are assumed to be paid for by a comprehensive health care system that pays for approved methods of dialysis as long as the patient lives. The system is part of a government health care insurance system that covers the cost of all necessary medical care but requires patients and families to cover the costs of access to care and other nonmedical costs of care. The investigation aims to include all alternatives that could provide favorable outcomes to patients while controlling the costs of the health insurance system.

Hemodialysis requires twice-weekly outpatient dialysis treatment that lasts an average of 3 hours. Hemodialysis results in hospitalization, on average, for 1 week per year as a result of complications. Based on extensive experience with hemodialysis, the life expectancy of the average person undergoing hemodialysis is estimated to be 10 years, with death occurring at the same rate throughout the follow-up period.

GREAT dialysis is a new method in which a dialysis device is implanted in the abdomen and thorax, and provides dialysis which is as good as the kidney's own dialysis for an average of 10 years. On average, surgery is assumed to be required every 10 years for replacement, with an average of 1 replacement per patient. There are no known side effects of GREAT dialysis except the 3% chance of death that results from the initial surgery and the 1% chance of death that results from the replacement surgery. Since GREAT dialysis is believed to function as well as the patient's own kidney, the life expectancy of the average person using GREAT dialysis is estimated at 20 years, except for those who die at surgery. However, since GREAT dialysis is a relatively new procedure, a low estimate of 10 years life expectancy was also made.

Utilities for hemodialysis have been established by asking hospitalized dialysis patients to rate the quality of their health. The average utility was 0.5, and this was used as the base-case utility for hemodialysis patients. Ninety-five percent of the patients had a utility between 0.9 and 0.3. These were used as the realistic high and realistic low estimates of utility. The utility for GREAT dialysis was set at 1 since, if successful, GREAT dialysis returns patients to their former states of health.

The costs of hemodialysis include yearly medical care costs of the procedure and the 1 week of hospitalization. The costs of GREAT dialysis include the medical care costs of the device and the surgery plus follow-up care for the initial implant and for one replacement. Future costs of hemodialysis and GREAT dialysis were discounted at 3%.

The investigators found that the incremental cost-effectiveness ratio of GREAT dialysis was –$2,000 per QALY compared with hemodialysis, reflecting increased QALYs and decreased costs. After performing one-way sensitivity analyses for utilities and life expectancy, a best case/worst case sensitivity analysis was conducted to see the impact of assuming that the utility of hemodialysis was 0.9 or alternatively 0.3, and the life expectancy of GREAT dialysis was 10 years instead of 20. The best case/worst case sensitivity analysis found that the incremental cost-effectiveness ratio for GREAT dialysis compared with hemodialysis varied from –$5,000 per QALY (best-case) to +$1,000 per QALY (worst case).

The investigators concluded that GREAT dialysis could save the system several billion dollars per year.

Based upon the sensitivity analysis, they also concluded that GREAT dialysis may increase costs as reflected in the worst case assumptions and therefore recommended that it not be included as a covered service. A reviewer of this article agreed that GREAT dialysis may cost more based on its use in this investigation, but argued that it should be covered since once implemented on a large scale, the costs would be lower. In addition, the reviewer suggested that GREAT dialysis should be used on all dialysis patients, including children.

Critique: Exercise No. 2

METHOD

- What type of decision-making investigation is being conducted?

The results of this investigation are expressed as incremental cost per QALY. Thus, the investigators were conducting a cost-utility study, or what we have called a cost-effectiveness analysis using QALYs.

- What is the study question and what target population does it address?

The investigation is addressing the costs and effectiveness of GREAT dialysis compared with hemodialysis for a population of adult patients who already need dialysis. Thus, the target population is the average adult who needs dialysis.

• From what perspective is the investigation being conducted?

As indicated by the investigators, both methods of dialysis are assumed to be paid for by a comprehensive health care system that pays for approved methods of dialyses as long as the patient lives. The payer is a government health care insurance system that covers the cost of all medical care but requires patients and families to cover the costs of access to care and other nonmedical costs of care. Thus, the perspective is that of a payer of comprehensive medical services and not a social perspective. A social perspective is slightly different since it would also include at least the short-term nonhealth care costs.

ASSIGNMENT

• What options are being evaluated?

The only options considered are GREAT dialysis and hemodialysis. Neither transplantation nor a combination of treatments is considered.

• Are the options relevant and the outcomes realistic?

If hemodialysis is commonly combined with transplantation, this alternative might have been included as well to ensure that the decision-making investigation reflected realistic decision-making. Similarly, if GREAT dialysis can be and is being combined with hemodialysis, that alternative would also be important.

• Is the time horizon appropriate?

The time horizon was the until the death of each patient. This is usually an appropriate time horizon for incorporating the timing of events.

ASSESSMENT

Figure 33.3 displays the decision tree used in this investigation, including the probabilities, utilities, and life expectancies.

• Are the probabilities, utilities, and costs precise and accurate?

The probabilities used for hemodialysis are based on extensive experience. However, since GREAT dialysis is a new procedure, much greater uncertainty exists regarding the probabilities of its outcomes. Thus, it would have been desirable to make realistic low and high estimates for the probabilities of favorable and adverse outcomes of GREAT dialysis. The investigators did include a low estimate for life expectancy for GREAT dialysis and low and high realistic estimates of utility for hemodialysis.

Asking patients undergoing the procedure to estimate their utilities is an acceptable method of obtaining utility scores. However, the utility of hemodialysis was estimated from inpatients undergoing dialysis. This is not the best group to use in estimating utilities because they may be more seriously ill than the group of patients undergoing outpatient hemodialysis. In general, those making life-changing

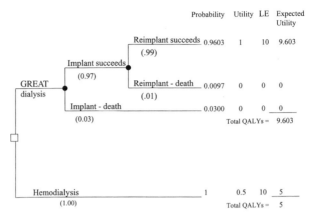

Figure 33.3. Decision tree used in the GREAT dialysis versus hemodialysis cost-effectiveness investigation.

decisions like the decision to undergo dialysis envision their utility as modestly lower than those who have already had the experience.

The investigators included medical care costs and future costs but did not include the nonmedical costs required from the patient or others, such as family members, to obtain the medical care.

RESULTS

• Are the results appropriately expressed in terms of cost-effectiveness ratios?

The investigators appropriately presented the results of effectiveness as QALYs and calculated an incremental cost-effectiveness ratio. Since hemodialysis is considered conventional therapy, it is appropriate to compare GREAT dialysis with hemodialysis.

• Is an appropriate sensitivity analysis conducted?

The use of a best case/worst case analysis is an acceptable method for conducting multiple-way sensitivity analysis. A Monte Carlo method could also have been used. It allows values to be varied in more realistic ways to produce a credibility interval. Additional one-way sensitivity analyses would ideally have been presented to indicate whether the results of GREAT dialysis are sensitive to such factors as the cost of GREAT dialysis and the time interval prior to replacement. Both factors may be subject to change as more experience is gained with GREAT dialysis.

• Is an appropriate method to discount for present value used?

The use of a 3% discount rate is the accepted discount rate, though the additional use of a 5% rate is also recommended. A more serious error is the discounting of costs without the discounting of effectiveness. Costs and effectiveness must be discounted at the same rate. Discounting of costs without discounting of effectiveness means that delaying use of a procedure is seen as desirable because each year the costs become less while the effectiveness remains the same. This is not realistic in the case of dialysis because delaying dialysis is usually not possible.

Discounting for effectiveness is important in this investigation not only because costs are discounted. GREAT dialysis carries a probability of death only during surgical implants, whereas hemodialysis carries a probability of death throughout the period of follow-up. This difference in the timing of the events implies that discounting needs to be conducted to compare the effectiveness of these two treatment alternatives.

INTERPRETATION

- Are the cost-effectiveness ratios correctly interpreted?

The investigators correctly concluded that the results of their base-case estimate showed that GREAT dialysis is cost-saving. If this base-case estimate was performed correctly, it can be used as the basis for interpreting the results of the investigation. Thus, it would have been acceptable for the investigators to declare GREAT dialysis not only cost-saving but cost-effective on the basis of the increased QALYs and decreased costs. They would need to limit this interpretation to the base-case conditions and the assumptions of this decision-making investigation.

- What definition is being used in this investigation to establish cost-effectiveness?

The investigators seem to be equating cost-saving and increased effectiveness with cost-effective, and seem to require the sensitivity analysis as well as the base-case estimates to demonstrate reduced costs and increased effectiveness. This is too difficult a criterion to meet. The results of the best case/worst case sensitivity actually strengthen the argument that GREAT dialysis is cost-effective compared with hemodialysis because even under the demanding condition of a worst case analysis, the incremental cost per QALY is not more than +$1,000. An increase of $1,000 for an additional QALY is considered cost-effective. Using cost reduction and increased effectiveness as the criterion for coverage is very demanding since new procedures that increase effectiveness while reducing costs are rare. Much more common are new procedures that increase costs while increasing effectiveness or that reduce costs while maintaining current levels of effectiveness.

EXTRAPOLATION

- How did the investigator extrapolate to similar populations? Were aggregate effects considered?

The investigators drew conclusions about the aggregate effects when they concluded that the use of GREAT dialysis would save the system several billion dollars per year.

- Did the reviewer extrapolate beyond the data?

The reviewer has extrapolated beyond the data. By concluding that changes in volume will alter the costs, they are making a statement about marginal costs as opposed to incremental costs. Marginal costs reflect the economies of scale or diseconomies of scale associated with the widespread use of a procedure. This extrapolation takes the reviewer beyond the data and thus carries assumptions that may or may not hold true. It is possible to argue for coverage of GREAT dialysis on the basis of the data contained within this investigation without having to extrapolate beyond the data.

- Did the reviewer extrapolate to other populations?

By drawing conclusions about children as well as adults, the reviewer extrapolated to another population. Children may or may not experience the same effectiveness and the same costs as adults undergoing GREAT dialysis. Extrapolation to children relies on a series of new assumptions that are not discussed as part of this investigation.

Summary

We have seen how decision-making investigators can quantitatively incorporate the benefits, harms, and costs of potential options. In doing this we have used decision trees to help structure the analysis. Decision trees allow us to incorporate probabilities, utilities, and life-expectancies to produce a measure of effectiveness known as quality adjusted life years or QALYs. Combining costs measured in dollars with effectiveness measured in QALYs allows us to develop summary measurements. A fully developed analysis is called a cost-utility analysis or a cost-effective analysis using QALYs. Incremental cost-effectiveness ratios comparing new interventions to standard or conventional treatments are key to determining whether treatments are cost-effective and which one is most cost-effective for a particular condition. Cost-effective ratio comparing options to the do-nothing or zero-cost-zero-effectiveness option can be helpful in comparing treatments for different conditions.

Cost-effectiveness analysis is not an end in itself. It may be a useful tool in developing guidelines as we will see in the next section.

A Guide to the Guidelines

V

34 Method

Guidelines attempt to synthesize the evidence in order to provide a wide range of recommendations for making decisions. The availability of recommendations for clinical practice is not new; they are as old as the teaching of medicine or even the Hippocratic oath. What is different about today's guidelines is the emphasis on evidence. In fact, the type of guidelines we are talking about have been called *evidence-based guidelines* or *evidence-based recommendations*.

When reviewing an evidence-based guideline, it is possible to use the M.A.A.R.I.E. framework to organize our approach and to help us identify the questions to ask. Figure 34.1 illustrates the application of the M.A.A.R.I.E. framework for reviewing guidelines.

Purpose of the Guideline

The movement to develop evidence-based guidelines was strongly motivated by the finding that clinicians in similar communities often have widely different practices for common or costly decisions. These range from if and when to do surgery to whom to hospitalize. From these investigations it was concluded that differences in practice not based on evidence result in unnecessary cost and unnecessary variations in quality. Only evidence could determine which practices were best, and only the development and acceptance of evidence-based guidelines could reduce these variations. These are the roots of the movement to develop evidence-based guidelines.

The original purposes for clinical guidelines were outlined by the Institute of Medicine[1] as follows:

1. Assisting clinical decision-making by patients and practitioners
2. Educating individuals or groups
3. Assessing and assuring the quality of care
4. Guiding allocation of resources for health care
5. Reducing the risk of liability for negligent care

Evidence-based guidelines were initially aimed at individual decision-making by individual clinicians. Today, evidence-based guidelines have been developed for the full range of clinical activity, from prevention though palliation. Perhaps as a reflection of the success of the evidence-based guidelines movement, today guidelines are being applied not only for the care of individual patients by individual clinicians but also for institutional and population-based decision-making. Institutional guidelines such as those for reducing the risk of anesthesia, preventing HIV infection after needle stick injury, or controlling SARS in a hospital setting are now widely used.

[1] Institute of Medicine, *Summary Guidelines for Clinical Practice: From Development to Use*, National Academy Press, 1992.

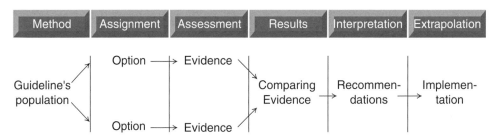

Figure 34.1. Application of M.A.A.R.I.E. framework to guidelines.

Community guidelines have become central to public health efforts to improve population health. Community guidelines are increasingly bringing to bear the evidence for effective intervention, such as those to control tobacco use, lead paint exposure, and childhood obesity. Guidelines for responding to crises from bioterrorism to environmental contamination are now accepted as standard operating procedures.

Thus, we begin our examination of guidelines by asking about a guideline's goal. What is it aiming to achieve, and at what level—the individual patient or clinician, the institution, or the community? Let us imagine that we were examining the following type of guideline.

> Colon cancer guidelines aim to establish indications and methods for screening those at average risk of colon cancer. They also aim to provide guidance for the advertising of aspirin use for prevention of colon cancer

This type of guideline aims at the individual clinical level when it addresses the goal of screening individual patients. When it addresses the issue of advertising of aspirin for prevention of colon cancer, it looks to the population or community level. Both of these approaches have the goal of reducing the mortality rate from colon cancer, but they aim to intervene in different ways. Thus, the first question we need to ask when looking at a guideline is: What is its goal and how does the guideline hope to achieve it?

Guideline's Target Population

As with the types of studies that we have examined, it is key to understand the target population for which the guideline is intended. Guidelines may be directed at narrowly defined groups or they may be directed at large numbers of individuals defined only by age or gender, as illustrated in the next example.

> Guidelines for screening for colon cancer are developed for the average male or female 50 years and older with or without a family history of colon cancer. They are not designed to apply to those with diseases that predispose them to colon cancer, such as ulcerative colitis or familial polyposis.

This description gives us a clear understanding of the target population for the guideline. It indicates that the guideline is designed for screening, which implies that it is aimed at asymptomatic patients. The target group is those 50 years and older, and applies to both those with and without a family history of colon cancer.

This is important because family history is a known risk factor for colon cancer, and the guideline might have excluded or treated this group separately.

In addition, the description indicates that the guideline does not apply to the much smaller group of individuals who are at increased risk because of predisposing diseases. It is important to appreciate from the beginning who is included and who is excluded. Guidelines, like investigations, usually have inclusion and exclusion criteria.

Guideline's Perspective

The guideline movement has spawned an increasing number of "players" who are rapidly developing guidelines, often to serve specific or even proprietary agendas. The vast array of guidelines and guideline developers makes it useful to classify them to get a better idea of the perspectives of the authors. We might classify guideline developers as follows:

- Government agencies that seek qualified and broadly representative individuals for a committee or task force to independently develop evidence-based guidelines. In the United States such agencies as the United States Preventive Services Task Force (Agency for Healthcare Research and Quality), the National Institutes of Health, and the Centers for Disease Control and Prevention have followed this approach.
- Professional societies such as the American College of Surgeons, the American College of Physicians, and many other clinically oriented professional societies
- Nonprofit patient-oriented groups such as the American Heart Association and the American Cancer Society
- For-profit and not-for-profit providers of care, including Kaiser-Permanente and national associations of health plans

Each of these organizations have their own approach, their own priorities, and at times their own biases. Thus, it is important to appreciate the authorship of the guideline so that the potential user can look for potential conflicts of interest that may subtly or not so subtly influence the way the guideline was developed or structured, as illustrated in the next example.

> Recommendations for colon cancer screening were made by a government task force, a society of endoscopists, and a national consumer-oriented cancer society. The endoscopists recommendations stress the use of colonoscopy, which allows examination of the entire colon. The consumer-oriented society stressed the use of occult blood testing and periodic sigmoidoscopy for patients who sought screening. The government task force recommended reaching as many patients as possible using a variety of options for screening.

Even assuming the best of intentions, different groups will interpret the evidence differently. Those with experience with and interest in a technical procedure such as colonoscopy are often inclined to recommend its use. Those who represent consumers will often emphasize satisfying the desires of those who seek care and minimizing the harm or discomfort for those who do. Broadly representative groups may seek to reach large numbers of individuals, hoping to benefit as many as possible. Those seeking to reach large number of individuals may leave open as many options for implementation as possible to circumvent the most controversial of issues, such as which it the best method for screening.

There is no universally accepted approach to developing and presenting guidelines. Perhaps the most structured and rigorous approach in widespread use was developed by the United States Preventive Services Task Force (USPSTF). We will utilize their approach throughout the "Guide to the Guidelines" section.[2]

Having defined the goal, the target population, and the perspective of guidelines, we will address the questions of assignment in the next chapter.

---

[2] "Current Methods of the U.S. Preventive Services Task Force: A Review of the Process," *Am. J. Prev. Med.* 20, suppl.3(2001): 21–35. This approach is also being used by the Task Force on Community Preventive Services developed by the Centers for Disease Control and Prevention.

35 Assignment

Assignment, as we have seen, implies that we are defining the groups being compared or the options being considered. Thus, assignment for guidelines implies that we examine which options for intervention are being considered; how the evidence is organized or structured; and what is considered relevant evidence and how is it being combined.

Options Being Considered

Guidelines should identify the options that are being evaluated as well as potential options that are being omitted, as illustrated in the following example.

> A group of colon cancer screening guidelines compare sigmoidoscopy, colonoscopy, and virtual colonoscopy. They do not consider double-contrast barium enema or occult blood testing.

These guidelines are explicit about which methods they include for consideration and which ones they omit. Often the guidelines will only indicate which options are considered and leave to the reader the task of recognizing which options are omitted. It is important to recognize the omissions as well as the inclusions because exclusion implies that the omissions are not recommended.

Structuring the Evidence

The method of organization of the evidence can take a number of forms. As we have seen, decision-making can be organized using a decision tree that defines the options, the decisions, and the outcomes of each decision, often including utilities of the outcomes as well as their probabilities. Use of a decision tree may at times guide the construction of a guideline. When that is the case, the decision tree should ideally appear in the guideline.

Often, however, other analytical frameworks and approaches are used. As we saw in chapter 19 on screening, the framework for evaluating a screening procedure should require fulfilling four criteria: substantial morbidity and mortality, early detection improves outcome, screening is feasible, and screening is acceptable and efficient.

The evidence for evidence-based guidelines may also be presented in a less structured format, often referred to as a *systematic review*. A systematic review is an effort to collect and present the research evidence to address specific clinical or public health questions. Systemic reviews may combine quantitative and qualitative methods, and often address a range of issues relevant to practice-based decision-making.

Thus, an article presenting an evidence-based guideline should indicate how the evidence is organized, as indicated in the following example:

> A systematic review of cohort and randomized clinical trials of cancer screening was conducted to address questions of indications for screening, methods for screening, costs of screening, and frequency of screening, as well as patient acceptance. A meta-analysis was used to examine whether there were differences in the effectiveness of different screening methods.

As this example illustrates, methods of presenting the evidence may be combined. Systematic reviews are often the starting point for collecting and presenting the evidence. The evidence may then be structured to address key questions using methods such as meta-analysis.[1]

Types of Evidence

It is key to explicitly state types of evidence being considered and how the evidence is being combined. Together, the types of evidence and their combination allow the reader to understand the criteria being used to decide between the options.

The types of evidence being considered are usually divided into benefits, harms, and financial costs.[2] These broad categories are usually adequate to include a wide range of important considerations. However, what is implied by each may need further definition. Do harms include the discomfort and anxiety of undergoing a procedure and waiting for the results? Do costs include consideration of reimbursement rates? Thus, the criteria in a guideline for colon cancer screening might look something like this:

> A guideline for colon cancer screening makes recommendations based upon the net effectiveness—that is, effectiveness minus the potential harm of the techniques. Issues of cost, patient acceptance, and provider reimbursement were not considered.

In addition to defining what is meant by benefits, harms, and costs, it is also important to understand how they are being combined. For instance imagine the following situation.

> In evaluating the options for colon cancer screening, the potential methods were first evaluated for net effectiveness—that is, their benefits and harms were considered. For the two methods that demonstrated the greatest effectiveness, cost was considered to determine which technique was recommended.

It is not unusual for developers of guidelines to separate issues of benefits and harms from those of costs. They may argue that there is no reason to consider costs unless an option reaches a certain level of effectiveness. This approach has the effect of excluding those options that have greatly reduced costs and modestly reduced effectiveness.

As we have seen, decision analysis and cost-effectiveness analysis are formal methods that can be used to combine considerations of benefits, harms, and costs. Decision analysis and cost-effectiveness analysis are built on what we have called

---

[1] There are a number of other methods for organizing and presenting data. Together, these have been called analytical frameworks. The Unites States Preventive Services Task Force, for example, has developed analytical frameworks for each of its areas of focus, i.e., screening, immunization, counseling, and chemoprevention.

[2] Not all considerations in decision-making relate directly to benefits, harms, and costs. Issues of ethics, for instance, may not directly relate to any of these outcomes. Guidelines can and should make as explicit as possible the types of evidence that are being considered.

expected utility. That is, when we use an expected-utility approach, we seek to maximize the net benefits for the average person.

Maximizing expected utility is not the only possible approach for combining the criteria. Other approaches can include minimizing the harm, maximizing the potential benefits, or a commonly used compromise approach that has been called *satisficing*. Satisficing implies that decision-making aims to achieve a good enough solution, often one that reduces the potential for major harms even if the average benefit is reduced. Let us see how satisficing may be implicitly used in developing guidelines, as illustrated in the following example.

> Colon cancer screening by flexible sigmoidoscopy was considered as an option to be performed by primary care physicians. However, when using this option, if a biopsy is needed, a repeat examination and biopsy by a gastroenterologist is strongly recommended.

Here, the option for flexible sigmoidoscopy does not allow primary care physicians to perform a biopsy even if this, on average, would reduce the cost or even increase the benefit. The potential for greater harm through perforation when the procedure is performed by those with less training and experience is presumable paramount in defining this option.

Thus the process of assignment is the process of defining the options, organizing the evidence and deciding how to decide. Once this process is complete, we can go on to the assessment process and look at the evidence itself.

36 Assessment

The process of assessment in examining guidelines requires us to look at the evidence for each of the options being considered. This process uses the criteria for making recommendations set forth in the assignment component. As part of the assessment process we need to look at the sources of the data, how the outcomes were measured, and how holes in the evidence were handled.

Sources of the Evidence

A guideline should identify the specific sources of evidence. In addition it should provide specific information that will allow assessment of the quality of the evidence. Specifically, the type of investigation, the number of participants, and the overall quality are important. This might be illustrated as follows:

> Evidence from a large randomized clinical trial has established the effectiveness and safety of screening for colon cancer. The trial demonstrated that fecal occult blood testing annually reduces the mortality from colon cancer for asymptomatic individuals 50 years and over regardless of their family history. Well-designed concurrent cohort studies suggest that sigmoidoscopy every 3 to 5 years in addition to fecal occult blood testing further reduces mortality. A large randomized clinical trial demonstrated that virtual colonoscopy is approximately as effective as colonoscopy in detecting polyps.

As we will see in Chapter 37 on results, the sources of the evidence will become important issues when the guideline developers attempt to score the strength of the evidence.

Measurement of Outcomes

The approach used to measure and incorporate harms, benefits, and costs should be outlined in guidelines, as in this example:

> Harms and benefits of screening for colon cancer were measured over the lifetime of the individual. Costs from a social perspective were taken into account only when options had approximately the same net effectiveness and also when considering the frequency of screening.

This guideline provides key information on how the measurements were conducted. It provides the time horizon for measurement, i.e., the lifetime of the individuals. It also indicates how costs were calculated—that is, using a social perspective. Guidelines are expected to make available far more details. However, these may not be readily available as part of a published article. Increasingly, however, these details should be available on a Web site.

Filling Holes in the Evidence

Evidence-based guidelines differ most dramatically from the traditional approach to recommendation in the way they treat expert opinion. In the traditional approach, experts informally reviewed the evidence and reached their own conclusions using their own approach. In evidence-based guidelines, quantitative evidence from well-conducted investigations is considered the most reliable form of evidence.

In evidence-based guidelines, expert opinion is itself considered a form of evidence. In terms of quality however, expert opinion is regarded as the least dependable form of evidence. Thus, expert option is often used only when there are holes in the evidence that cannot be filled in by available investigations or other data.

Since expert opinion is itself considered a form of evidence, evidence-based guidelines often use a systematic process for collecting and incorporating expert opinion. Rather than selecting one particular expert, they may use a process designed to determine whether there is agreement among experts. If there is little or no agreement, guidelines may develop a realistic range of values based upon expert opinion.

Two basic approaches to obtaining expert opinions have been called the *consensus conference* and the *Delphi approach.* The consensus conference approach, originated by the National Institutes of Health, aims to bring together face-to-face a broad range of experts to determine whether they can agree upon a predefined set of questions. Every effort is made to define those issues in which they can reach agreement. Using a consensus conference approach, when agreement is not possible, the range of realistic values might be defined.

In the Delphi approach a representative group of experts is again included. However, in this approach the participants never meet each other and their identities are not known to each other. The approach begins by having each participant address the questions posed, followed by formal feedback of all the responses to the participants. Each participant then may change their response or further justify their initial opinion. The process is continued until the participants have reached a consensus or made it clear that a range of opinions exist.

Let us see how these approaches to incorporating expert opinion might be used in the development of evidence-based guidelines, as in the following example.

> The evidence on colonoscopy's harms in practice were not available in the literature. A majority of an expert group using a Delphi approach believed that use of colonoscopy as an initial screening method would result in a probability of perforation of approximately 1 per 1,000 uses. Based on the Delphi approach, this best-guess estimate of the probability of perforation along with low and high realistic estimates were obtained.

Expert opinion here has been translated into what we previously called best-guess and realistic high and realistic low estimates. While expert opinion is not always converted into quantitative evidence, this example illustrates the degree to which evidence-based recommendations regard expert opinion as a form of data that needs to be systematically collected and presented.

37 Results

The results component of evidence-based guidelines consists of the synthesis of the evidence upon which recommendations can be based. Thus, when looking at results, we will focus on the strength of the evidence, the methods for addressing uncertainties in the evidence, and the options that were eliminated on the basis of the evidence.

Scoring the Strength of the Evidence

The overall quality of the evidence can be judged using the following key criteria:

1. Design and conduct of the investigations that produced the evidence
2. Relevance of the investigations to the target population
3. Coherence of the evidence or the absence of gaps in the evidence

We will refer to these criteria as design/conduct, relevance, and coherence. Let us see what is meant by each of these criteria.

The developers of guidelines need to begin by assembling the available investigations related to potential recommendations. As with a meta-analysis, it is important that they undertake a complete search of the available evidence.

Developers of guidelines often score or grade the research evidence using a hierarchy of research types, starting with the highest grade evidence:

- Randomized clinical trials
- Concurrent cohort studies
- Retrospective cohort studies and case-control studies

Lower grades of evidence use what is called a *time series*. In a time series there is no simultaneous control group. The study group after an intervention may be compared with its condition before the intervention, or the study group may be compared to historical controls. One form of time series is exemplified by the introduction of penicillin in the 1940, in which the dramatic results compared to previous treatment, at least in the short run, made clear the effectiveness of penicillin.

In evidence-based guidelines the lowest grade of evidence is reserved for respected authorities, descriptive studies, case reports, and even the report of expert committees.

Meta-analyses are often graded based on the types of investigations included in the meta-analysis. Thus a meta-analysis made up exclusively of randomized clinical trials would be considered stronger than a meta-analysis made up of retrospective cohort studies or case-control studies.

Design and Content

It is important to recognize, however, that the type of study design alone does not ensure the quality of the investigation. While concurrent cohort studies by definition lack randomization, their size and the efforts to identify and adjust for confounding variables may make up for this inherent limitation. Likewise, the inherent tendencies for biases in retrospective cohort studies and case-control studies may be partially or fully overcome by good study design. Thus, the authors of guidelines need to consider both the design and conduct of the investigations that produce the evidence used in evidence-based guidelines. Table 37.1 outlines the system of categorizing study design and conduct that has been used by the United States Preventive Services Task Force when grading the evidence.

Thus, in developing evidence-based recommendations, the first step is to determine the degree to which the key studies have study design types high in the hierarchy of research designs and are well-conducted studies. The USPSTF refers to this evaluation as determining *aggregate internal validity.* Specifically, aggregate interval validity is the degree to which the studies provide valid evidence for the population and the setting in which it is conducted.

Table 37.1. *Hierarchy of research designs*

Category of study design	Type of study design	Issues in conduct of the study
Category I	Evidence obtained from at least one properly randomized clinical trial	Statistical power, success of randomization, success of masking, completeness of follow-up, and clinical importance of the outcomes measured
Category II-1	Evidence obtained from well-designed studies without randomization (concurrent cohort studies)	Statistical power, comparability of study and control groups, completeness and length of follow-up, clinical importance of outcomes measured, adjustment for potential confounding variables
Category II-2	Evidence obtained from well-designed retrospective cohort or case-control studies	Comparability of cases and controls, biases in assessment, completeness of assessment, adjustment for potential confounding, variables, potential for reverse causality
Category II-3	Evidence obtained from multiple time series with vs. without the intervention, or dramatic results in uncontrolled experiments (such as the results of the introduction of penicillin treatment in the 1940s) could also be regarded as this type of evidence (dramatic changes in rates).	Quality of historical comparisons— short term before-and-after comparisons with clear-cut outcome measurements are more reliable.
Category III	Opinions of respected authorities based on clinical experience, descriptive studies, and case reports, or reports of expert committees	Was a method used to establish a consensus of expert opinion—i.e., was it representative of expert experience?

(Adapted from Agency for Healthcare Research and Quality, U.S. Preventive Services Task Force Guide to Clinical Preventive Services, Vol. 1, AHRQ Pub. No. 02-500.)

Table 37.2. *Factors affecting relevance of the evidence*

Factor	Meaning	Example
Patient relevance—biological analogy	Are there biological reasons to believe that the results obtained in a study will be different in another population?	Data on colon cancer might be extrapolated from men to women, but data on coronary artery disease might not be.
Patient relevance—demographic, risk, and clinical differences	Were the populations studied different from the populations for which the intervention is intended in ways that may affect the results?	Studies on older, severely ill patients may not apply to younger, generally healthy individuals.
Intervention relevance—relationship of the intervention to clinical practice	Was the intervention method used in the investigation similar to those routinely available or feasible in typical practice?	An investigation that used special equipment to monitor the patients, special incentive to increase adherence to treatment, or special methods to reduce or detect side effects may not be directly relevant to use in clinical practice.
Intervention relevance—relationship of the investigation's setting to clinical practice	Were the special characteristics of the research setting likely to affect the results?	Were differences such as availability of consultants, 24-hour coverage, or increased attention as part of research likely to alter the outcome in the usual clinical setting?

(Adapted from Agency for Healthcare Research and Quality, U.S. Preventive Services Task Force Guide to Clinical Preventive Services Vol. 1, AHRQ Pub. No. 02-500.)

Relevance

In addition to evaluating the quality of the investigations, it is also important to evaluate their relevance. Relevance refers to the degree to which the intervention studied is investigated in groups or populations that are similar to the populations of interest—that is, the target population for whom the intervention is intended. The USPSTF calls the evaluation of relevance *aggregate external validity.*[1]

Expert opinion may be needed to evaluate relevance. However, the process should begin by examining the evidence itself. To evaluate the relevance of an investigation, guideline developers need to ask such questions as: Are the types of patients studied and the methods used typical of the types of patients and methods that are encountered in typical clinical practice? For example, primary care practice if the intervention is designed for primary care. Table 37.2 summarizes the types of factors that can affect the relevance of an investigation and gives an example of each factor.

[1] The United States Preventive Services Task Force is interested in the applications of preventive services to primary care. Thus, they define aggregate external validity as the extent to which the evidence is relevant and generalizable to the population and conditions of typical primary care practice.

Coherence

Finally, in addition to evaluating the study design/conduct and relevance of the evidence, it is important ask what we will call coherence questions—does the evidence fit together? Coherent evidence requires that we ask:

- Are there gaps in the evidence or does the evidence hold together as a convincing chain demonstrating efficacy or contributory cause?
- Has it been demonstrated that the intervention actually improves important health outcomes?

We have already looked at these issues when we explored the criteria for efficacy. Thus, high-quality evidence should provide evidence of association, prior association, and altering the cause alters the effect. Investigations that fulfill the supportive or adjunct criteria we discussed in the Studying a Study section criteria may bolster the arguments for efficacy or causation when the definitive criteria are not established.

Ideally we want to be sure that clinically important endpoints are affected and not just early surrogate endpoints unless these surrogate endpoint can be shown to correlate closely with important clinical endpoints.

Grading System

Guideline developers thus need to combine considerations of design/conduct with questions of relevance and coherence to produce an overall measurement of the strength of the evidence. A grading system for the overall evidence has been used by the USPSTF. It classifies the overall quality of the evidence as:

- Good
- Fair
- Poor

Table 37.3 outlines the definition of each category of quality and the meaning of the category. When these summary judgments regarding the quality of the evidence are used, the reader of the guidelines needs to appreciate the types of reviews and conclusions that should lie behind the final score. For instance, image the following conclusions about the evidence:

> All available evidence was formally reviewed. The authors of the guidelines concluded that the quality of the evidence was good.

A conclusion of good evidence implies that a systematic effort was made to identify the evidence; the evidence was derived from high quality study types; and the investigations were well conducted. It also implies that the studies' populations were relevant to the guidelines, and the evidence produced a coherent conclusion that the intervention has effectiveness in practice. Thus, behind the increasingly common summary statement of good, fair, and poor quality lie a great deal of careful review plus, at times, considerable amounts of subjective judgment.

Table 37.3. *Grading the overall quality of the evidence*

Overall quality of the evidence	USPSTF definition	Meaning
Good quality	Evidence includes consistent results from well-designed, well-conducted studies in representative populations that directly assess effects on health outcomes.	When considering the design/conduct of the investigations, the relevance of the studies, and the coherence of the evidence, a convincing case for effectiveness in practice can be made.
Fair quality	Evidence is sufficient to determine effects on health outcomes, but the strength of the evidence is limited by the number, quality, or consistency of the individual studies, generalizability to routine practice, or indirect nature of the evidence on health outcomes.	When considering the design/conduct of the investigations, the relevance of the studies, and the coherence evidence, there are no fatal flaws or holes in the evidence that invalidate a conclusion of effectiveness in practice.
Poor quality	Evidence is insufficient to assess the effects on health outcomes because of limited number or power of studies, important flaws in their design or conduct, gaps in the chain of evidence, or lack of information on important health outcomes.	When considering the design/conduct of the investigations, the relevance of the studies, and the coherence of the evidence, there are fatal flaws or holes in the evidence that invalidate a conclusion of effectiveness in practice.

(Adapted from Agency for Healthcare Research and Quality, U.S. Preventive Services Task Force Guide to Clinical Preventive Services Vol. 1, AHRQ Pub. No. 02-500.)

Addressing Uncertainties

Because of the inherent limitation of the evidence and the need for subjective opinion when grading the evidence, it is important that guideline developers make efforts to address the uncertainties that inevitably remain.

As we saw in our discussion of decision analysis and cost-effectiveness analysis, one method for addressing the remaining uncertainties is sensitivity analysis. At times guidelines may be subjected to formal sensitivity analysis, especially when they are built upon decision trees or other formal quantitative decision models, as illustrated in the next example.

> The net effectiveness of virtual colonoscopy is not sensitive to whether or not the procedures were conducted every 5 or every 10 years. However, conducting virtual colonoscopy screening more frequently than every 5 years would substantially increase the costs, while conducting the screening less often than every 10 years would substantially reduce the net effectiveness.

More often, the remaining uncertainties are addressed subjectively, as illustrated in the next example.

> The success of colonoscopy as a screening technique for colon cancer is believed to be dependent on the availability of skilled colonoscopists who can rapidly and reliably examine the entire colon. Estimates of the number of currently available colonoscopists and the number that could be expected in the future based on current reimbursement rates led to the conclusion that colonoscopy was not an option that could be currently recommended for general use in screening.

Behind this type of result are a series of quantitative and subjective judgments that address the uncertainties regarding the usefulness of colonoscopy as a screening technique. This type of informal sensitivity analysis is often used to draw conclusions despite the uncertainty that remains.

Eliminating Options

The process of examining the results ends with an effort to determine whether any of the options being considered can be eliminated from further consideration. Eliminating options, like addressing uncertainties, may be done formally or informally.

The formal approach to elimination of options asks whether any of the options can be eliminated by what are called *dominance* and *extended dominance.* Let us see what we mean by dominance and extended dominance in the next example.

> When cost and net effectiveness were considered, double-contrast barium enema every 3 to 5 years was more expensive and less effective than flexible sigmoidoscopy every 3 to 5 years. Thus, double-contrast barium enema was eliminated from further consideration. Sigmoidoscopy every year was eliminated because it was more expensive and no more effective than sigmoidoscopy every 3 to 5 years plus fecal occult blood testing every year.

When one option is more effective and less expensive than another option, it is said to be dominant. The less effective and more expensive option is dominated by the more effective and less expensive option. Thus, the dominated option can be eliminated from further consideration, as illustrated in the example above for double-contrast barium enema.

Extended dominance usually implies that two options are approximately equally effective, but one options costs more to produce the same effect. The option that costs less is said to have extended dominance. Thus, in this example sigmoidoscopy every 3 to 5 years has extended dominance over sigmoidoscopy every year, and yearly sigmoidoscopy can be eliminated from further consideration.[2]

In summary, the results component of the M.A.A.R.I.E. framework for guidelines looks at the quality of the evidence, the efforts to incorporate remaining uncertainty, and the elimination of options. The results component is the basis for producing the evidence-based guidelines. However, before accepting these guidelines, we need to go on to examine the components of interpretation and extrapolation.

---

[2] This definition of extended dominance implies that net effectiveness is more important than cost as an initial criteria. Only if effectiveness is approximately equal is cost then taken into account. This reflect the approach often used in guideline development, though it is possible to envision an approach to extended dominance in which cost is considered first due to a fixed budget.

38 Interpretation

Interpretation asks us to look at the meaning of the guidelines for those for whom they are intended, the target population. To interpret the guidelines we need to look at the system used to score the strength of the recommendation. As we will see, this scoring system incorporates not only the quality of the evidence but the magnitude of the potential impact. In interpreting the recommendations we also need to look at what type of recommendation is being made and what assumptions are required to make the recommendations.

Strength of the Recommendation

Recommendations require more than quality evidence. They require conclusions about the magnitude of the impact on health outcomes. When the quality of the evidence is fair or good, then it is important to also make a judgment about the magnitude of the health benefit that can be expected for the average person for whom the service or intervention is recommended. Thus we need to ask not only does it work, but how well does it work? That is, does it have an important impact?

The magnitude of the effect may be classified in quantitative terms using measures such as odds ratios or relative risk, number needed to treat or lives saved, or quality adjusted life years. Any of these measures may be used, depending on the circumstances.

These quantitative measures are used by the USPSTF and other guideline developers as the basis for grading the magnitude of the effects:

- substantial
- moderate
- small
- zero/negative

Unfortunately, there are no accepted rules for what fulfills each of these grades. Thus, there is a role for subjective judgments. To better understand this process, let us take a look at how an intervention might be classified as substantial.

The overall grade needs to take into account both the harm and the benefit to produce a score for the net benefit (benefit minus harm). However, in classifying the magnitude of the effect, it is often useful to separately score the magnitude of the benefit and the magnitude of the harm.

The benefit may be substantial from an individual perspective if it has a large impact on an infrequent condition that poses a major burden at the individual patient level. PKU screening of newborn infants is an example of this type of impact.

Alternatively, the benefit may be considered substantial if it has at least a small relative impact on a frequent condition in a substantial population. Reducing coronary artery disease by increasing physical activity may be an example of this type of impact.

The magnitude of a harm may be substantial because it occurs frequently, such as the side effects of many medications. Alternatively, it may be substantial even when infrequent because of its life-threatening potential, such as anaphylaxis, aplastic anemia, or life-threatening arrhythmia.

In addition, when considering the harms of an intervention, the authors of the guideline need to define which harms are considered relevant. For instance, the USPSTF defines harms as including direct harm from the service, such as side effects and complications. It also takes into account what it calls the indirect harm, such as the consequences of increased follow-up testing and screening, psychological effects, and loss of insurability.

Scoring the overall magnitude of the intervention then requires the guideline authors to follow the basic steps we outlined in decision analysis. That is, they need to measure the benefits, measure the harms, and place a utility on the outcomes.

Thus, in making evidence-based recommendations it is often important to incorporate utilities. But whose utility? The USPSTF uses utilities reflecting the "general values of most people." When these are thought to vary greatly and when the variation is thought to affect the recommendation, then no recommendation is made for or against routine provision of the service.

Table 38.1 summarizes the approach used by the USPSTF.

Now we have seen the rather complicated steps that are needed to score the quality of the evidence and strength of the recommendation. Despite the complicated nature of the process, the net benefit may be presented using an overall grade of A, B, C, D, or I. Just as in many educational institutions, these overall grades reflect scores obtained along the way as well as a bit of subjective judgment. Like grades in courses, there is a category for incomplete, what is called "I" for insufficient. Table 38.2 indicates the grading categories used by the USPSTF. Notice that when the evidence it poor, the magnitude of the net benefit is "I".

Thus, behind the grading of the recommendation is considerable evidence as well as judgment. Increasingly, recommendations are presented with these letter scores, as illustrated in the next example.

> A recommendation for screening for colon cancer for all those over 50 received an overall grade of A. Several options were recommended as possible screening methods.

Note here that it is the overall recommendation for screening that receives the grade of A. The recommendation may go on to indicate the positive and negative aspects of different techniques but may not necessarily grade these or recommend one method over another.

Types of Recommendations

Classification of the recommendations is usually linked with specific implications for implementation. Recommendations may be classified as:[1]

- Standards
- Guidance
- Alternatives

[1] The term "guideline" is often used instead of guidance. Since "guideline" also refers to the overall set of recommendations its use in this context may cause confusion. The term "option" is often used rather than "alternative." Because "option" is used to indicate one particular intervention, it will not also be used to indicate that more than one option may be chosen.

Table 38.1. *Criteria for making evidence-based recommendations*

Criteria	Definition	Comments
Quality of the evidence	The overall evidence is classified as good, fair, or poor using the previous criteria to measure quality.	If the evidence is poor, there is no need to further consider recommendation. The recommendation is classified as "I" (insufficient evidence).
Magnitude of the benefit	The magnitude of the effect is classified as substantial, moderate, small, or zero/negative.	The benefit may be substantial from an individual perspective if it: • Has a large impact on an infrequent condition that poses a significant burden at the individual patient level (e.g., detection of PKU), or • Has at least a small relative impact on a frequent condition in a substantial population (e.g., reducing coronary artery disease).
Magnitude of the harm	The magnitude of the harm judged as substantial, moderate, small, or zero/negative.	Harm includes: • Direct harms are side effects and complications. • Indirect harms include consequences of follow-up testing and screening, psychological effects, and loss of insurability.
Net benefit	Combine the magnitude of the benefit and the magnitude of the harm plus the utility of the potential outcomes. Classify net benefit as substantial, moderate, small, or zero/negative	The USPSTF uses utilities reflecting the "general values of most people." When these are thought to vary greatly and when the variation is thought to affect recommendation, then no recommendation is made for or against routine provision of the service.

(Adapted from Agency for Healthcare Research and Quality, U.S. Preventive Services Task Force Guide to Clinical Preventive Services Vol. 1, AHRQ Pub. no. 02-500.)

"Standards" imply that the intervention is intended for routine use when specific conditions are met, i.e., it is expected that it will be implemented. Clinically, standards may be seen as indications. The implication is that a standard "must" be implemented.[2]

"Guidance" implies that the decision whether or not use an intervention depends on the presence or absence of indications plus contraindications. The implication of guidance is that an intervention "should" be performed unless a contraindication is present.

"Alternatives" imply that there is more than one potential intervention, none of which can be generally recommended over the others. The choice between intervention is made on the basis of individual preference. Thus, the implication of alternatives is that the intervention "may" be used.

---

[2] At times, standards may imply that an implementation must not be performed.

Table 38.2. *Classification of recommendations*

Quality of the evidence	Net benefit substantial	Net benefit moderate	Net benefit small	Net benefit zero/negative
Good	A	B	C	D
Fair	B	B	C	D
Poor	I	I	I	I

(Adapted from Agency for Healthcare Research and Quality, U.S. Preventive Services Task Force Guide to Clinical Preventive Services Vol. 1, AHRQ Pub. no. 02-500.)

The following example demonstrates how standards, guidance and alternatives can be presented in a guideline.[3]

> Screening for colon cancer is indicated for all those 50 years and over. It should generally employ a method that effectively screens both the proximal and distal colon and rectum. This may include yearly screening for fecal occult blood plus flexible sigmoidoscopy every 3 to 5 years, colonoscopy every 10 years, or virtual colonoscopy every 5 to 10 years.

This guideline incorporates standards, guidance, and alternatives. Screening is expected for all men and women 50 years and older. This implies that screening "must" be offered. Guidance is provided, recommending that a method of screening "should" be used that effectively screens both the proximal and distal colon plus the rectum. The use of "should" implies that contraindications to a complete screening of the colon may exist. Finally the guideline states three alternatives that "may" be used, implying that any of these methods fulfill the intent of the guideline.

The USPSTF has created a more formal set of levels of recommendation. These aim to address whether or not a service should be "routinely provided." Services that are routinely provided may be included in "periodic health examinations" or they may be "delivered in other contexts such as illness visits." Table 38.3 indicates the implications of the grades of A, B, C, D, and I.

Underlying Assumptions

The recommendations made as part of guidelines usually require the authors to make a number of assumptions related to the decision-making process employed by the users of guidelines. Thus, before completing the interpretation component we need to see if we can identify key assumptions and ask whether these are realistic.

As we saw in our review of decision analysis and cost-effectiveness analysis, quantitative decision-making requires the investigators to make a series of assumptions, many of which aim to simplify the process and enable the investigators to obtain the needed evidence. When the assumptions that underlie the evidence are not realistic, we need to question the meaning or interpretation of the guideline. While this may be the situation with any of the assumptions, two key assumptions are frequently violated. We will refer to these as the discounting and the risk-taking assumptions.

---

[3] Standards, guidance, and alternatives can be seen as having legal and financial implications. The implications of guidelines for malpractice and insurance coverage are still evolving and controversial. However, guidelines are increasingly being linked to coverage and liability decisions.

Table 38.3. *Levels of recommendation*

Levels of Recommendation	Action	Justification	Implications
A	USPSTF strongly recommends that clinicians routinely provide the service to eligible patients.	Good evidence of substantial health benefit	This category represents an evidence-based recommendation to provide the service on a routine basis to all those for whom it is intended.
B	USPSTF recommends that clinicians routinely provide the service to eligible patients.	The quality of the evidence is good or fair and the net benefit is at least moderate.	In this category a priority may be placed on A over B level services considering constraints of time and resources, i.e., costs.
C	The USPSTF makes no recommendation for or against routine provision of the service.	There is at least fair evidence but the balance of benefits and harms is too close to justify a general recommendation.	Clinicians may choose to offer the service on other grounds. For instance, an individual patient may be expected to gain greater benefit than the average patient observed in studies, or an individual patient's values or utilities are unusual enough to justify the service.
D	The USPSTF recommends against routinely providing the service to asymptomatic patients.	There is at least fair evidence that the service is ineffective (has zero net benefit) or that harms outweigh benefits.	This category represents an evidence-based recommendation not to provide the service on a routine basis.
I	The USPSTF concludes that the evidence is insufficient to recommend for or against routinely providing the service.	The evidence is classified as poor or conflicting and the balance of benefits and harms cannot be determined.	This category implies that an evidence-based recommendation cannot be made and decisions whether or not to provide the service must be made on grounds other than scientific evidence.

(Adapted from Agency for Healthcare Research and Quality, U.S. Preventive Services Task Force guide to clinical preventive services vol. 1, AHRQ Pub. no. 02-500.)

Discounting Assumption

As we have discussed as part of decision analysis and cost-effectiveness analysis, most people would prefer to receive $100 today rather than one year from now. This is true even if you are protected against inflation (and deflation). Not only is a dollar generally worth more today than next year, but so are the benefits of health. In general we'd rather pay off a $100 debt in one year rather than today, and we'd rather delay bad outcomes or harms if we can. This process of taking time into account is called discounting.

When formally synthesizing quantitative evidence, it is assumed that the discount rate used for benefits, harms, and cost is the same. As we have seen, the use of different discount rates artificially either encourages or discourages the use of a particular intervention. For instance, if we place a higher discount rate on benefits than we do on harms and costs, we will encourage the immediate use of interventions with immediate benefits and discourage the use of ones with delayed benefits.

Evidence-based studies and recommendations generally assume a 3% to 5% discount rate per year. A 5% discount rate implies that a benefit received, a harm suffered, or a cost paid one year from now has only 95% of the value as one that occurs in the immediate future.

Despite the fact that evidence-based studies use a relatively low discount rate and require the use of the same discount rate for benefits, harms, and costs, clinicians and patients may not agree with these rules. Let us see how this might happen, and the implications.

> Image that you have a disease that results in a 20% probability of death each year for two years. You have a choice between two options. In Option #1 you wait until the beginning of year #2 to take the treatment. Option #2 is given now, at the beginning of year #1. The interventions are identical except for the timing of the deaths and the occurrence of side effects that only occur with Option #2. Look at Figure 38.1 and choose Option #1 or Option #2.

Did you select Option #2? Many, if not most, people do. Selecting Option #2 implies that your discount rate is more than 10%, perhaps far more. That is, you place a greater value on benefits that occur immediately and less value on harms that occur in the future compared to the 3% to 5% discount rate used in evidence-based studies.

Option #1

Year #1	Year #2
20% death from	0% death from
the disease	the disease

Treat

Option #2

Year #1	Year #2
0% death from	20% death from
the disease	the disease
	and
	2% death from side effects

Treat

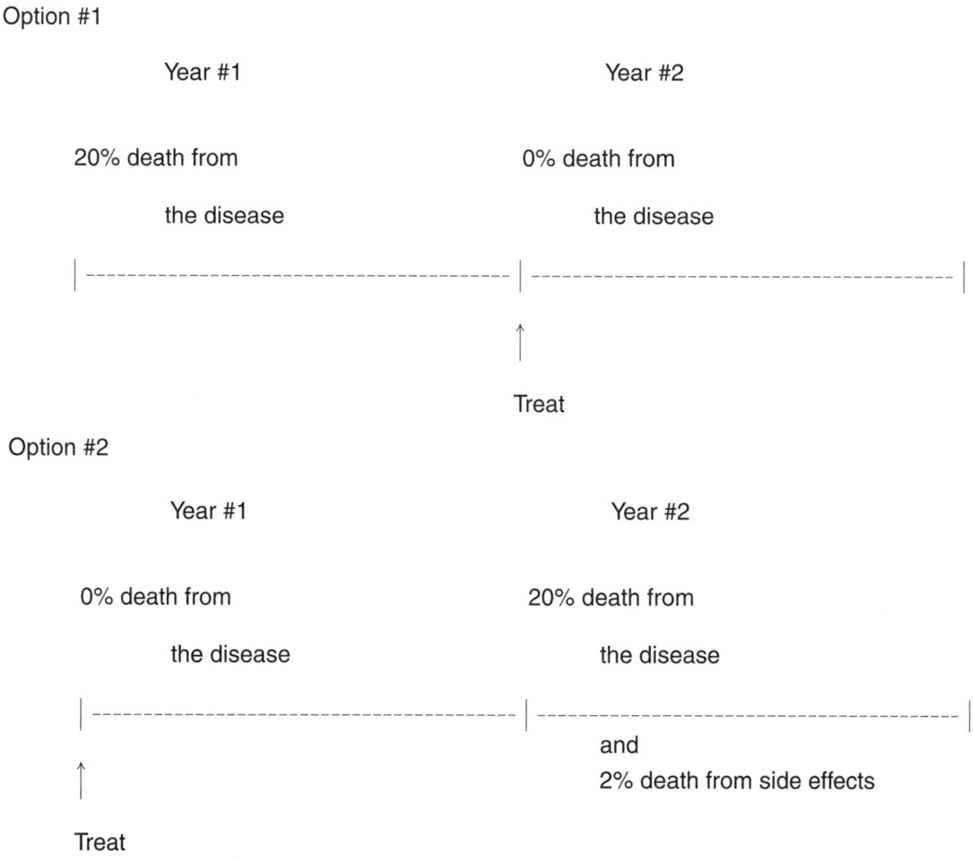

Figure 38.1. Comparison of two interventions.

Thus we need to recognize that many guidelines take a longer-term view than taken by individual patients or clinicians. Even when the development of guidelines complies with all of the recommended procedures for their development, they may not be consistent with the priorities of the decision-makers who often place great importance on short-term benefits.

Risk-Taking Assumptions

In addition to assuming a uniform discount rate for benefits, harms, and costs, guideline development often assumes what has been called *risk-neutrality*. Risk neutrality implies that decision-makers prefer the outcome that maximizes the probability of an outcome times its utility, i.e., its expected utility. This assumption is frequently violated because decision-makers do not seek only to maximize expected utility, they often make decisions suggesting that they are *risk-seeking* and at other times they are *risk-avoiding.*

Individual have their own patterns of risk-seeking and risk-avoiding; however, for most people the desire to take or avoid risk is very dependent on the type of situation and is thus predictable. To better understand this phenomenon, let us take a look at two situations that begin with different utilities.

Situation A
Let us imagine that you have coronary artery disease and have a reduced quality of life that has a utility of 0.8 compared to your previous state of full health that had a utility of 1.0. Imagine that you are offered the following pair of options. You can select only one of the options. Which do you prefer?

#1 Select a treatment with the following possible outcomes:
 50% chance of raising the quality of your health (your utility) from 0.8 to 1.0
 50% chance of reducing the quality of your health (your utility) from 0.8 to 0.6

#2 Refuse the above treatment and accept a quality of your health (your utility) of 0.8

Situation B
Let us imagine that you have coronary artery disease and have a reduced quality of life that has a utility of 0.2 compared to your previous state of full health that had a utility of 1.0. Imagine that you are offered the following pair of options. You can select only one. Which do you prefer?

#1 Select a treatment with the following possible outcomes:
 10% chance of raising the quality of your health (your utility) from 0.2 to 1.0
 90% chance of reducing the quality of your health (your utility) from 0.2 to 0.1

#2 Refuse the above treatment and accept a quality of your health (your utility) of 0.2

Did you answer # 2 in Situation A and # 1 in Situation B? Most, but not all, people do. To understand this exercise you need to appreciate that in terms of the evidence, as defined by expected utility, Option #1 and Option #2 are identical in each situation. That is, it is a "toss-up" between these two options when only probabilities and utilities are included, as demonstrated in Fig. 38.2 and Fig. 38.3. Thus, the evidence does not argue for one option over the other. The choice is really depend on your risk-taking attitude.[4]

---

[4] A minority of individual prefer Option #1 in both situations A and B. These individuals choose to take a risk even when confronted with a situation in which most people are risk-avoiders. These individuals have at times been termed risk-takers. Alternatively, a minority of individuals prefer Option #2 in both situations A and B. These individuals choose to avoid risk even when confronted with a situation in which most people would be risk-seekers. These individuals have at times been termed risk-avoiders.

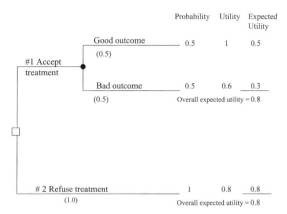

Figure 38.2. Decision tree for situation A showing that Option #1 and Option #2 are a toss-up in terms of expected utility.

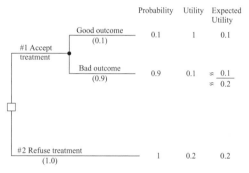

Figure 38.3. Decision tree for situation B showing that Option #1 and Option #2 are a toss-up in terms of expected utility.

What does it mean to choose Option #2 in Situation A and Option #1 in Situation B? In Situation A we begin with a utility of 0.8. For many people this is a tolerable situation and they do not want to take any chances that they may be reduced to a lower, intolerable utility. Thus they want to guarantee continuation at a tolerable level of health. This can be called the "guarantee effect."

In Situation B we begin with a utility of 0.2. For many people this is an intolerable situation. These people are usually willing to take their chances of getting even worse in the hopes of a major improvement in their health. When the quality of life is bad enough, most people are willing to take their chances and "go for it." This risk-taking behavior can be called the "long-shot effect."

Thus risk-seeking and risk-avoiding choices are both common, defensible, and reasonably predictably. Risk-seeking choices are particularly prominent among the severely ill, while risk-avoiding choices are particularly common among the healthy or asymptomatic.

Thus, it is important to recognize that recommendations that carry even a low probability of death or serious harm may be rejected by patients in generally good health. An option that carries a substantial probability of death or serious harm may be sought out by those who are seriously ill.

We need to recognize that most recommendations are made on the assumption of risk-neutrality, and decision-makers, be they clinicians or patients, often are not risk-neutral when they make decisions. It is not surprising that even the most formally constructed guidelines may not always make intuitive sense to patients and clinicians.

In this chapter we have examined the meaning of guidelines in terms of the strength of the recommendations, their implications for use, and the need to examine key assumptions of discounting for time and risk-taking. Now let us turn our attention to the implementation of guidelines, their extrapolation into practice.

39 Extrapolation and Questions to Ask

Extrapolation

Implementation of guidelines in clinical or public health practice requires us to ask how guidelines should be implemented; for what populations the guideline should be used; and whether there is a process for updating or revising the guidelines.

Implementation in Target Population

Issues of implementation may include methods for organizing the delivery of services, promoting the services to those most in need, documenting efforts to offer the service, etc.

The process of implementation of guidelines may be presented as an algorithm. Algorithms are usually constructed to provide a step-by-step decision-making process that is displayed as a graphical flowchart. Algorithms allow a visual display of the decision-making process recommended in a guideline. Algorithms may be quite complex. Regardless of the complexity, algorithms are constructed by using a set of rules much like the rules used in the construction of decision trees.

In algorithms:

- an ellipse states or defines the decision to be made
- six-sided figures incorporate questions that need to be answered
- boxes indicate an action that needs to be taken

By tradition, algorithms begin at the top and move down, indicating the ordering of the process.

As illustrated in Fig. 39.1, algorithms usually pose an issue such as: Should this patient be screened for colon cancer? They then ask specific question to determine whether a particular individual is a candidate for screening. This algorithm could be extended to decide between the potential forms of screening and what to do if the patient decides not to have a screening test.[1]

Methods for implementation also include issues that occur before or after the issues addressed by algorithms. For instance, how should patients be sought for screening or how should the decision be documented. Let us take a look at these types of issues in the next hypothetical example.

> Priority in screening programs for average-risk individuals should be on widely covering the population with at least one screening intervention rather than repeatedly screening the same individuals. Thus a reminder system should be implemented to identify and remind all those 50 years and over who have not received a recommended colon cancer screening test to make an appointment.

---

[1] Algorithms are often used to allow delegation of implementation to those with less training or experience. Algorithms are also used to clarify the underlying thinking process built into guidelines, identify possibilities that are not addressed by guidelines, or to teach the approach included in guidelines. Algorithms are only one method for implementation of guidelines.

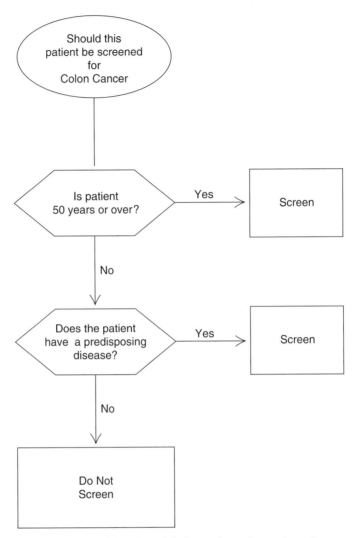

Figure 39.1. A simple algorithm that might be used to select patients for screening for colon cancer.

Algorithms usually address what to do when confronted with an individual patient. This implementation issue goes further. It addresses what should be done to identify patients and offer them screening. This type of implementation issue implies that organized health care delivery systems carry a responsibly that extends beyond a responsibility for those who present for care. This broadened responsibility may be incorporated into the methods for implementation.

At the other end of the process are issues of implementation related to documentation of what has or has not been done, as illustrated in the following hypothetical example.

Patients who are seen in primary care practice for other purposes should be advised to undergo a screening procedure at approximately age 50. Documentation that this advice was provided should be included in the patient's medical record. Those who indicate they do not wish to undergo screening should be asked to sign a release indicating that they have understood the recommendation and do not wish to undergo screening.

Thus, the processes for implementing guidelines goes beyond the guidelines themselves. They ask us to extrapolate guidelines into practice. When extrapolating into practice, we need to recognize that it is possible to extend the recommendations to those who were not included in the initial target population. Thus, we need to examine the extent to which guidelines are extended beyond the target population.

Implementation Beyond the Target Population

When actually implementing a guideline, as with extrapolation of investigations, it is important to consider whether the guideline is being extrapolated beyond the target population. This may be done by extending the recommendations to those at lower risk, perhaps younger or healthier patients, or to other countries or regions that have different prevalence or severity of a disease, as illustrated in the next example.

> The colon cancer screening guideline developed for the United States are also recommended for other developed countries with a high mortality rate from colon cancer, but were not recommended for less-developed countries and for populations with lower mortality rates from colon cancer.

This type of extrapolation is intentionally cautious. It is going beyond the data but recognizing the dangers of extrapolating conclusions between societies with very different distributions of disease and resources. A recommendation for widespread use of colon cancer screening would have requires a long list of questionable assumptions.

Review and Revision

As we have seen, the development of guidelines usually requires assumptions for which there is little or no data. In addition, uncertainty is often addressed by a subjective process such as the use of expert opinion. As time passes, evidence may be available that addresses these assumptions. In addition, new options may be available that have increased benefits or decreased harms or costs. Thus, it is important when examining a guideline to determine its publication date.

Guidelines should include a process and timetable for revision, as illustrated in the next example.

> Review of this guideline should occur after adequate evidence is available to assess the benefits, harms, and costs of virtual colonoscopy. The evidence of effectiveness of colonoscopy every 10 years compared to sigmoidoscopy every 3 to 5 years plus fecal occult blood testing every year should be reviewed in 5 years to determine whether use of these methods continues to be recommended.

The rapid pace of change that is going on in health and health care requires that most guidelines be formally reviewed either when specific data is available or on a set timetable. When a guideline is out-of-date, the reader of the guideline needs to be very cautious in accepting its conclusions.

As we have seen, guidelines have become a key method for integrating evidence into practice. The use of the M.A.A.R.I.E. framework can help us organize our approach to reviewing guidelines and help us identify their uses and limitations.

Questions to Ask: A Guide to the Guidelines

The following questions to ask can serve as a checklist when reading evidence-based guidelines.

Method: Guideline's purpose and target population

1. **Purpose:** What is the purpose of the guidelines?
2. **Target population:** What is the target population for whom the guidelines are intended?
3. **Perspective:** What is the perspective of the authors of the guideline?

Assignment: Options and evidence being considered

1. **Options:** What options are being considered?
2. **Structuring the evidence:** How is the evidence organized? e.g., Systematic review, meta-analysis, decision tree, etc.
3. **Types of evidence:** What types of evidence are being considered and how are they being combined?

Assessment: Presenting the evidence

1. **Sources of evidence:** What sources of evidence are used?
2. **Measurement of outcomes:** How are the outcomes measured?
3. **Filling holes in the evidence:** How are holes in the evidence addressed? e.g., expert opinion, consensus, conference, Delphi method, etc.

Results: Synthesizing the evidence

1. **Scoring the strength of the evidence:** Is a scoring system used to grade the strength of the evidence?
2. **Addressing uncertainties:** How are remaining uncertainties addressed? e.g., sensitivity analysis, subjective judgment, etc.
3. **Eliminating options:** What approach is used to eliminate options?

Interpretation: Making recommendations

1. **Strength of the recommendation:** Is a scoring system used to grade the strength of the recommendation?
2. **Types of recommendations:** What types of recommendations are made? e.g., standards, guidance, alternatives, etc.
3. **Underlying assumptions:** What assumptions are made in the recommendations? e.g., discounting, risk-taking, etc.

Extrapolation: Implementation

1. **Implementation in target population:** Do the recommendations include methods for implementation in the target population?
2. **Implementation beyond the target population:** Are recommendations made for implementation beyond the target population?
3. **Review and revision:** Is a timetable and an approach to revision of the guidelines presented?

Selecting a Statistic

VI

40 Basic Principles

The "Selecting a Statistic" section presents a method for organizing and understanding the use statistical techniques. It is designed to provide a step-by-step approach for selecting and interpreting commonly used statistical techniques. The following chapters present the components of the flowchart of statistics. The final chapter puts it all together in summary form and walks you through an example. To gain practice using the flowchart, the Studying a Study Online Web site at **www.StudyingaStudy.com** provides eight exercises that illustrate the use of the flowchart.

A series of basic principles underlie the choice of statistical techniques. As we have stressed, statistics have three purposes in the analysis of the results of health research:

1. Estimation: To make estimates of the strength of relationships or the magnitude of differences, i.e., effect size
2. Inference: To perform statistical significance testing. These tests allow us to draw inferences about a population from samples obtained from the same population, taking into account the influence of chance.
3. Adjustment: To adjust for the influence of confounding variables and interactions on the estimates and inferences.

In the "Selecting a Statistic" section, our goal is to provide insights about how statistics can be used to serve these purposes.

We must first recognize that the measurements taken on individuals in an investigation are a subset or *sample* of a larger group of individuals who might have been included in the investigation. This larger group is called the *population*.[1]

If we can plot the frequency with which different measurement values occur in the population, this provides a graphic representation of the *population's distribution of data*. A population's distribution of data tells us how frequently various data values occur in the larger population from which samples are drawn for observation (Fig. 40.1). Biostatisticians use the term *describe a distribution* when referring to the presentation of data on the larger population. Data in this graphic form, however, are difficult to communicate.

Rather than describing a population distribution graphically, statistical methods are concerned with summarizing as simply as possible the population's distribution of data. Every type of distribution of data has a limited number of summary values called *parameters* that are used to completely describe the particular distribution of

---

[1] In health research, we usually think of measurements being taken on persons rather than on animals or objects. This might lead us to the mistaken impression that the statistical use of the term "population" is the same as its use to describe a politically or geographically distinct collection of persons. Although the term "population" in statistics might be that type of collection, it is not limited to such. Rather, a population is defined as the collection of all possible measurements (not necessarily of persons) from which a sample is selected.

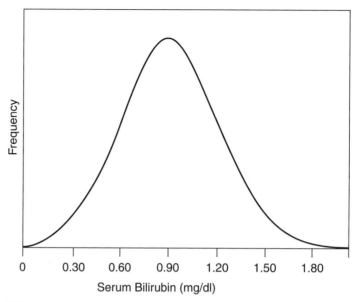

Figure 40.1. A hypothetical population distribution for serum bilirubin measurements.

data. For example, to completely describe a *Gaussian distribution,*[2] two parameters are needed—one measuring what is called *location* and the other measuring what is called *dispersion* or spread of the data. Two examples of these parameters are the *mean*[3] (the distribution's location along a continuum, or more specifically, its center of gravity) and the *standard deviation*[4] (the dispersion or spread of the distribution as indicated by how far from the mean individual measurements occur). Figure 40.2 shows a Gaussian distribution with the mean (μ) indicated as the measure of the distribution's location and the standard deviation as the measure of dispersion.

To demonstrate what is meant by the location of a distribution, let us assume that the mean serum bilirubin in the population is 1.2 mg/dL instead of 0.9 mg/dL. Figure 40.3 shows what the Gaussian distribution of serum bilirubin would be in this case.

Notice that the general shape of the distribution in Fig. 40.3 is unaltered by changing the mean, but the position of the center of gravity of the distribution is moved 0.3 mg/dL to the right.

If we changed the dispersion of the distribution in Fig. 40.2, however, the shape of the distribution would be altered without changing its position. For example,

---

[2] The Gaussian distribution is also known as the *normal distribution*. We avoid using that term because "normal" has an alternative meaning clinically. The Gaussian distribution is the most commonly assumed population distribution in statistics.

[3] The term *average* is often used as a synonym for the mean. In statistical terminology, these are not the same thing. A mean is calculated by summing all the measurements and dividing by the number of measurements. An average, on the other hand, is calculated by multiplying each of the measurements by particular values, called weights, before summing them. That sum is then divided by the sum of the weights. A mean is a special type of average in which the weight for every measurement is equal to 1.

[4] The standard deviation (σ) is the square root of the variance (σ^2). The variance is equal to the mean square deviation of data (χi) from the mean (μ). Therefore, the population standard deviation is equal to the square root of: $\Sigma(\chi i - \mu)^2 \sigma \div N$

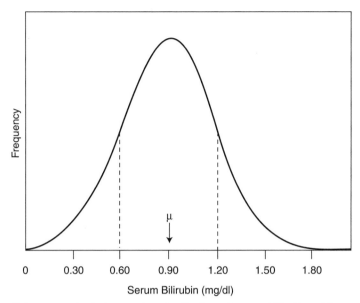

Figure 40.2. A hypothetical Gaussian distribution of serum bilirubin with a mean of 0.9 mg/dL and a standard deviation of 0.3 mg/dL. The broken lines indicate values equal to the mean ± 1 standard deviation.

compare the distribution in Fig. 40.2 to Fig. 40.4, in which the standard deviation has been changed from 0.3 mg/dL to 0.4 mg/dL.

We seldom are able to observe all the possible measurements in a population. That is, we are not able to fully describe a population. Using measurements observed in a sample from the larger population, however, we can calculate numerical

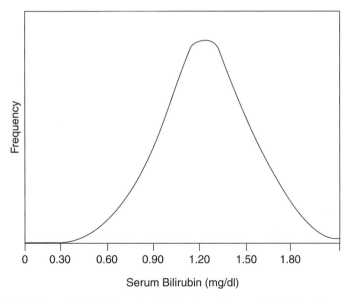

Figure 40.3. A hypothetical Gaussian distribution of serum bilirubin with a mean of 1.2 mg/dL and a standard deviation of 0.3 mg/dL. Comparison of this distribution with Fig. 40.2 shows what is meant by different locations of a population's distribution of data.

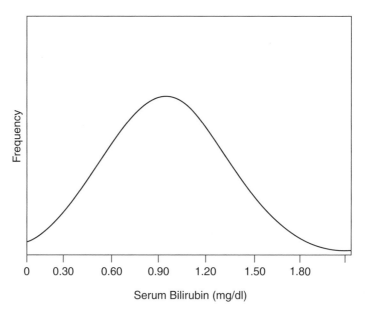

Figure 40.4. A hypothetical Gaussian distribution of serum bilirubin with a mean of 0.9 mg/dL and a standard deviation of 0.4 mg/dL. Comparison of this distribution with Fig. 40.2 shows what is meant by different dispersions of a population's distribution of data.

values to estimate the value of the larger population's parameters. These samples' estimates of a population's parameters are the focus of statistical methods. In fact, those estimates are called *statistics*. A single statistic used to estimate the numerical value of a particular population's parameter is known as a *point estimate*. These point estimates are the statistics we use to make estimates of the strength of relationships or magnitude of differences in the population.

As we have seen, a sample is a subset of all possible measurements from a population. For all statistical methods, it is assumed that the sample is a randomly chosen subset of the population from which it is drawn or obtained. Although random subsets can be obtained in several ways, in this section we consider only the simplest (and most common), called a *simple random sample*. In a simple random sample, all measurements in the population have an equal probability of being included.[5] Chance alone, then, dictates which measurements are actually included.

When a population's parameters are estimated using a sample's statistics, chance selection of the particular measurements to be actually included in the sample influences how close the sample's estimate is to the actual numerical values of the population's parameters. Unfortunately, we can never know how closely a particular statistic correctly reflects its corresponding population's parameter because we would have to measure the entire population to know the actual value of the parameter. What we can determine, however, is how much the statistics are expected to vary on the basis of chance variations among random samples. That knowledge forms the basis of statistical inference, or statistical significance testing.

[5] In a general sense, a *random sample* implies that any one individual in the population has a known probability of being included in the sample. Here, we are limiting those known probabilities to the condition that they are all equal to each other. Thus we are using a simple random sample.

The framework of statistical inference was described in Section I, "Studying a Study." We noted that statistical significance testing is performed under the assumption that the null hypothesis is true. The null hypothesis provides us with the hypothetical value with which our observed estimates can be compared. For instance, an odds ratio and a relative risk have a null hypothesis that their value is 1, while a difference has a null hypothesis that its value is 0.

We also noted in Section I that the bottom line in statistical significance testing is the *P* value.[6] *P* values are calculated from research observations or data by first converting the sample's estimate to an appropriate *standard distribution*. We use standard distributions to simplify calculations because the *P* values corresponding to any location in these distributions can be obtained from statistical tables. Much of what we consider to be the methodology and mathematics of statistics is related to converting estimates to a standard distribution in order to obtain *P* values.[7]

As we discussed in Section I, an alternative to using statistical significance testing to investigate the influence of chance on sample estimates is to calculate an interval estimate or confidence interval.[8] Within a confidence interval, we have a specified degree of confidence (often 95%) that the larger population's parameter value is included.[9] Commonly, confidence intervals are found by algebraically rearranging calculations used to perform statistical significance tests.[10]

When performing statistical significance tests or calculating confidence intervals, a *one-tailed* or a *two-tailed* procedure can be used. A two-tailed statistical significance test or confidence interval is used whenever the researcher cannot be sure whether the population's parameter is greater than or smaller than the value implied by the null hypothesis. That is the usual circumstance, but occasionally one encounters *one-tailed* statistical significance tests or confidence intervals in the health research literature. A one-tailed test or confidence interval is applicable when the investigator is willing to assume that the direction of the relationship being studied is known and analysis is concerned only with examining the size or strength of the relationship.

To illustrate the distinction between one- and two-tailed statistical procedures, imagine a randomized clinical trial in which we measure diastolic blood pressure for a group of individuals before and after treatment with an antihypertensive drug that has previously been demonstrated to be effective. Before examining the data resulting from the study, we might assume in our hypothesis that diastolic pressure will decrease when patients are on the drug. In other words, we might assume that it is impossible for the drug to cause an increase in diastolic blood pressure. With

---

[6] Recall that the *P* value is the probability of obtaining a sample at least as different from that indicated by the null hypothesis as the sample actually obtained if the null hypothesis truly describes the population. It is not, as often assumed, the probability that chance has influenced the sample observations. That probability is equal to 1 (i.e., we are certain that chance has influenced our observations).

[7] Examples of standard distributions include the standard normal, Student's *t*, chi-square, and *F* distributions. These distributions are discussed in later chapters.

[8] This interval is sometimes referred to as *confidence limits*. In statistical terminology, confidence limits are the numerical values that bound a confidence interval.

[9] In classic statistics, an *interval estimate* means that if we examine an infinite number of samples of the same size, a specified percentage (e.g., 95%) of the interval estimates would include the population's parameter. A more modern view among statisticians is that this is tantamount to assuming there is a specified chance (e.g., 95%) that the value of the population parameter is included in the interval. The latter interpretation is usually the one of interest to the health researcher.

[10] When confidence intervals are calculated from the same data as statistical significance testing, they are said to be *test-based*.

that assumption, statistical significance testing or confidence interval calculation can be one-tailed and the statistical power of our analysis increased. If, on the other hand, our study hypothesis is that a new antihypertensive drug will lower diastolic blood pressure, statistical significance testing or confidence interval calculation should be two-tailed. This is because we consider it to be possible, even though it might be unlikely, that a new antihypertensive drug would cause an increase in diastolic blood pressure. Notice that it is tempting for an investigator to use a one-tailed test because it increases the statistical power. Thus, one need to be cautious and thoroughly justify any use of one-tailed tests.

Selecting Statistical Methods

Let us take a look at the issues we need to address when selecting a statistical technique or evaluating a statistical technique used in a research article. When selecting a specific statistical method, statisticians think about *variables*. Variables represent data in the statistical method. For example, if we included measurements of age in our research, age would be represented by one of the variables in our statistical analysis. Once we understand what the variables are, we must make two decisions: (a) what is the function of each variable and (b) what type of data is represented by each of those variables. First, let us see what we mean by the function of a variable.

Most statistical methods distinguish between two potential functions *dependent* and *independent* variables. These are indications of the function of a variable in a particular analysis. Usually, a collection of variables that is designed to investigate a single study hypothesis contains only one dependent variable. That dependent variable can be identified as the variable of primary interest, or the outcome, or the endpoint of a study. Remember that in a case-control study, however, the dependent variable is the previous characteristic that is being assessed. We generally wish to test hypotheses or make estimates, or both, about that one dependent variable. There may be more than one outcome in an investigation; however, we usually analyze one outcome at a time.[11]

On the other hand, the collection of variables might contain no, one, or several independent variables. The independent variables reflect the study hypothesis plus potential confounding variables which need to be taken into account when hypotheses are to be tested and estimates are to be made. In addition, independent variables may include variables that examine the interactions between two independent variables.

To illustrate the distinction between dependent and independent variables, consider a cohort study in which the relationship between smoking and the probability of coronary artery disease is investigated. Suppose only two variables are measured on each individual: smoking (vs. not smoking) and coronary artery disease (vs. no coronary artery disease). To analyze those data, we first recognize that our primary interest is to test a hypothesis about the probability of coronary artery disease. Thus, coronary artery disease is the dependent variable. Further, we wish

---

[11] The use of statistical methods for adjustment and subsequent statistical significance testing has traditionally been the end of the process. It is advisable however, to regard the process as a first step in which the most important variables affecting an outcome are recognized. Once this is accomplished the investigator may also include additional variables that combine two of the existing variables to examine potential interactions between the variables. To be included, an interaction variable needs to be statistically significant which is quite unusual.

to compare the probability of coronary artery disease among smokers and non-smokers. Hence, smoking status is the independent variable.

After identifying the one dependent variable, the number of independent variables determines the category of statistical methods that is appropriate to use. For instance, if we are interested in estimating the probability of coronary artery disease in a community without regard to smoking status or any other characteristic of individuals, we would apply statistical procedures known as *univariable analyses*. These procedures are applicable to a set of observations that contains one dependent variable and no independent variables. To examine the probability of coronary artery disease relative to smoking status, however, we would use methods called *bivariable analyses*. These methods are applied to collections of observations with one dependent variable and one independent variable. Finally, if we were interested in the probability of coronary artery disease for individuals of various ages, genders, and smoking habits, we would apply *multivariable analyses*.[12] These methods are used for sets of observations that consist of one dependent variable and more than one independent variable. Multivariable methods are frequently used to accomplish our third goal of statistical methods: to adjust for the influence of confounding variables.

Health research investigations often include several sets of variables. For example, suppose we have conducted a randomized clinical trial in which subjects received either drug X or a placebo and are cured or not cured of a particular disease. Because we were concerned about the influence of age and gender on cure (i.e., we were concerned that age and gender differences might be confounding variables), we included them in our research records. Therefore, our study contains four variables: treatment (drug X or placebo), cure (yes or no), age, and gender. The collection that includes all four variables would have cure as the variable of interest; thus, cure would be the dependent variable. Treatment, age, and gender would be independent variables, reflecting our interest in examining cure relative to the specific treatment received and the subject's age and gender.

Even before testing hypotheses about cure, however, we would likely be interested in whether randomization achieved similar age distributions in the two treatment groups. The collection of variables that would allow us to compare age distributions contains age as the dependent variable and treatment group (drug X or a placebo) as the independent variable. Here age is the variable of interest and treatment is the condition under which we are assessing age. Thus, here the independent and dependent variables are reversed. The decision about which is the dependent variable and which is the independent variable depends on the question being asked.

Types of Data

In order to select a statistical technique, we not only need to characterize the function of the variables in an analysis, we must determine the type of data contained in

---

[12] A common error in the use of statistical terminology is to refer to procedures designed for one dependent variable and more than one independent variable as *multivariate analyses*. This term, however, properly refers to procedures designed for more than one dependent variable. The use of multivariate procedures, such as discriminate analysis, is typically rare in health research. Discriminant analysis, however, may be used when there is only one outcome being measured but it is represented by nominal data that must be represented by more than one nominal variable. Note that multivariate procedures are not included in the flowchart.

the measurement of each variable. To categorize types of data, the first distinction we make is between *continuous* and *discrete* data.

Continuous data are defined as data that provide the possibility of observing any of an infinite number of equally spaced numerical values between any two points in its range of measurement. Examples of continuous data include blood pressure, serum cholesterol, age, and weight. For each of these variables, we can choose any two numerical values and imagine additional intermediate measurements that would be, at least theoretically, possible to observe between those values. We might, for instance, consider the ages of 35 and 36 years. We could think of different ages between 35 and 36 that are distinguished by the number of days since a person's 35th birthday or the number of hours or minutes since that birthday. Theoretically, there is no limit to how finely we can imagine time being measured. Notice, however, that continuous data do not need to have an infinite range of possible values but rather an infinite number of possible values within their range. That range may, and usually does, have a lower and an upper boundary. Age is a good example. The lower boundary is zero, and it is difficult to imagine individuals much older than 120 years.

Discrete data, on the other hand, can have only a limited number of values in their range of measurement. Examples of discrete data include number of pregnancies, stage of disease, and gender. For each of these variables, we can generally select two values between which it is not possible to imagine other values. For instance, there is no number of pregnancies between two and three pregnancies.

In practice, the distinction between continuous and discrete data is often unclear. For one thing, no variables exist for which we can actually measure an infinite number of values.[13] We solve this problem by recognizing that, if a great number of measurements can be made and if the intervals between measurements are uniform, then the measurements are nearly continuous. This, however, creates another source of confusion in that it allows data that are theoretically discrete to be redefined as continuous. For example, the number of hairs on one's scalp is certainly discrete data: We cannot imagine observing a value between 99,999 and 100,000 hairs. Even so, the number of possible numerical values within the entire range of the number of hairs is very great. Can we consider such a variable to be composed of continuous data? Yes, for most purposes that would be entirely appropriate.

Data can be defined further by their scale of measurement. Continuous data are measured on scales, called *ratio* or *interval scales*,[14] that are defined as having a uniform interval between consecutive measurements. As opposed to continuous data, some types of discrete data measurements are made on an *ordinal scale*. Data on an ordinal scale have a specific ranking or ordering, as do continuous data, but the interval between consecutive measurements is not necessarily known or constant. A common sort of variable measured on an ordinal scale is an ordering of the stage of disease. We know, for instance, that stage 2 is more advanced than stage 1, but we cannot assert that the difference between the two stages is the same as the difference between stage 3 and stage 2.

---

[13] For example, we might imagine but could not determine blood pressure in picometers of mercury. So, in reality, all data are discrete.

[14] The distinction between the ratio scale and the interval scale is that the former includes a true zero value whereas the latter does not. Certain types of discrete data, such as counts, have uniform intervals between measurements and, therefore, are measured in ratio or interval scales. Other types of discrete data, however, are measured either on an ordinal or a nominal scale.

If we are unable to apply any ordering to discrete data, then we say that the data were measured on a *nominal scale*. Examples of characteristics composed of nominal scale discrete data are treatment, gender, race, and eye color. Additional data that we treat as nominal data include measurements with two categories even though they might be considered to have an innate order because one is clearly better than the other (e.g., alive vs. dead).

Note that the term "nominal variable" can be confusing. In its common use, a nominal variable is a characteristic, such as gender or race, that has two or more potential categories. From a statistical point of view, however, one nominal variable is limited to only two categories. Thus, race or eye color should be referred to as nominal data that require more than one nominal variable for inclusion in statistical procedures. The number of nominal variables required is equal to the number of categories of the nominal data minus one. Thus, if we have data on gender with two genders, we require only one nominal variable, but if we have data on race with five races we require four nominal variables.

Thus, for purposes of selecting a statistical procedure or interpreting the result of such a procedure, it is important to distinguish between three categories of variables:

1. Continuous variables: includes continuous data, such as age, and discrete data that contain a great number of possible values, such as number of hairs;
2. Ordinal variables: includes discrete data that can be ordered one higher than the next and with at least three and at most a limited number of possible values, such as stages of cancer;
3. Nominal variables: includes discrete data that cannot be ordered, such as race, and dichotomous data that can assume only two possible values, such as dead or alive.

The order in which those categories are listed indicates the relative amount of information contained in each type of variable. That is, continuous variables contain more information than ordinal variables, and ordinal variables contain more information than nominal variables. Thus, continuous variables are considered to be at a higher level than ordinal or nominal variables.

Measurements with a particular level of information can be rescaled to a lower level. For example, age (measured in years) is a continuous variable. We could legitimately rescale age to be an ordinal variable by defining persons as being children (0–18 years), young adults (19–30 years), adults (31–45 years), mature adults (46–65 years), or elderly adults (>65 years). We could rescale age further to be a nominal variable. For instance, we might simply divide persons into two categories: young and old, or children and adults. We cannot, however, rescale variables to a higher level than the one at which they were actually measured.

When we rescale measurements to a lower level, we lose information. That is, we have less detail about a characteristic if it is measured on a nominal scale than we do if the same characteristic was measured on an ordinal or continuous scale. For example, we know less about a woman when we label her a mature adult than we do when we say that she is 54 years old. If an individual is 54 years old and we measured age on a continuous scale, we could distinguish that person's age from another individual who is 64 years old. However, if age was recorded on the ordinal scale above, we could not recognize a difference in age between those individuals.

Loss of information, when rescaled measurements are used in statistical procedures, has the consistent effect, all else being equal, of increasing the Type II error rate. That is to say, rescaling to a lower level reduces statistical power, making it harder to establish statistical significance and, thus, to reject a false null hypothesis. What we gain by rescaling to a lower level is the ability to circumvent making certain assumptions, such as uniform intervals, about the data that are required to perform certain statistical tests. Specific examples of tests that require and those that circumvent such assumptions will be reviewed in greater detail in following chapters in this section.

Thus far, we have reviewed the initial steps that must occur in selecting a statistical procedure. These steps are:

1. Identify one dependent variable and all independent variables, if present, on the basis of the study question.
2. Determine for each variable whether it represents continuous, ordinal, or nominal data.

Having completed these steps, we are ready to begin the process of selecting a statistic.

The Flowchart

The remaining chapters of this section are arranged as branches of a flowchart designed to facilitate selection and interpretation of statistical methods. Most statistical procedures that are frequently encountered in health research have been included.

To begin use of the flowchart (Fig. 40.5), an investigator must first determine which of a set of variables is the dependent variable. If the set contains more than one dependent variable, an investigator can analyze the data using one of the dependent variables at a time.[15] If the set seems to contain more than one dependent variable, the data may address more than one study hypothesis. In that case, the relevant dependent variable and independent variables for a specific study hypothesis should be identified.

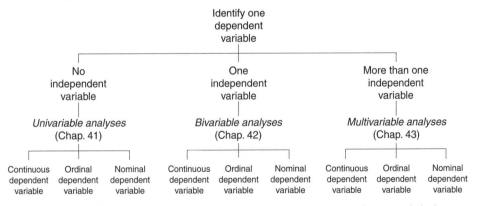

Figure 40.5. Flowchart to determine the chapter and division that discuss statistical procedure relevant to a particular set of variables.

[15] Alternatively, an investigator can use multivariate procedures such as discriminant analysis or factor analysis.

Once a single dependent variable has been identified, the investigator identifies the remaining variables as the independent variables. The investigator can use the number of independent variables in the investigation to locate the chapter that discusses this number of independent variables, i.e., no, one, or more than one. Each chapter contains three major divisions. The first is concerned with sets of variables in which the dependent variable is continuous. The second division addresses ordinal dependent variables, and the third addresses nominal dependent variables. Within each division, techniques for continuous, ordinal, and nominal independent variables, if available, are discussed.

As a reader of the literature, it is possible for you to use the flowchart in reverse. That is, you can identify a statistical technique or procedure used in a research article. You can then locate this procedure at or near the end of the flowchart. This will allow you to work backward through the flowchart to better understand whether the technique is appropriate and what type of question it addresses.

41 Univariable Analysis

If a set of measurements contains one dependent variable and no independent variables, the statistical methods used to analyze these measurements are a type of *univariable analysis*. Three common uses of univariable analysis methods are found in the health literature. The first use is in descriptive studies (e.g., case series) in which only one sample has been examined. For example, a researcher might present a series of cases of a particular disease, examining various demographic and pathophysiologic measurements on those patients.

The second common application of univariable analysis is when a sample is drawn for inclusion in a study. For example, before randomization in a randomized clinical trial, we might want to perform measurements on the entire sample chosen for study. That is, we may want to determine the mean age and percentage of women in the group selected to be randomized before they are assigned to a study or control group.

Usually, in descriptive studies and when examining one sample, the interest is in point estimation and confidence interval estimation rather than statistical significance testing. Tests of hypotheses are possible in the univariable setting, but one must specify, in the null hypothesis, a value for a population's parameter. Often, it is not possible to do this in a univariable analysis. For example, it is difficult to imagine what value would be hypothesized for prevalence of hypertension among individuals in a particular community.[1]

The third application of univariable analysis is one in which such a hypothesized value is easier to imagine. That is the case in which a measurement, such as diastolic blood pressure, is made twice on the same, or very similar, individuals, and the difference between the measurements is of interest. In that application, it is logical to imagine a null hypothesis stating that the difference between measurements is equal to zero. Thus, the difference in diastolic blood pressure measurements is the dependent variable. Even though the difference, by its nature, is a comparison of groups, differences themselves are not compared between any groups. Therefore, there is no independent variable. When comparing two measurements of the same characteristic on the same, or very similar, individuals, we are dealing with a univariable problem. Thus, in an investigation using paired data in which the measurement on each pair constitutes one observation, the data are analyzed using univariable methods. Thus in univariable analysis the data may come from one individual or from two individuals who are paired as part of the study design.

In Chapter 40 we learned that the first steps in choosing a statistical procedure are:

---

[1] At first, it may seem that a null hypothesis might state that the prevalence in a particular community is equal to the prevalence in some other community or the prevalence estimated in another study. It is important to keep in mind, however, that the value suggested for a population's parameter in a null hypothesis must be known without error. That will not be true unless all members of the comparison community were included in the calculation of prevalence.

1. Decide which variable is the dependent variable.
2. Determine how many, if any, independent variables the set of observations contains.
3. Define the type of data represented by the dependent variable as being continuous, ordinal, or nominal.

Now we are ready to use the first of our flowcharts. Each flowchart in the chapters in this section begins at the top by indicating the types of variables used for the dependent and independent variables (if any). They then indicate the estimate, point estimate, or the measurement used to summarize the data. At the bottom of each flowchart is the general category of statistical technique that is most frequently used to calculate confidence intervals or test hypotheses by statistical significance testing. A box in between indicates the name of the general category of statistical procedures that identify the approach being used.

Continuous Dependent Variable

If we follow the flowchart in Fig. 40.5 down to univariable analyses, we can continue by using Fig. 41.1. If we are interested in a continuous dependent variable, we are led to the mean.[2] The mean is the point estimate of interest when we have a continuous dependent variable and no independent variable. Next we note "paired tests" enclosed in a box followed by "Student's t test" that is underlined. In this and subsequent components of the flowchart, boxes indicate, if applicable, general categories of statistical methods, and underlining indicate specific procedures that are used for statistical significance testing or calculating confidence intervals.

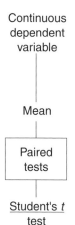

Figure 41.1. Flowchart to select a univariable statistical procedure for a continuous dependent variable (continued from Fig. 40.5).

---

[2] In univariable analysis of a continuous dependent variable, data are usually assumed to come from a population with a Gaussian distribution. Therefore, the mean is commonly used to measure location. The sample's estimate of the population's mean is usually the estimate of primary interest. The flowchart focuses on our interest in the mean. Dispersion of Gaussian distributions is measured by the standard deviation or, alternatively, by the standard deviation squared, which is called the *variance*. Estimates of the standard deviation and the variance or other measures of dispersion are not listed in the flowcharts. Estimates of dispersion are usually used to take into account the role of chance in estimating the location of the population's distribution. They are not, by themselves, frequently estimates of primary interest.

To calculate a confidence interval for the mean of a sample, the *Student's t distribution* is most often used. The Student's *t* distribution is a standard distribution to which means of continuous dependent variables are converted to make calculations easier.[3]

The Student's *t* distribution allows us to derive confidence intervals based on the observed mean and the *standard error.* The standard error measures the spread or dispersion in the mean that we would expect if all possible samples of the same size as the one actually obtained were drawn from the population. The standard error of a mean becomes smaller as the sample's size grows larger. More specifically, the standard error is equal to the standard deviation divided by the square root of the sample's size. Thus, the larger the sample's size the more closely the sample's mean can be expected to be to the population's mean.

The standard error is used with the Student's *t* distribution in calculating interval estimates for means of continuous variables. The confidence interval for a mean is equal to the sample's estimate of the mean $\pm$ the Student's *t* value for the desired level of confidence multiplied by the standard error. For a 95%, two-tailed estimate, the Student's *t* value is approximately equal to 2 for sample sizes of 20 or more. By adding and subtracting a value equal to twice the standard error to the point estimate of the mean, one can determine an approximate confidence interval when the sample size is 20 or greater. That is tantamount to saying, with 95% confidence, that the population's mean lies within the interval limited by the sample mean $\pm$ two standard errors.[4] For example, if we read in a research report that the mean $\pm$ the standard error for serum cholesterol in a sample is equal to 150 $\pm$ 15 mg/dL, we can be 95% confident that the population mean lies within the approximate interval from 120 to 180 mg/dL.

As we discussed at the beginning of this chapter, there is a special case of a univariable analysis in which statistical significance testing is applicable. The most common example is a study in which a continuous dependent variable is measured twice in the same individual. For instance, we might measure blood pressure before and after a patient receives an antihypertensive medication. If our interest is not really in the actual measurements before and after treatment but rather in the difference between those measurements, we have a paired design. This is a univariable problem because the dependent variable is the difference between measurements and no independent variable exists. By using a paired design and having each individual serve as their own control, we have attempted to remove the influence of variation between subjects in the initial, or baseline, measurement.

A Student's *t* distribution is used to test hypotheses or construct confidence intervals for continuous data from a paired design in the same way it is used for other univariable analyses. Although the statistical procedures used to analyze data

---

[3] The Student's *t* distribution is like the Gaussian distribution, but it requires an additional parameter known as *degrees of freedom.* The purpose of degrees of freedom in the Student's *t* distribution is to reflect the role of chance in estimation of the standard deviation. Use of the Student's *t* distribution to make interval estimates for means or for statistical significance testing recognizes the fact that the standard deviation is estimated from the sample. That is, the standard deviation is not precisely known. The degrees of freedom for a univariable sample of a continuous variable equals the sample's size minus one.

[4] Other confidence intervals can, likewise, be estimated by considering multiples of the standard error. More than 99% of possible sample estimates of the mean are included within the range of the population mean $\pm$ 3 standard errors. This assumes that the population of all possible means has a Gaussian distribution. This is in fact the case for a large number of samples. This can be demonstrated by using the central limit theorem.

collected in a paired design are no different from other univariable procedures, they are often given separate treatment in introductory statistics texts. In those cases, the procedure for examining the mean difference in data from a paired design is called a *paired* or *matched Student's t test*.[5]

The sample mean $\pm$ the standard error communicates how confident we can be in our estimate of the population's mean. Remember that the standard error is an indicator of the dispersion of all sample means that might be obtained by sampling the population repeatedly, each time obtaining a sample of the same size.

Rather than the sample mean $\pm$ the standard error, we often see univariable data presented as the sample mean $\pm$ the standard deviation. The sample mean $\pm$ the standard deviation addresses a different issue. The standard deviation estimates, using the sample's data, the dispersion of measurements in the larger population. That is, the dispersion of the one particular sample's data is the best available estimate we have available of the actual dispersion in the larger population. Approximately 95% of the data values in a population distribution occur within the range of the population mean $\pm$ 2 standard deviations.[6]

Therefore, when using univariable statistical procedures for a continuous dependent variable, we may be interested in estimating the location of the population's mean and, thus, in the observed mean and standard error. Alternatively we may be interested in estimating the dispersion of measurements in the population and, thus, in the observed mean and standard deviation.

Ordinal Dependent Variable

Univariable statistical methods for ordinal dependent variables are presented in Fig. 41.2. Unlike continuous variables, we do not assume a particular distribution of population data, such as a Gaussian distribution, for ordinal variables. Methods used for ordinal variables are, thus, referred to as *distribution-free* or *nonparametric*. It is important to realize, however, that these procedures are not assumption-free. For example, we continue to assume that our sample is randomly sampled or representative of some population of interest.

Because we are not assuming a particular distribution of the population's data measured on an ordinal scale, we cannot estimate the population's parameters that summarize the distribution. As a substitute we can identify the location of ordinal data along a continuum. We can do that with the *median*. The median is the midpoint of a collection of data, selected so that half the values are larger and half the values are smaller than the median.[7] The median will equal the mean when the

---

[5] It is important to recognize that the matched Student's *t* test is actually only applicable when pairing is applied. The use of the term "matching" is confusing because it may also apply to the situation when participants in an investigation are chosen to ensure balance between groups by age, gender, or other factors. We referred to this type of matching as group matching. Paired or matched statistical methods are not applicable when group matching has occurred.

[6] About two-thirds of the population data occur within the mean ± 1 standard deviation, and more than 99% occur within the mean ± 3 standard deviations. To apply these interpretations, we assume that the population's data have a Gaussian distribution.

[7] No theoretical population distribution has the median as its measure of location, but it can be used as an estimate of the mean of a Gaussian distribution. The median circumvents an assumption we make when calculating the mean. That assumption is that intervals between measurements in a distribution are known and uniform. Since the median is calculated using only the relative rank or order of the measurements, the same median would be estimated regardless of whether or not those intervals are known or uniform. Therefore, we can use the median to estimate the mean of a population of continuous data.

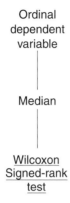

Ordinal
dependent
variable

Median

Wilcoxon
Signed-rank
test

Figure 41.2. Flowchart to select a univariable statistical procedure for an ordinal dependent variable (continued from Fig. 40.5). In this and subsequent components of the flowchart, the underlining indicates the name of the most commonly used procedure for significance testing and calculation of confidence intervals.

population has a symmetric distribution, as illustrated in Fig. 41.3A, but not when the distributions are asymmetrical as illustrated in Fig. 41.3 B and C.

Looking at the bottom of the flowchart in Fig. 41.2, we see *Wilcoxon signed-rank test* underlined. This is the statistical significance test that would be used to test the null hypothesis that the median equals zero in a univariable analysis. For instance in an investigation of the estimated stage of disease before and after a surgical staging procedure, the null hypotheses may be zero change in stage.

Nominal Dependent Variable

A single *nominal dependent variable* represents data in which a condition exists or, by default, that it does not exist. Examples of nominal dependent variables include dead/alive, cured/not cured, and disease/not disease. The amount of information contained in a single nominal dependent variable is quite limited compared with continuous dependent variables, such as age, or with ordinal dependent variables, such as stage of disease.

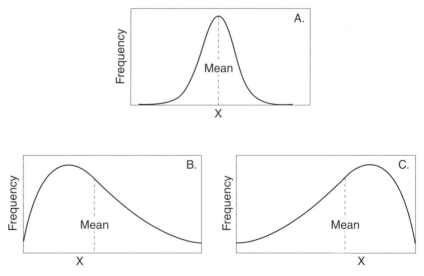

Figure 41.3. Location of the mean for (**A**) symmetric and (**B, C**) asymmetric distributions. X indicates the location of the median.

For each measurement or observation of a variable composed of nominal data, we determine only the presence or absence of the condition. For example, we might determine whether an individual in a sample has a particular disease. For a sample consisting of more than one observation, we can estimate the *frequency,* the number of times the condition occurs in the population. For instance, we can estimate the number of persons in the population with a particular disease. Most often, we are interested in the frequency relative to the total number of observations. If we divide the number of times a particular condition is observed in a sample by the total number of observations in that sample, we have calculated the *proportion* of observations in the sample with the condition. A proportion calculated from the sample's observations is a point estimate of the proportion of the population with the condition. An equivalent way to interpret the sample's proportion is that it estimates the *probability* of the condition occurring in the population. Two commonly encountered proportions or probabilities in health research are prevalence and case fatality.

Probabilities do not have a Gaussian distribution. They are assumed to have either a *binomial* or *Poisson distribution*. A binomial distribution is generally applicable to any probability calculated from nominal data when the observations are independent of one another. By independent, we mean that the result of one observation does not influence the result of another. The binomial distribution is a standard distribution that can be used to calculate *P* values for statistical significance tests and to calculate confidence intervals.

A Poisson distribution is a special case of a binomial distribution that is used when the nominal event, such as disease or death, is rarely observed and the number of observations or potential events is great. The Poisson distribution is computationally simpler than the binomial distribution. It generally provides a good approximation of the binomial distribution when the number of individuals observed with the condition is less than or equal to 5 and the total number of individuals in a sample is greater than or equal to 100. Thus Poisson distribution is commonly used for rates of disease.

Calculating confidence intervals or performing statistical significance tests for nominal dependent variables becomes feasible when the binomial and Poisson distributions can be approximated by the Gaussian distribution. This is often called a *normal approximation,*[8] and it can be performed if the number of individuals with a condition, i.e., the event, is greater than 5 and the number of observations, i.e., the potential events, is greater than 10.

Rates

In statistical terminology, the term *rate* is reserved to refer to a measurement which includes a measure of time. We have called this a true rate. It is important to distinguish a rate from a proportion. Rates, unlike proportions, are affected by

---

[8] In a normal approximation to a binomial or Poisson distribution, we only need to estimate the probability of observing the event because the standard error is calculated from that probability. This is unlike using the Gaussian distribution for continuous variables where we must make separate estimates of location and dispersion. As a result, it is not necessary or even appropriate to use the Student's *t* distribution to take into account, through degrees of freedom, the precision with which dispersion has been estimated. Rather, the standard normal distribution is used. Thus, one can calculate the confidence interval of a proportion using a Poisson distribution if one knows only the frequency of the event. The rule of three is a special case of this 95% confidence interval when the frequency of the event is 0.

the length of time that is used in measuring the events. The key to identifying a rate or true rate is to ask whether the number of events is affected by the duration of observation, i.e., more events occur in 2 years than 1 year. The most common measurement of interest in health research that meets the statistical definition of a rate is the incidence rate.

Because diseases usually occur infrequently per unit of time, rates are often assumed, in univariable analysis, to have a Poisson distribution. Statistical significance tests and determination of confidence intervals for rates usually rely on a normal approximation. Thus, procedures for rates are the same as those used for probabilities, except that statistical significance testing and confidence interval determinations, if performed, use the Poisson distribution or its normal approximation.

Figure 41.4 summarizes the decisions that need to be made when choosing which measurement to use for estimation and for statistical significance testing or calculating confidence intervals with one nominal dependent variable. To continue down the flowchart we need to determine whether the measurement is a true rate, i.e., it is affected by time or a proportion, i.e., it is not affected by time. The underlined procedures at the bottom of the flowchart indicate those used for statistical significance testing and calculating confidence intervals.

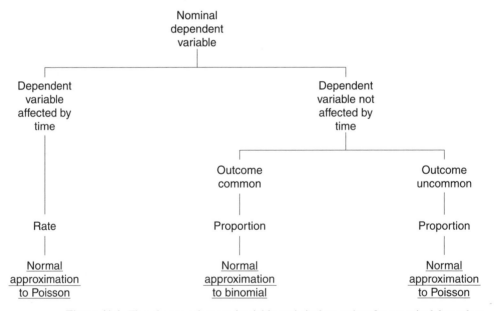

Figure 41.4. Flowchart to select a univariable statistical procedure for a nominal dependent variable (continued from Fig. 40.5).

42 Bivariable Analysis

In bivariable analysis, we are concerned with one dependent variable and one independent variable. In addition to determining the type of dependent variable being considered, it is necessary, when choosing an appropriate statistical procedure, to identify the type of data represented by the independent variable. The criteria for classifying independent variables are the same as those previously discussed for dependent variables, for example, nominal data such as race. If the data is represented by more than one independent variable, bivariable analysis is not used.

Methods for univariable analysis are largely concerned with calculating confidence intervals rather than statistical significance testing. The reason for that emphasis is that appropriate null hypotheses for univariable analyses are, except for observations from paired samples, difficult to imagine. This limitation does not apply to bivariable or multivariable analyses. In general, the null hypothesis of no association between the dependent and independent variables is relevant to bivariable analyses.

Continuous Dependent Variable

Figure 42.1 summarizes the steps in the flowchart that are needed when we have one continuous dependent variable and one independent variable. Note that we do not consider a continuous dependent variable associated with an ordinal independent variable. The reason for this omission is that no statistical procedures are available to compare a continuous dependent variable associated with an ordinal independent variable without converting the continuous variable to an ordinal scale.

Nominal Independent Variable

A nominal independent variable divides dependent variable values into two groups. For example, suppose we measured bleeding time for women who were birth control pill (BCP) users and nonusers. The dependent variable, bleeding time, is continuous; the independent variable, BCP use/nonuse, is nominal. The nominal independent variable divides bleeding time into a group of bleeding time measurements for BCP users and for BCP nonusers. We have sampled bleeding time from a population that contains a group of BCP users and a group of BCP nonusers.[1]

Two methods of sampling independent variables are important in this example.[2] The first method is *naturalistic* or *representative sampling*. In the example of

---

[1] A universal assumption in statistics is that our observations are the result of random sampling. This assumption applies to the dependent variable, but it is not necessarily assumed by statistical tests for sampling of independent variables.

[2] There is actually a third method of sampling independent variables. That method is similar to purposive sampling, but instead of selecting observations that have specific independent variable values, the researcher randomly assigns a value, such as a dose, to each subject. This third method of sampling is used in experimental studies. Note that the term "representative" may imply naturalistic sampling if it refers to the independent variable and implies that the distribution of values of the independent variable in an investigation's sample reflects the distribution in the larger population.

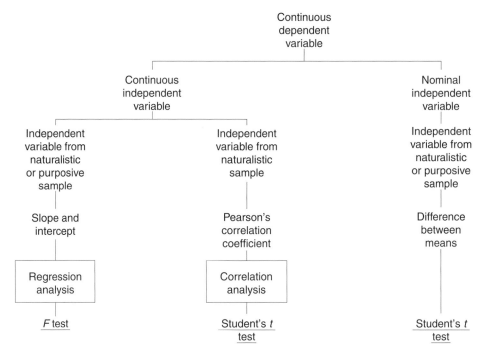

Figure 42.1. Flowchart to select a bivariable statistical procedure for a continuous dependent variable (continued from Fig. 40.5).

bleeding time, naturalistic sampling would imply that we would randomly sample, for example, 200 women from a large population and then determine who is a BCP user or a BCP nonuser. If our sampling method was unbiased, the relative frequencies of BCP users compared with BCP nonusers in our sample would be representative of the frequency of BCP use in the population.

The second method is *purposive sampling*. If we used a purposive sample to study bleeding time, we might identify 100 women who are BCP users and 100 women who are BCP nonusers, and who fulfill the investigation's inclusion and exclusion criteria. Because the researcher determines the number of BCP users and nonusers, the relative frequency of individuals with the nominal condition, birth control pill use, is not representative of the relative frequency in the population.

Thus, the distinction between naturalistic and purposive sampling is whether or not the distribution of the independent variable in the sample is representative of the distribution of that variable in the population. In naturalistic sampling, it is representative; in purposive sampling, it is not. Naturalistic sampling is often used in cohort studies. Purposive sampling is common in case-control studies and randomized clinical trials. As we shall see later in this chapter, the method used to sample the independent variable affects our options for appropriate statistical techniques or the statistical power of the technique chosen.

In bivariable analysis, such as the association between birth control pill use and bleeding time, we are interested in a way in which we can compare bleeding times between BCP users and nonusers. In the comparison of means, our interest is generally in their difference.[3] For example, we may be interested in the difference between mean bleeding times for BCP users and nonusers.[4] Calculating confidence intervals and statistical significance testing involving differences between means use the Student's t distribution, as indicated at the bottom right of Fig. 42.1.

The appropriateness of using the Student's t distribution in statistical significance testing and calculation of confidence intervals is not affected by the method of sampling the independent variable. However, the statistical power of those procedures is greatest when the number of observations is the same for each category of the independent variable. That is, we would have the greatest chance of demonstrating statistical significance for a true difference in mean bleeding times among 200 women if we used purposive sampling to select 100 BCP users and 100 BCP nonusers.

Continuous Independent Variable

We are often interested in using the measurement of a continuous independent variable to estimate the measurement of a continuous dependent variable.[5] As an example, suppose that we are interested in evaluating the relationship between the dosage of a hypothetical drug for treating glaucoma and intraocular pressure. Specifically, we would like to estimate the intraocular pressures (dependent variable) we expect to be associated in the population with various dosages of the drug (independent variable).

Some types of questions that can be addressed about estimation of the continuous dependent variable depend on how the continuous independent variable was sampled. Regardless of whether naturalistic or purposive sampling was used, however, we can construct a linear equation to estimate the mean value of the dependent variable (Y) for each value of the independent variable (X). This is called *regression analysis* or *linear* regression. In our example, the dependent variable is the mean intraocular pressure, and the independent variable is the dosage of medication. A linear equation in a population is described by two parameters: a *slope* (b) and an *intercept* (a).

$$Y = a + bX$$

The intercept estimates the mean of the dependent variable when the independent variable is equal to zero. Therefore, the intercept for the linear equation for intraocular pressure and dosage would estimate the population's mean intraocular

---

[3] The reason for this interest is that differences between means tend to have a Gaussian distribution, whereas other arithmetic combinations, such as ratios of means, do not.

[4] The standard error for the difference between means is calculated from estimates that combine the variances from each of the groups being compared. To calculate the standard error for the difference in mean bleeding times, we would combine our estimates of the variance in bleeding times among BCP users and the variance among BCP nonusers. Specifically, this standard error is equal to the square root of the sum of the variances of the distributions of each group mean divided by the sum of the sample sizes. Knowing that, we can more fully understand why we cannot use univariable confidence intervals as a reliable surrogate for bivariable tests of inference. Comparison of univariable confidence intervals is equivalent to adding standard errors of two samples. That is not algebraically equivalent to the standard error of differences between means.

[5] The term predict rather than estimate is often used. We have avoided the term predict because it implies the ability to extrapolate from independent data to dependent data even when the dependent data is not known or is outside the range of values included in the investigation.

pressure for individuals not receiving the drug. The slope of a linear equation tells us the amount the mean of the dependent variable changes for each unit change in the numerical value of the independent variable. The slope of the equation that relates intraocular pressure to the dosage of drug estimates how much intraocular pressure decreases for each unit increase in dosage.

If we are interested in this sort of estimation, we need to calculate two point estimates from our sample's observations: the intercept and the slope. To obtain these estimates, we most often use *least-squares regression*. This method selects numerical values for the slope and intercept that minimize the distances or, more specifically, the sum of the differences squared between the data observed in the sample and those estimated by the linear equation.[6]

Rather than consider the intercept and the slope separately, however, we can consider the linear equation as a whole as the estimate of interest. To do this, we examine the amount of variation in the dependent variable that we are able to explain using the linear equation divided by the amount of variation that we are unable to explain with the linear equation.

In the example of medication to treat elevated intraocular pressure, we would divide the variation in intraocular pressure that is explained by knowing medication dosage by the variation in intraocular pressure that is left unexplained. Then we can perform statistical significance testing on the null hypothesis that the data contained in the regression equation do not add to our ability to explain the value of the dependent variable (intraocular pressure), given a value of the independent variable (medication dosage). We use the *F* test to test the null hypothesis in regression analysis, as indicated on the left side of Fig. 42.1.

In investigations such as the one examining mean intraocular pressure and dosage of a medication to treat glaucoma, we usually assign dosages that are not representative of all dosages that could have been selected. In other words, we seldom can use naturalistic sampling to investigate a dose-response relationship. It is appropriate to use linear regression methods regardless of whether a naturalistic or a purposive sampling method is used to obtain values of the independent variable. When a method of sampling, such as naturalistic sampling, is used to obtain a sample of an independent variable that is representative of the larger population, it is possible to use another category of statistical techniques known as *correlation analysis*.

Correlation analysis might be used, for example, if we randomly sampled individuals from a population and measured both their quantity of salt intake and their diastolic blood pressure. Here, both the independent variable (salt intake) and the dependent variable (diastolic blood pressure) have been randomly sampled from the population and thus are representative of all those who could have been included. The distribution of quantities of salt intake in our naturalistic sample is representative, on average, of the population's distribution of salt intake.

The distinction between the dependent and the independent variables is less important in correlation analysis than it is in other types of analyses. The same results are obtained in correlation analysis if those functions are reversed. In our example, it does not matter, from a statistical point of view, whether we consider

---

[6] The differences between the observed numerical values of the dependent variables and those estimated by the regression equation are known as *residuals*. Residuals indicate how well the linear equation estimates the dependent variable.

diastolic blood pressure or salt intake as the dependent variable when performing a correlation analysis.[7]

In correlation analysis, we measure how the dependent and independent variables' values change together. In our example, we would measure how consistently an increase in salt intake is associated with an increase in diastolic blood pressure. The statistic that is calculated to reflect how closely the two variables change together is called their *covariance*. The most commonly used correlation coefficient for two continuous variables is known as *Pearson's correlation coefficient*. Pearson's correlation coefficient is the ratio of covariance to the square root of the product of the variances of the individual variables, and is symbolized by r. This correlation coefficient is a point estimate of the strength of the association between two continuous variables. This is an important distinction between regression analysis and correlation analysis. Regression analysis can be used to estimate dependent variable values from independent variable values but does not estimate the strength of the relationship between those variables in the population. Correlation analysis estimates the strength of the relationship in the population but cannot be used to estimate values of the dependent variable corresponding to values of the independent variable. Thus correlation analysis and regression analysis can provide complementary information.

The correlation coefficient has a range of possible values from -1 to $+1$. A correlation coefficient of zero indicates no relationship between the dependent and independent variables. A positive correlation coefficient indicates that as the value of the independent variable increases, the value of the dependent variable increases. A negative correlation coefficient indicates that as the value of the independent variable increases, the value of the dependent variable decreases.

Interpreting the strength of association between the dependent and independent variables is facilitated if we square the correlation coefficient to obtain the *coefficient of determination* (R^2). If we multiply the coefficient of determination by 100%, it indicates the percentage of variation in the dependent variable that is explained by or attributed to the value of the independent variable.[8] The coefficient of determination can be thought of as a measure for continuous variables parallel to attributable risk percentage for nominal variables because it addresses how much variability in the dependent variable can be attributed to the independent variable. It is appropriate to use the coefficient of determination only when the independent variable, as well as the dependent variable, is sampled using representative or naturalistic sampling.

One of the most common errors in interpretation of statistical analysis is to incorrectly use the correlation coefficient to make point estimates for a particular population. That is, the correlation coefficient is sometimes used even though the independent variable's values are not sampled by a method that ensures, on average, that the sample will be representative of the population. Using this approach can create an artificially high correlation coefficient due to sampling only extreme values of the independent variable.

---

[7] When performing regression analyses or correlation analyses, we make a series of assumptions. These are referred to as random sampling of the dependent variable, homogeneity of variances or homoscedasticity, linear relationship between dependent and independent variables, and independent variable measured with perfect precision.

[8] The term "explain" is used here because it is widely used. "Explain" should not imply a cause and effect relationship, correlation is really a form of association.

Ordinal Dependent Variable

In Fig. 42.2, note that we do not consider an ordinal dependent variable associated with a continuous independent variable because before we can include the data from a continuous independent variable, it must be converted to the ordinal scale. This is similar to the situation we discussed with a continuous dependent variable in an analysis with an ordinal independent variable. No statistical procedures are commonly used to compare an ordinal dependent variable with a continuous independent variable without making such a conversion.

Nominal Independent Variable

As indicated in Fig. 42.2, the *Mann-Whitney test* is a statistical significance test applicable to one nominal independent variable and an ordinal dependent variable. It is also applicable to a continuous dependent variable converted to an ordinal scale. This might be done to circumvent some of the assumptions of the Student's *t* test. The null hypothesis considered in a Mann-Whitney test is that the two groups do not differ in location in the population. Because this is a nonparametric test, no parameter of location is specified in the null hypothesis. The difference between medians is indicated in parenthesis to indicate that it may be used as a point estimate even though it is not specified in the null hypothesis.

Ordinal Independent Variable

If the independent variable represents ordinal or continuous data converted to an ordinal scale, we can estimate the strength of the association between the dependent

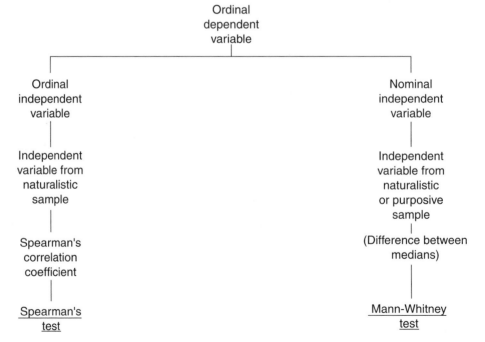

Figure 42.2. Flowchart to select a bivariable statistical procedure for an ordinal dependent variable (continued from Fig. 40.5).

and independent variables using a method parallel to correlation analysis. In the case of ordinal variables, the most commonly used correlation coefficient is *Spearman's correlation coefficient*. That coefficient can be calculated without making many of the assumptions necessary to calculate the coefficient described for continuous variables. It is important to remember, however, that any correlation coefficient must be determined from samples in which both the dependent and the independent variables are representative of a larger population. In other words, we must use naturalistic sampling. There is no nonparametric test that releases us from this assumption. This considerably limits the ability to use correlation methods.

As with a correlation coefficient calculated for two continuous variables, we can perform statistical significance testing and calculation of confidence intervals. For Spearman's correlation coefficients we accomplish this using Spearman's test. We can also use the square of the Spearman's correlation coefficient to provide a nonparametric estimate of the coefficient of determination, the percentage of the variation in the dependent variable that is explained by the independent variable. In contrast to Pearson's coefficient of determination, Spearman's coefficient of determination tells us the percentage change in the dependent variable's category rank that can be explained by changes in the category rank of the independent variable.[9]

Nominal Dependent Variable

Bivariable statistical methods for nominal dependent variables are presented in Fig. 42.3.

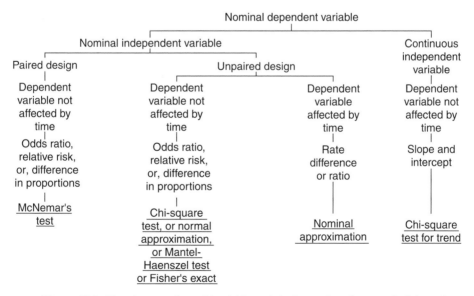

Figure 42.3. Flowchart to select a bivariable statistical procedure for a nominal dependent variable (continued from Fig. 40.5).

---

[9] Note that if continuous data is converted to ordinal data and a Spearman's correlation coefficient is calculated, it will often be larger than the corresponding Pearson's correlation coefficient. This is due to the fact that correlation coefficients for ordinal data are attempting to estimate a category of ordinal data rather than a particular value as in the correlation coefficient for continuous data, i.e., Pearson's correlation coefficient.

Nominal Independent Variable: Paired Design

If investigators are interested in collecting information on a nominal dependent variable and a nominal independent variable, they have the choice of a paired or an unpaired design. If appropriately constructed, a paired design may have more statistical power than a corresponding unpaired design. Remember that pairing is the special type of matching in which both the dependent and independent variables are measured on each individual in a pair of two similar individuals, and the observations on the pair are analyzed together. Alternatively, an individual may serve as her own control, and data from the same individual can be used twice in the analysis.

As indicated in Fig. 42.3, the odds ratio or relative risk are commonly used point estimates for estimating the strength of the relationship in a paired design. To conduct statistical significance tests on pairs of data, *McNemar's test* is used. Related methods can be used to calculate confidence intervals from paired observations.

Nominal Independent Variable: Unpaired Design

In bivariable analysis of an unpaired nominal dependent variable, we first determine whether the dependent variable is affected by time. Affected by time implies that an increase in the length of observation results in a greater probability of observing the outcome. This distinction is especially important when study subjects are observed for different lengths of time. If the denominator variable is not affected by time, we may use a proportion or probability and obtain either a relative risk or a difference in proportions, or alternatively, we can calculate an odds ratio. If the dependent variable is affected by time, we use a rate, or what we have called a true rate, and obtain either a difference or a ratio.

From a statistical significance testing point of view, the choice to use a ratio or a difference usually does not matter. In fact, in bivariable analysis, the same statistical significance tests are used regardless of whether the point estimate is a ratio or a difference. This is suggested by the fact that the null hypothesis that a difference is equal to 0 is equivalent to the null hypothesis that a ratio is equal to 1. When a ratio is equal to 1, the numerator must be equal to the denominator; thus, the difference between the numerator and the denominator must be equal to 0.

In bivariable analysis of nominal independent and dependent variables from an unpaired design, we are likely to encounter a variety of statistical significance testing methods. As in univariable analysis of a nominal dependent variable, these methods are of two general types: exact methods and normal approximations. The exact method for bivariable proportions is the *Fisher's exact* procedure.[10] Two commonly used approximation methods for proportions are the *normal approximation* and the *chi-square test*.[11] Rates are most often analyzed using a normal approximation. Statistical significance tests and calculation of confidence intervals for the odds ratio are usually based on the *Mantel-Haenszel test*, also a normal approximation.

---

[10] The Fisher's exact procedure is used when any of the frequencies predicted by the null hypothesis for a 2×2 table are less than 5.

[11] Actually, the normal approximation and the chi-square procedures are equivalent in bivariable analysis. The square root of the chi-square statistic is equal to the normal approximation statistic.

Ordinal Independent Variable

When an investigation includes a nominal dependent variable and ordinal independent data, the ordinal independent data needs to be converted to nominal data. Remember that ordinal data with multiple potential categories will require more than one nominal variable. It will require one less than the number of potential categories of the ordinal data. Thus this type of analysis is actually a form of multivariable analysis and will be discussed in Chapter 43.

Continuous Independent Variable

When we have a continuous independent variable that is not affected by time and a nominal dependent variable, we are able to consider the possibility that a trend exists for various values of the independent variable. For example, we might be interested in examining the study hypothesis that the proportion of individuals who develop stroke increases in a linear fashion as the diastolic blood pressure increases versus the null hypothesis that no linear relationship exists between those variables. This same sort of hypothesis is considered in simple linear regression with the exception that here we have a nominal dependent variable rather than a continuous dependent variable, as indicated on the right side of Fig. 43.3. Rather than a simple linear regression, we perform a *chi-square test for trend*.[12]

We have now examined the commonly used statistical methods for analyzing one dependent variable and one independent variable. Often, however, we will be interested in more than one independent variable. In these situations, we will use multivariable techniques, as discussed in the next chapter.[13]

---

[12] Even though we have a special name for the test used to investigate the possibility of a linear trend in a nominal dependent variable, we should realize that a chi-square test for trend is very similar to a linear regression. In fact, the point estimates in the most commonly used methods to investigate a trend are the slope and intercept of a linear equation that are identical to the estimates we discussed for linear regression. Point estimation of the coefficients in a chi-square test for trend is identical to estimation in a simple linear regression. For inference and interval estimation, a slightly different assumption is made that causes confidence intervals to be a little wider and P values to be a little larger in the chi-square test compared with linear regression. That difference decreases as the sample size increases. Also note that here we are using a very specific meaning of the term "trend." Trend is often used less rigorously to imply that the data suggests a relationship even though the results are not statistically significant.

[13] Note that when nominal data have more than two categories, more than one nominal variable is required to represent the data. When nominal data are used as independent variables, multivariable analysis, as explained in Chapter 43, is used. When more than one nominal variable is required for the dependent variable, special multivariate techniques, such as discriminant analysis, are needed. These techniques are beyond the scope of this book. Note, however, that the chi-square test can be used for more than one nominal dependent variable.

43 Multivariable Analysis

In multivariable statistics,[1] we have one dependent variable and two or more independent variables. The independent variables may be measured on the same scale or on different scales. For example, all the independent variables may be represented by continuous data, or alternatively, some may be represented by continuous data and some may be represented by nominal data. When one characteristic such as race requires more than one independent nominal variable, multivariable analysis is also used.

Only nominal and continuous independent variables are indicated in a number of flowcharts that follow. In these situations, ordinal independent variables can be included in multivariable analysis, but they must first be converted to a nominal scale.[2]

There are three general advantages to using multivariable methods to analyze health research data. First, this approach allows investigation of the relationship between a dependent variable and an independent variable while controlling for or adjusting for the effect of other independent variables. This is the method for removing the influence of confounding variables in the analysis of health research data.

For example, if we were interested in diastolic blood pressure of persons receiving various dosages of an antihypertensive drug, we may want to control for the potential confounding effects of age and gender. To adjust for these potential confounding variables in the analysis of results, we would use multivariable analysis with diastolic blood pressure as the dependent variable and with dosage, age, and gender as independent variables.

Investigators thus seek to include confounding variables in their analysis of results. In doing this, they need to carefully choose which variables to include, because confounding variables themselves may be associated with each other. For instance, older patients might generally receive lower doses of medication. When two independent variables are associated and thus share information, we say that *multicollinearity* is present. Often it is necessary for an investigator to include only one of the variables that demonstrate multicollinearity. Much of the decision-making in multivariable techniques is related to which variables to include and which to exclude from the analysis of results.[3]

---

[1] Multivariable analysis is often referred to as *multivariate analyses*. True multivariate analysis refers to analyses in which there are more than one dependent variable. These forms of analyses are rarely used in medicine or public health.

[2] Multivariable analyses also allow inclusion of interaction terms. Traditionally, interaction terms, unlike confounding variables, need to be statistically significant before they can be entered into a multivariable analysis. Tests for interaction generally have low statistical power. Thus, despite the fact that interactions are common, the inclusion of interaction terms is relatively uncommon. Use of P values greater than 0.05 have been suggested as a way of addressing this issue.

[3] Some indication of the existence of shared information by independent variables can be obtained by examining bivariable correlation coefficients for those variables, but the best method to evaluate the existence of multicollinearity is to inspect regression models that include and exclude each independent variable. If regression coefficients change substantially when a variable is included compared to when it is excluded, multicollinearity exists.

The second advantage of multivariable statistical methods is that they may allow us to perform statistical significance tests on several variables while maintaining a chosen probability of making a Type I error. In other words, at times we may use multivariable analysis to avoid the multiple comparison problem introduced in Section I, "Studying a Study."

To recall the multiple comparison problem, imagine that we have many independent variables that we compare with a dependent variable using a bivariable method such as the Student's t test. Although in each of those bivariable tests we permit only a 5% chance of making a Type I error, the chance that we would commit at least one Type I error among all those comparisons would be somewhat greater than 5%. We call the chance of making a Type I error for any particular comparison the *testwise error*. The chance of making a Type I error for at least one comparison is known as the *experimentwise error*. Bivariable analyses control the testwise error rate. Many multivariable methods, on the other hand, are designed to maintain a consistent experimentwise Type I error rate. That is, at times multivariable procedures are in and of themselves capable of taking into account multiple comparison issues.

Two types of null hypotheses are examined in most multivariable methods of analysis that are designed to avoid the multiple comparison problem. The first is known as the *omnibus null hypothesis*. This null hypothesis addresses the relationship between the dependent variable and the entire collection of independent variables as a unit. A drawback of the omnibus null hypothesis is that it does not allow investigation of relationships between the dependent variable and each of the independent variables individually. This is accomplished by the second type of null hypotheses addressed in *partial tests* or *pairwise tests*.

A third advantage of multivariable methods is that they often allow the investigator to accomplish estimation, inference, and adjustment using one statistical procedure. Thus, depending on the type of method, odds ratios or life tables may be produced directly from the statistical procedures. At times, however, this may limit the choice of point estimate that can be produced from a particular form of analysis.

Because of these advantages of multivariable methods, they are frequently used to analyze health research data. Let us now take a closer look at these methods and the ways they can be interpreted.

Continuous Dependent Variable

Figure 43.1 summarizes the steps that are needed when we have one continuous dependent variable and two or more independent variables.

Nominal Independent Variables

In bivariable analysis of a continuous dependent variable and a nominal independent variable, the independent variable has the effect of dividing the dependent variable's values into two subgroups. In multivariable analysis, we have more than one nominal independent variable, and thus we are able to divide dependent variable values into more than two subgroups. The most common methods to compare

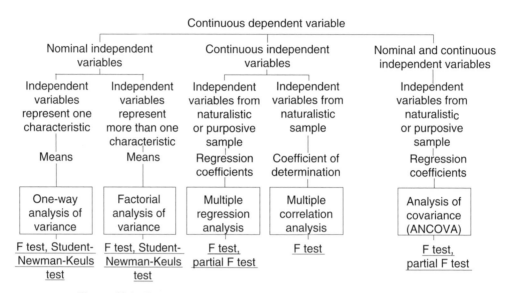

Figure 43.1. Flowchart to select a multivariable statistical procedure for a continuous dependent variable (continued from Fig. 40.5).

means of the dependent variable among three or more subgroups are forms of a general statistical approach called *analysis of variance (ANOVA)*.[4]

The simplest type of ANOVA is one in which nominal independent variables are used to separate the nominal dependent data into subgroups. For example, suppose we are interested only in the relationship between fasting blood glucose and race, defined as white, black, or other. "Other" is when the race is not white or black. We now have to consider three subgroups of race (white, black, and other) for which we determine fasting blood glucose. This type of ANOVA is known as a *one-way* ANOVA.[5] The omnibus null hypothesis in a one-way ANOVA is that the means of the subgroups are all equal to one another. In our example, the omnibus null hypothesis would be that mean fasting blood glucose for whites is the same as for blacks and for persons of other races.

In order to use one-way ANOVA, we need to assume that it is impossible for an individual to be included in more than one category. For example, in health research, we perhaps artificially usually regard races as mutually exclusive categories. For each individual, we record a single race. Thus, it is impossible, in this context, for an individual to be considered both white and black.

Now let us imagine that we are interested in both race and gender. When we use both race and gender, these individual characteristics are not mutually exclusive. For example, an individual can be of either gender regardless of his or her race. It is necessary, therefore, to have another way in which subgroups can be

[4] It seems incongruous that a method to compare means should be called an analysis of variance. The reason for this name is that ANOVAs examine the variation between subgroups, assuming that the variation within each of the subgroups is the same. If the variation between subgroups exceeds the variation within those groups, the subgroups must differ in location, measured by means.

[5] When only one nominal independent variable is being considered, we are comparing only two subgroups, and the one-way ANOVA is exactly the same as a *t* test for bivariable analysis.

defined by nominal independent variables when we wish to utilize more than one characteristic.

Commonly, the solution is to segregate those characteristics into *factors*. A factor is a collection of one or more nominal independent variables that define mutually exclusive, but topically related, categories or characteristics. For example, suppose we have two independent variables defining race and one independent variable defining gender in our sample of persons for whom we measure fasting blood glucose levels. The three independent variables in this example actually represent two separate factors: race and gender. We can define 6 subgroups among which we wish to compare mean fasting blood glucose levels: white males, white females, black males, black females, other males, and other females. The type of ANOVA that considers two or more factors is known as a *factorial ANOVA*.

With factorial ANOVA, we can test the same sort of omnibus null hypothesis tested in a one-way ANOVA. In our example, the null hypothesis would be that mean level of fasting blood glucose is the same in white females as it is in white males, black females, black males, other females, and other males. In addition, we can test hypotheses about the equality of means of fasting blood glucose levels between the subgroups within a given factor. That is, we can examine the separate effect of different races on mean level of fasting blood glucose and the effect of gender on mean level of fasting blood glucose. The statistical tests that are used to examine the factors separately are often called tests of *main effects*. All these null hypotheses in ANOVAs are tested using an F test.

The results of examining a main effect take into account possible confounding relationships of the other factors. In our example, we would test the null hypothesis that the fasting blood glucose mean levels for the three race subgroups are all equal by using an ANOVA test of the main effect of race. That test would control for any differences in distribution of genders among the racial groups. Thus, factorial ANOVA allows us to take advantage of the ability of multivariable analysis to control for multiple confounding variables.[6]

In addition, ANOVAs also address the second advantage, dealing with the multiple comparison problem. In ANOVAs, the omnibus null hypothesis maintains an experimentwise Type I error rate equal to α, usually 5%. It is seldom enough, however, to know that differences exist among means within a factor without knowing specifically in which category the means differ. That is, it is not enough to know that mean fasting blood glucose level differs by race without knowing the contribution of specific races to the difference.

---

[6] To interpret tests of main effects, it is assumed that the factor has the same relationship with the dependent variable regardless of the level of other factors. That is, we assume that the difference between the fasting blood glucose means in blacks, whites, and other races is the same regardless of whether the individual is a male or a female. This is not always the case. For example, females might have a higher fasting blood glucose level than do males among white subjects, but females and males might be similar or, in a greater extreme, males might have higher fasting blood glucose level than do females among black subjects. If this sort of relationship exists between factors, we say that an *interaction* exists between gender and race. In clinical and epidemiological terminology, we might say that a *synergy* or *effect modification* exists between race and gender in determining fasting blood glucose levels. In addition to testing for main effects, factorial ANOVAs can be used to test hypotheses about interactions. Additional interaction variables for race and gender would tell us, for instance, how much more the fasting blood glucose level differs for black women than would be expected by adding the effect of being black to the effect of being female.

To examine the subgroup means in greater detail, we use pair-wise tests.[7] Note that in several places in Fig. 43.1 the underlined test used for statistical significance tests of the omnibus hypothesis is followed after a comma by the statistical significance test used for pair-wise comparisons. The most widely used pair-wise test for sets of observations that include a continuous dependent variable and more than one nominal independent variable is the *Student-Newman-Keuls test*. As indicated in Fig. 43.1, after using the *F* test, this test is used for pair-wise statistical significance testing for one-way and factorial ANOVA. This test allows examination of all pairs of subgroup means while maintaining an experimentwise Type I error rate of $\alpha = 0.05$. An algebraic rearrangement of the Student-Newman-Keuls test allows us to calculate confidence intervals for the dependent variable for each value of the independent variables.

Continuous Independent Variables

When the independent variables in a study are represented by continuous data, we can choose between two approaches that correspond to approaches discussed in Chapter 42 in which we considered regression analysis and correlation analysis. Most often, we are interested in estimating values of the dependent variable corresponding to specific independent variable values. In bivariable analysis, we used linear regression to estimate the value of the dependent variable given the value of the independent variable. When we have more than one continuous independent variable, we use *multiple regression analysis*.[8]

In multiple regression, the mean of a continuous dependent variable is estimated by a linear equation that is like the one in simple linear regression except that it includes two or more continuous independent variables.

$$Y = a + b_1X_1 + b_2X_2 + \ldots + b_iX_k$$

For example, suppose we are interested in estimating plasma cortisol levels based on total white blood cell (WBC) count, body temperature, and urine production in response to a water load. To investigate that relationship, we measure cortisol (μg/dL), WBC count (10^3), temperature (°C), and urine volume (mL) in 100 patients. Using multiple regression, we might estimate the following linear equation:

$$\text{Cortisol} = -36.8 + 0.8 \times \text{WBC} + 1.2 \times \text{temperature} + 4.7 \times \text{urine volume}$$

As in ANOVA, multiple regression allows testing of an omnibus hypothesis that has an overall Type I error rate usually set a 5%. The null hypothesis in multiple regression is that the entire collection of independent variables cannot be used to estimate values of the dependent variable. An *F* test is used to evaluate the statistical significance of the multiple regression omnibus null hypothesis. Suppose that, in our example, we find a statistically significant *F*. This implies that, if we know the

---

[7] In ANOVA, these pair-wise tests are often called *á posteriori tests*. The reason for that terminology is that some pair-wise tests, especially the older tests, require a statistically significant test of the omnibus hypothesis before the pair-wise test can be used.

[8] Note that the use of a continuous dependent variable in regression method requires fulfillment of a series of assumptions including Gaussian distribution of the dependent variable and *homoscedasticity* or equality of the variance, i.e., equal variance of the dependent variable values in the population for each value of the independent variable. Statistical methods called *transformation* may be used to help satisfy both of these two assumptions.

WBC count, temperature, and urine volume for a particular patient, then we can do better than chance in estimating the value of that patient's plasma cortisol level.

In addition to interest in the omnibus hypothesis in multiple regression, it is most often desirable to examine relationships between the dependent variable and specific independent variables. One way in which those relationships are reflected is in the regression coefficients associated with the independent variables. *Regression coefficients* are estimates of the bs in the regression equation. That is, they are point estimates that can directly be used to estimate the magnitude of the relationship. The results of multiple regression analysis allow point estimation and calculation of confidence intervals for those coefficients. Unfortunatly the magnitude of the regression coefficients cannot be directly compared because they depend on the units of measurement.

Calculation of confidence intervals and statistical significance testing for coefficients associated with specific independent variables in multiple regression is parallel to pairwise analyses in ANOVA. In ANOVA, however, pairwise analyses were designed to maintain an experimentwise Type I error rate equal to α. In multiple regression, the testwise Type I error rate equals α, but the experimentwise error rate is influenced by the number of independent variables being considered. Thus multiple regression, unlike ANOVA, is susceptible to the multiple comparison problem.

The more independent variables examined in multiple regression, the greater the likelihood that at least one regression coefficient will appear to be statistically significant even though no relationship exists between those variables in the larger population being sampled. Therefore, in multiple regression, statistically significant associations between the dependent variable and independent variables that were not expected to be important before the data were examined should be interpreted with some skepticism.

If all the continuous independent variables in a set of observations are the result of naturalistic sampling from some population of interest, we might be interested in estimating the strength of the association between the dependent variable and the entire collection of independent variables. This is parallel to our interest in bivariable correlation analysis. As indicated in Fig. 43.1, in multivariable analysis, the method used to measure the degree of association is called *multiple correlation analysis*. The result of multiple correlation analysis can be expressed as a *multiple coefficient of determination* (as distinguished from its square root called the *multiple correlation coefficient*).

It is important to keep in mind that these statistics reflect the degree of association between the dependent variable and the entire collection of independent variables. For instance, suppose that in our example we obtain a multiple coefficient of determination equal to 0.82. This means that 82% of the variation in plasma cortisol among patients can be explained by knowing WBC count, temperature, and urine volume. The statistically significant F test associated with the test of the omnibus null hypothesis in multiple regression analysis also tests the null hypothesis that the population's multiple coefficient of determination equals zero. Confidence intervals for coefficients of determination can be derived from these same calculations. These measures can be and often are calculated whenever a multiple regression method is used. However, they may not accurately indicate the percentage of the variation explained unless all of the independent variables are the result of naturalistic or representation sampling.

Nominal and Continuous Independent Variables

Often, an investigator is faced with a set of observations in which some of the independent variables are continuous and some are nominal. For example, suppose an investigator conducted a study designed to explain cardiac output on the basis of energy output during exercise. Further, she expect the relationship between cardiac output and energy output to be different for the two sexes. In this example, the set of observations would contain cardiac output, a continuous dependent variable; energy output, a continuous independent variable; and gender, a nominal independent variable.

To examine a data set that contains a continuous dependent variable and a mixture of nominal and continuous independent variables, the investigator uses an *analysis of covariance (ANCOVA)*. The continuous independent variables in ANCOVA are related to the dependent variable in the same way that continuous independent variables are related to the dependent variable in a multiple regression. Similarly, the nominal independent variables are related to the dependent variable in the same way nominal independent variables are related to the dependent variable in ANOVA. Therefore, ANCOVA is a hybrid method containing aspects of both multiple regression and ANOVA.

With ANCOVA, the investigator deals with nominal data, such as gender, using an *indicator* or *dummy variable,* which is given a numerical value of 0 or 1. Indicator variables allow us to create two regression lines that differ only by their intercept. An indicator variable for gender would tell us how much the estimate of cardiac output differs between males and females.

Ordinal Dependent Variable

Figure 43.2 summarizes the steps that are needed when we have one ordinal dependent variable and two or more independent variables. In univariable and bivariable analyses, statistical methods are available to analyze ordinal dependent variables and to allow an investigator to convert continuous dependent variables to an ordinal scale when the data does not fulfill the assumptions necessary to use the statistical methods designed for continuous dependent variables. This also is true of multivariable methods for ordinal dependent variables.

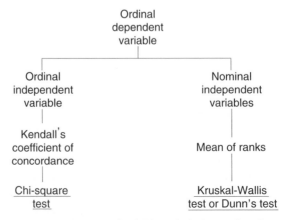

Figure 43.2. Flowchart to select a multivariable statistical procedure for an ordinal dependent variable (continued from Fig. 40.5).

Ideally, we would like to have methods for ordinal dependent variables that parallel all the important multivariable methods for continuous dependent variables: ANOVA, ANCOVA, and multiple regression. Unfortunately, this is not the case. The only well-accepted multivariable procedures for ordinal dependent variables are ones that can be used as nonparametric equivalents to certain ANOVA designs. Thus, Fig. 43.2 is restricted to methods that can be used with nominal independent variables or, alternatively, with ordinal independent variables. Continuous independent variables must be converted to an ordinal or nominal scale to use these methods.

Methods for an ordinal dependent variable may be used when the data does not satisfy the assumptions required to utilize the data as continuous data. Let us reconsider the previous example of fasting blood glucose levels measured among persons of three race categories (black, white, and other) and of both genders. Our interest was in determining the independent effects of race and gender on blood sugar.

To analyze the data, we used a factorial ANOVA. If we were concerned about fasting blood glucose levels satisfying the assumptions of the ANOVA,[9] we could convert the data to an ordinal scale by assigning relative ranks to fasting blood glucose measurements. That is, the measured level of blood glucose would no longer be used. Rather, the 100 patients would be given a blood glucose rank from 1 to 100. Then, we could apply the *Kruskal-Wallis test* or alternatively *Dunn's test* to those converted data. These tests are appropriate for performing statistical significance testing on an ordinal dependent variable and two or more nominal independent variables with either a one-way or factorial design. Nonparametric procedures also are available to make pairwise comparisons among subgroups of the dependent variable.

As indicated in Fig. 43.2, when all the independent variables are represented by ordinal data and the dependent variable is also represented by ordinal data, *Kendall's coefficient of concordance* can be used as a nonparametric multiple correlation analysis. When the analysis includes both ordinal and nominal independent variables, the ordinal variables need to be rescaled to nominal variables and the Kruskal-Wallis test used.

When using multivariable methods designed for ordinal dependent variables to analyze sets of observations that contain a continuous dependent variable which the investigator has converted to an ordinal scale, we should keep in mind a potential disadvantage. The nonparametric procedure has less statistical power than does the corresponding parametric procedure. This is true for all statistical procedures performed on continuous data converted to an ordinal scale. Thus, if the assumptions of a parametric statistical procedure are fulfilled, it is advisable to use this parametric procedure to analyze a continuous dependent variable rather than a parallel nonparametric procedure.

Nominal Dependent Variable

In health research, we are often interested in outcomes measured as dependent variables such as live/die, cure/not cure, or disease/no disease measured as nominal data. Further, because of the complexity of health phenomena, it is most

---

[9] The assumptions for ANOVA and ANCOVA are the same as those previously labeled in the footnote 7 on regression analysis in Chapter 42.

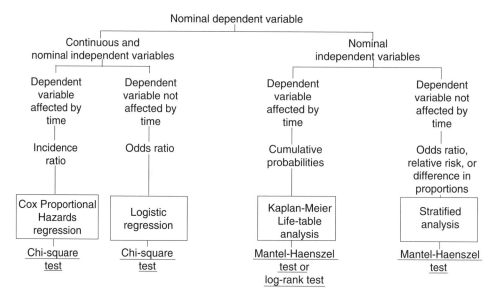

Figure 43.3. Flowchart to select a multivariable statistical procedure for a nominal dependent variable (continued from Fig. 40.5).

often desirable to measure a large number of independent variables, to control for confounding variables and to investigate the possibility of interaction or synergy between variables. Consequently, multivariable analyses with nominal dependent variables are frequently used in the analysis of health research data.

We have separated multivariable statistical procedures for nominal dependent variables into two groups: those that are useful when the independent variables are all nominal and those that are useful for a mixture of nominal and continuous independent variables (Fig. 43.3). The analyses in the first group are restricted to nominal independent variables or variables converted to a nominal scale. The analyses in the second group, on the other hand, can be used with nominal and continuous independent variables. There are no well-established methods to include ordinal independent variables unless they are converted to a nominal scale.

Nominal Independent Variables

When we analyze a nominal dependent variable and two or more nominal independent variables, we are interested in measures that are the same as those of interest in bivariable analysis of a nominal dependent variable and a nominal independent variable. For example, we might be interested in proportions (probabilities), rates, or odds. In multivariable analysis of nominal dependent and independent variables, however, we are interested in these measures of disease occurrence while adjusting for the other independent variables.

For example, suppose we are interested in comparing the probability or prevalence of asthma among coffee drinkers and subjects who do not drink coffee. Here, prevalence of asthma is the variable of interest and, therefore is the nominal dependent variable. Asthma (yes or no) is the nominal independent variable. We would want to adjust for the potential confounding effect of cigarette smoking.

To do that, we might include another nominal independent variable that identified cigarette smokers versus nonsmokers.

When we have two or more independent variables in a data set and they are all nominal, or are converted to a nominal scale, the general approach to adjust for independent variables is often a *stratified analysis*. As described in Section I, "Studying a Study," stratified analysis methods involve separating observations into subgroups defined by values of the nominal independent variables thought to be confounding variables. In our example of asthma prevalence and coffee consumption, we would begin a stratified analysis by dividing our observations into two groups: one composed of smokers and one composed of nonsmokers.

Within each subgroup we would calculate a separate estimate of the prevalences of asthma for coffee drinkers and nondrinkers. Those separate estimates are known as *stratum-specific point estimates*. The stratum-specific point estimates are combined using a particular system of weighting the stratum-specific estimates. That is, we would combine the information from each stratum, using a method to determine how much impact each stratum-specific estimate should have on the combined estimate.[10] The resulting combined estimate is considered to be an adjusted or standardized point estimate for all strata combined with the effects of the confounding variable taken into account.

In the flowchart (Fig. 43.3), we have indicated two types of nominal dependent variables: those that are and those that are not affected by time. Being affected by time implies there are multiple times at which participants are observed to assess outcomes and that the frequency with which an outcome is observed is influenced by the duration of follow-up. In addition, different individuals are observed for different periods of time. When a dependent variable is affected by time we say that it is *time-dependent*.[11]

In Chapter 9 we saw that a randomized clinical trials often fulfill these criteria and that life-table methods are be used when individuals are followed for varying periods of time. As we will see shortly, there is more than one way to produce a life table.[12]

If the dependent variable is affected by time and the independent variables include data containing observations from persons followed for various periods of time, we must use special statistical procedures to take into account differences

[10] The system of weighting stratum-specific estimates is an important way in which different stratified analysis methods differ. In direct standardization, the weighting system is based on the relative frequencies of each stratum in some reference population. The most useful weighting systems, from a statistical point of view, are those that reflect the precision of stratum-specific estimates. This may be accomplished by using the inverse of the variance as the weight.

[11] The dependent variable in randomized clinical trials and concurrent cohort studies is often time dependent, and independent variables are often obtained over varying lengths of time. Data for independent variables are often collected over differing lengths of time due to loss to follow-up, development of the endpoint such as death, or late entry into the study resulting in a short period of observation when the investigation is stopped. When data is collected for a shorter length of follow-up, we say that is has been *censored,* regardless of the reason.

[12] Dependent variables that are affected by time can cause problems in interpretation if the groups being compared differ in their lengths of follow-up, which is often the case. These problems can be circumvented if we consider incidence rate as the appropriate estimate for the dependent variable because the incidence rate has a unit of time in the denominator and, thus, takes length of follow-up into account. Unfortunately, incidence rate is a measurement that can be confusing to interpret. When length of follow-up differs, incidence rates need to be expressed as cases per person-year. Most people find it difficult to intuitively understand what "cases per person-year" implies. By contrast, it is much easier to understand *risk*. Risk is the proportion of persons who develop an outcome over a specified period of time. Thus, risk measures what is called the *cumulative probability* of developing the outcome.

in follow-up time. When all independent variables are nominal, the methods we use are types of *life-table analysis*. The most commonly used method is called the *Kaplan-Meier life table*.

These methods consider periods of follow-up time, such as 1-year intervals, as a collection of nominal independent variables. Each 1-year interval is used to stratify observations in the same way data are stratified by categories of a confounding variable such as age group. Cumulative survival,[13] which is equal to 1 minus the cumulative probability of death, is determined by combining these adjusted probabilities of surviving each time period.

Continuous and Nominal Independent Variables

In health research using a nominal dependent variable we are often interested in both continuous and nominal independent variables.[14]

Methods of analysis that permit simultaneous investigation of continuous and nominal independent variables and their interactions are parallel in their general approach to multiple regression discussed earlier. The methods we use here, however, are different from multiple regression in three ways. The first difference, as the Figs. 43.1 and 43.3 indicate, is that multiple regression is a method of analyzing continuous dependent variables, while we are now concerned with nominal dependent variables.

The second difference is that most of the methods for nominal dependent variables do not use the least-squares method used in multiple regression to find the best fit for the data. Most often, nominal dependent variable regression coefficients are estimated using the *maximum likelihood method*.[15]

The third difference is perhaps the most important to health researchers interpreting the results of regression analysis of nominal dependent variables. Although this type of analysis provides regression coefficient estimates and their standard errors, the remainder of the information resulting from the analysis is unlike that in multiple regression. These regressions do not provide us with any estimates parallel to correlation coefficients. Thus, without a coefficient of determination, it is not possible to determine the percent of variation in the dependent variable that is explained by the collection of independent variables.

For outcomes affected by time, the most commonly used regression method is the *Cox proportional hazards regression* or *Cox regression*. In this approach, the collection of independent variables and, at times, their interactions, are used to estimate the incidence ratio[16] of the nominal dependent variable,[17] such as the

---

[13] Life tables were originally designed to consider the risk of death, but they can be used to calculate the risk of any irreversible outcome that can occur only once.

[14] The stratified analysis approach appeals to many researchers because it appears to be simpler than other analyses. However, this approach does have some shortcomings. Stratified analysis is designed to examine the relationship between a nominal dependent variable and one nominal independent variable while controlling for the effect of nominal confounding variables. It does not allow for a straightforward examination of more than one independent variable, investigation of interactions or synergy, consideration of continuous or ordinal confounding variables without converting them to a nominal scale, or estimation of the importance of confounding variables. These are often features of great interest to health researchers.

[15] The maximum likelihood method chooses estimates for regression coefficients to maximize the likelihood that the data observed would have resulted from sampling a population with those coefficients.

[16] The term *hazard* is most often used as a synonym for incidence in the Cox model.

[17] Actually, Cox regression predicts the natural logarithm of the ratio of the incidence adjusted for the independent variables divided by the incidence unadjusted for those variables.

incidence of death. Thus Cox regression can be thought of as producing adjusted relative risks.

Algebraic combination of the coefficients for a particular Cox regression equation can be used to estimate and plot the survival curve—that is, a life table—for a set of independent variable values. When all the independent variables are nominal, the Cox regression estimates survival curves that are very similar to those resulting from Kaplan-Meier life-table analysis. However, Cox regression is able to incorporate continuous as well as nominal independent variables. Cox regression can thus be used to construct the equivalent of a life table that has been adjusted for multiple independent variables. Cox regression can in and of itself address our three basic questions of statistics: estimation, inference, and adjustment.

In a life-table the magnitude of the difference between groups can be estimated by using the percentage survival from the end (right side) of the survival curves. Inference (statistical significance testing) can be performed comparing the survival curves taking into account all of the data. Finally, Cox regression has the advantage of incorporating the adjustment for confounding variables. Thus, the Cox regression is increasingly used in health research.

As indicated in Fig. 43.3, nominal dependent variables that are not affected by time are frequently analyzed using a multivariable approach called *logistic regression*. The dependent variable in logistic regression is the natural logarithm of the odds of group membership. Thus, odds ratios are the estimate obtained from logistic regression regardless of the type of investigation. We can, therefore, view logistic regression as a method of adjusting odds ratios for nominal and continuous confounding variables. Logistic regression is now widely used in health research, thus increasing the importance of the odds ratio as a point estimate used in cohort studies and randomized clinical trials as well as case-control studies.[18]

Now that we have completed our overview of univariable, bivariable, and multivariable analyses, let us put the process together in the final chapter and see how we can use the combined flowchart.

---

[18] In recent years a method known as *generalized regression models* are increasingly being used. This method combines logistic regression methods for nominal or dichotomous outcomes with multiple regression methods for continuous outcomes.

44 Selecting a Statistic Flowchart

In this chapter, the entire flowchart that is required for selecting a statistic is presented. To gain practice using each of the branches of the flowchart, try out the eight exercises on the Studying a Study Online Web site at **www.StudyingaStudy.com.**

This summary flowchart can be used in two ways. One way is to start at the top as we have done previously, and begin with Fig. 44.1 and trace the flowchart down to discover what types of statistical procedures are appropriate for a particular investigation. As a reader of the literature rather than a researcher you can use the flowchart starting at the bottom. That is, you can identify a statistical technique used in an investigation and can work backward up the flowchart to understand the questions being asked by the technique and the types of data for which it is appropriately used.

To illustrate the use of the flowchart, we will start at the top in Fig. 44.1 and identify one dependent variable. We then ask whether we are dealing with 0, 1, or more than 1 independent variables. Next, we must decide the type of data represented by the dependent variable (continuous, ordinal, or nominal). After we make these decisions, we will encounter a figure number that will guide us to the next flowchart element that is applicable to our data.

Each of the subsequent flowchart components is constructed in a similar way. If the data contain independent variables, we will need to identify the type of data represented by each one.[1] If special restrictions or assumptions are required for a statistical procedure, we will need to decide if the data satisfy these restrictions. If these restriction are not fulfilled or no statistical procedures are available for the type of data represented by one or more of the variables, it is often possible to convert the variables to a lower-level scale and consult the flowchart for an option that is consistent with the converted variables. That is, when the restrictions on a statistical procedure are not fulfilled, continuous variables can be converted to ordinal variables and ordinal variables can be converted to nominal variables. Remember, however, that this results in some loss of statistical power.[2]

Following down the flowchart, we come to a summary measurement or point estimate that is useful for our data. This is followed, if applicable, by a general classification of statistical procedures that are enclosed in a box. At the very bottom, we encounter the name of the procedures that are most commonly used for both statistical significance testing and calculation of confidence intervals on data sets like the one we are examining. These are underlined.

---

[1] Remember that for statistical purposes, a nominal variable refers to only two categories of a characteristic. If a characteristic has k categories, $k - 1$ nominal variables will be needed. If more than one nominal variable is needed to represent the independent variable, then multivariable analysis is needed.

[2] For instance, the use of correlation analysis is restricted to situations in which naturalistic sampling has been used. Fulfillment of the assumptions of Gaussian distribution and homoscedasticity of the dependent variable are required for the use of continuous dependent variables. A transformation of the data, however, may allow an investigator to fulfill these assumptions. Even though nonparametric procedures have a lower statistical power, at times the loss of statistical power may be quite modest.

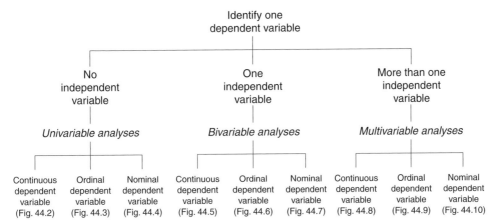

Figure 44.1. Master flowchart to determine which of the subsequent flowcharts are applicable to a particular data set.

When using the flowchart, note the following:

1. Additional conditions that need to be satisfied to use a type of statistical procedure are shown immediately after the type of independent variables, such as pairing or affected by time.[3]
2. Terms enclosed in a box indicate a general classification of statistical procedures.
3. When a comma alone appears between two underlined statistical significance tests, the first test is used to evaluate the omnibus null hypothesis, whereas the second test is used in pairwise comparisons. An "or" indicates alternative test that may be used.

Remember that the flowchart, starting at the top, is applicable to researchers who are interested in selecting a statistical procedure for a set of data. More often, as readers of the health research literature, we are interested in checking that a procedure selected by others is an appropriate one. The flowchart can be used to assist in that process by first finding the name of the selected procedure at the bottom of the flowchart and tracing the flowchart backward to determine whether the procedure is a logical choice for the data set being analyzed.

Let us consider an example of how to use the flowchart of statistics in Fig. 44.1 through Fig. 44.10. Together these figures represent the overall Selecting a Statistic flowchart presented in Chapters 40 through 43. To see how the flowchart can be used, consider the following research study.

A randomized clinical trial of a new vitamin supplement is designed to test the hypothesis that the new supplement will reduce the chance that the mother will deliver a second child with spina bifida. The study was conducted by randomizing 1000 women who had previously delivered a child with spina bifida to the new

---

[3] These conditions need to be distinguished from assumptions about the data itself. Remember that pairing is the special type of matching in which one study individual is paired with one control individual and the pair is analyzed as a unit. Affected by time implies that an increase in the duration of observation results in a greater probability of observing the outcome, and individuals are observed for different lengths of time.

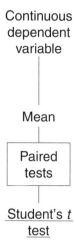

Figure 44.2. Flowchart to select a univariable statistical procedure for a continuous dependent variable.

treatment study group and 1000 other women who had previously delivered a child with spina bifida to the conventional treatment/control group. All women were in their first trimester of pregnancy. The study and control groups were similar except that the control group had an average age of 32 years compared to 28 years for the study group. Maternal age is believed to be a risk factor for spina bifida. Spina bifida was assessed at the time of birth.

To use the flowchart, we start with Fig. 44.1. The first step is to identify one dependent variable. The dependent variable is the characteristic of primary interest for which the investigation is trying to estimate a value or test a hypothesis. In this investigation, we are testing the hypothesis that the new prenatal vitamins will prevent spina bifida. The presence or absence of spina bifida is the dependent variable.

Moving down the flowchart in Fig. 44.1, we come to the next question that must be addressed: How many independent variables does this investigation include? The independent variables represent all the other data that we wish to include in the analysis. In this study, we need to include treatment (vitamin supplement or conventional treatment) and age. Age is included because it is a potential confounding variable. Thus, we have more than one independent variable and can move down Fig. 44.1 to multivariable analysis. The next question will require us to select one

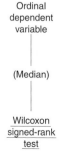

Figure 44.3. Flowchart to select a univariable statistical procedure for an ordinal dependent variable.

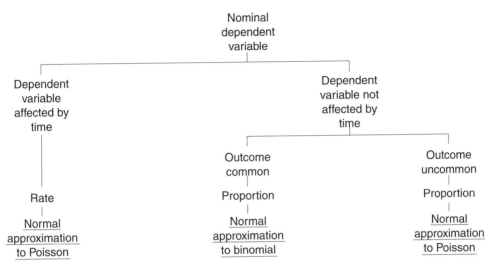

Figure 44.4. Flowchart to select a univariable statistical procedure for a nominal dependent variable.

of the following figures (Figs. 44.8 through 44.10) that display the remainder of the flowchart.

The next question is "What type of dependent variable do we have?" Because the presence or absence of spina bifida is the dependent variable, we have one nominal dependent variable. This brings us to the end of Fig. 44.1 and leads us to Fig. 44.10. Thus, Fig. 44.1 guides us to one of the subsequent flowcharts.

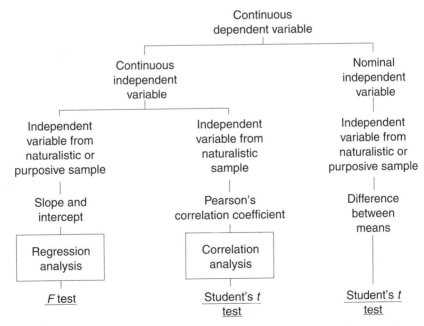

Figure 44.5. Flowchart to select a bivariable statistical procedure for a continuous dependent variable.

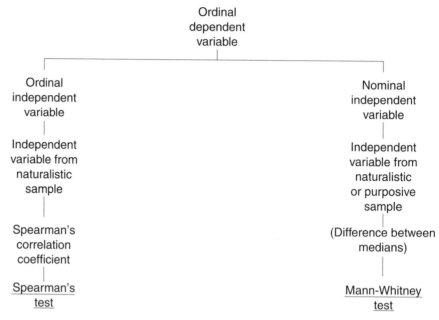

Figure 44.6. Flowchart to select a bivariable statistical procedure for an ordinal dependent variable.

Turning to Fig. 44.10, on page 368 we see all the methods we have discussed for one nominal dependent variable. We now ask whether this investigation has only nominal independent variables or whether it has both continuous and nominal independent variables. In this investigation, the independent variables are treatment group and age. The treatment group has only two categories; therefore,

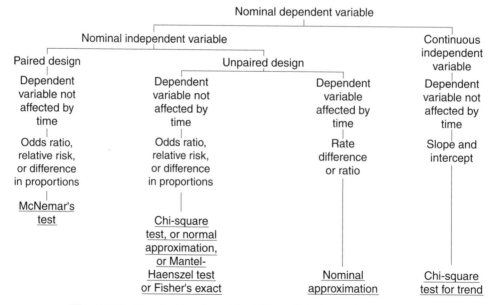

Figure 44.7. Flowchart to select a bivariable statistical procedure for a nominal dependent variable.

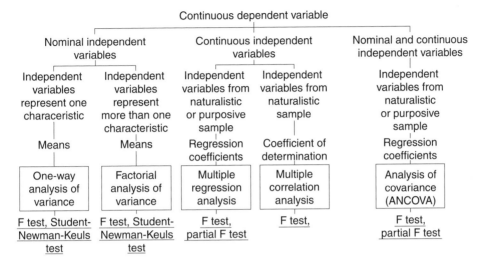

Figure 44.8. Flowchart to select a multivariable statistical procedure for a continuous dependent variable.

it is a nominal variable. Age is a continuous variable. Thus, having both nominal and continuous variables, we can proceed down the left side of the flowchart in Fig. 44.10.

Now we need to decide whether the dependent variable, delivery of a child with spina bifida, is affected by time. Being affected by time requires that there are multiple times that participants are observed to assess outcomes. This is often the situation in randomized clinical trials. However, here we are only assessing outcome once at the time of birth. Thus, there is only one assessment point, and the dependent variable is not affected by time.

This leads us to the odds ratio as our estimate of the strength of the relationship between the treatment group and the occurrence of spina bifida. Proceeding down the flowchart in Fig. 44.10 we come to the general category of statistical techniques known as *logistic regression* (enclosed in the box). The estimate of the strength of the relationship here is the odds ratio. As indicated by the underlined chi-square test, statistical significance testing and confidence intervals are performed on the odds ratio using a chi-square method.

Having worked through the flowchart starting at the top, we have seen the type of investigation in which logistic regression can be used. When logistic regression

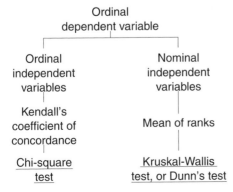

Figure 44.9. Flowchart to select a multivariable statistical procedure for an ordinal dependent variable.

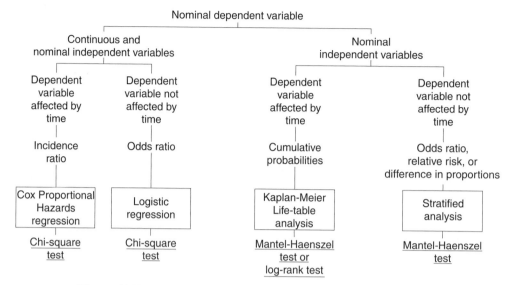

Figure 44.10. Flowchart to select a multivariable statistical procedure for a nominal dependent variable.

is used in an investigation, we can now appreciate the conditions under which its use is appropriate. When logistic regression is used, we expect to see a nominal dependent variable and continuous as well as nominal independent variables. The odds ratio will be the resulting point estimate and the outcomes will only be measured once for each participant, i.e., they are not time-dependent. This is what we mean by using the flowchart in reverse.

When we read in the health literature that a statistical procedure has been used, we can look near the bottom of Figs. 44.2 through 44.10 and locate that procedure, such as logistic regression. Then we can move up the flowchart and identify the types of data and any special conditions that are necessary for its use.

The Selecting a Statistic flowchart is designed to be a practical guide to help identify and understand the use of the most common statistical procedures. Used along with the Questions to Ask in the last chapter of each section, it can help you read the medical evidence.

Now you need some practice. It's time to try out the exercises and journal articles included in the Studying a Study Online Web site at **www. StudyingaStudy.com**. A little practice and you'll find that using the M.A.A.R.I.E. framework and Selecting a Statistic flowchart can become second nature and even an enjoyable part of your professional practice.

Glossary

Accuracy   Without systematic error or bias; on average the results approximate those of the phenomenon under study.

Actuarial Survival   The actuarial survival is an estimate of life expectancy based on a cohort or longitudinal life table. The 5-year actuarial survival estimates the probability of surviving 5 years, and may be calculated even when there are only a limited number of individuals actually followed for 5 years.

Adjustment   Techniques used after the collection of data to take into account or control for the effect of known or potential confounding variables and interactions. (*Synonym:* control for, take into account, standardize)

Affected by Time   A measurement is affected by time if an increase in the duration of observation results in a greater probability of observing the outcome, and individuals are observed for different lengths of time. A variable that is affected by time is said to be time-dependent.

Aggregate Impact   The overall impact of an intervention on the entire population of individuals to whom it is directed.

Aggregate External Validity   As used by the United States Preventive Services Task Force, the extent to which the evidence is relevant and generalizable to the population and conditions of typical primary care practice.

Aggregate Internal Validity   As used by the United States Preventive Services Task Force, the degree to which the studies used to support an evidence-based recommendation provide valid evidence for the populations and the settings in which they were conducted.

Algorithm   An explicit, often graphic presentation of the steps to be taken in a making a decision such as diagnosis or treatment. An algorithm may be used to present evidence-based guidelines using a standardized graphical approach.

Allocation Concealment   In a randomized clinical trial, the inability of the individual making the assignment to predict the group to which the next individual will be assigned.

Allocation Ratio   In a randomized clinical trial the proportion of participants intended for each study and control group.

Alternative Hypothesis   In statistical significance testing, the actual choices are between the null hypothesis and an alternative hypothesis. The alternative hypothesis states that a difference or association exists.

Analysis of Covariance (ANCOVA)   Statistical procedures for analysis of data that contain a continuous dependent variable and a mixture of nominal and continuous independent variables.

Analysis of Variance (ANOVA)   Statistical procedures for analysis of data that contain a continuous dependent variable and more than one nominal independent variable. ANOVA procedures include one-way and factorial ANOVA.

Analytical Study   All types of investigations that include a comparison group within the investigation itself (e.g., case-control, cohort, and randomized clinical trials).

Appropriate Measurement   A measurement that addresses the question that an investigation intends to study, i.e., one that is appropriate for the study question. (*Synonym:* construct validity, content validity)

Artifactual Differences or Changes   Differences or changes in measures of occurrence that result from the way the disease or condition is measured, sought, or defined.

Assessment   The determination of the outcome or endpoint of the study and control groups.

Assessment Bias   A generic term referring to any type of bias in the assessment process. Recall, report, and instrument errors are specific types of assessment bias.

Assignment   The process by which individuals become part of a study group or control group.

Association   A relationship among two or more characteristics or other measurements beyond what would be expected by chance alone. When used to establish criterion number one of contributory cause, association implies that the two characteristics occur in the same individual more often than expected by chance alone. (*Synonym:* individual association)

At-Risk Population   The population that is represented in the denominator of most rates—that is, those who are at risk of developing the event being measured in the numerator. In the context of risk factors, the at-risk population may be referred to as those with the risk factors.

Attributable Risk Percentage   The percentage of the risk, among those with the risk factor, that is associated with exposure to the risk factor. If a cause-and-effect relationship exists, attributable risk is the percentage of a disease that can potentially be eliminated among those with the risk factor if the effect of the risk factor is completely eliminated. (*Synonym:* attributable risk, attributable risk [exposed], etiological fraction [exposed], percentage risk reduction, protective efficacy ratio)

Averaging Out   The process of obtaining overall expected utilities for a decision tree by adding together the expected utilities of each of the potential outcomes included in the decision tree.

Base-Case Estimate   The estimate used in a decision-making investigation that reflects the investigators' best available or best-guess estimate of the relevant value of a particular variable. High and low estimates reflect the extremes of the realistic range of values around the base-case estimate.

Bayes' Theorem   A mathematical formula that can be used to calculate posttest probabilities (or odds) based on pretest probabilities (or odds) and the sensitivity and specificity of a test.

Bayesian   An approach to statistics that takes into account the preexisting probability (or odds) of a disease or a study hypothesis when analyzing and interpreting the data in the investigation.

Bias   A condition that produced results which depart from the true values in a consistent direction. (*Synonym:* systematic error)

Binomial Distribution   A mathematical distribution that is used to calculate probabilities for populations composed of nominal data.

Biological Plausibility   An ancillary, adjunct, or supportive criteria of cause-and-effect which implies that the relationship is consistent with a known biological mechanism.

Bivariable Analysis   Statistical analysis in which there is one dependent variable and one independent variable.

Blind Assessment   The evaluation of the outcome for individuals without the individual who makes the evaluation knowing whether the subjects were in the study group or the control group. (*Synonym:* masked assessment)

Blind Assignment   Occurs when individuals are assigned to a study group and a control group without the investigator or the subjects being aware of the group to which they are assigned. When both investigator and subjects are "blinded" or "masked," the study is sometimes referred to as a double-blind study. (*Synonym:* masked assignment)

Calibration   An estimate used in prediction rules that measures performance of a test, risk factor, or other variable to summarize its performance not only on the average participant but on participants whose characteristics are far from the average.

Carry-Over Effect   A phenomenon that may occur in a cross-over study when the initial therapy continues to have an effect after it is no longer being administered. A "wash-out" period is often used to minimize the potential for a carry-over effect.

Case-Control Study   A study that begins by identifying individuals with a disease (cases) and individuals without a disease (controls). The cases and controls are identified without knowledge of an individual's exposure or nonexposure to factors being investigated. (*Synonym:* retrospective study)

Case Fatality   The number of deaths due to a particular disease divided by the number of individuals diagnosed with the disease at the beginning of the time interval. The case fatality estimates the probability of eventually dying from the disease.

Case-Mix Bias   A form of selection bias that may be created when treatments are selected by clinicians to fit characteristics of individual patients.

Central Limit Theorem   The principle that regardless of the distribution of the data in a population, the mean values calculated from samples tend to have a Gaussian distribution. This tendency increases as the size of the sample increases.

Censored Data   Data is censored when collection of data is terminated at a particular point in time and it is not known whether or not the outcome subsequently occurred. Data may be censored due to loss to follow-up, or termination of the investigation.

Chance Node   A darkened circle in a decision tree that indicates that once a decision is made, there are two or more outcomes that may occur by a chance process. These potential outcomes are displayed to the right of the chance node.

Chi-Square Distribution   A standard mathematical distribution that can be used to calculate P values and confidence intervals in a variety of statistical procedures for nominal dependent variables.

Chi-Square Test   A statistical significance test that can be used to calculate a P value for a nominal independent and a nominal dependent variable. The chi-square test is one of a large number of uses of the chi-square distribution.

Chi-Square Test for Trend   A statistical significance test that is used for a nominal dependent variable and a continuous independent variable.

Coefficient of Determination   The square of a correlation coefficient. This statistic when appropriately used indicates the proportion of the variation in one variable (the dependent variable) that is explained by knowing the value of one or more other variables (the independent variables).

Cohort   A group of individuals who share a common exposure, experience, or characteristic. (*See:* cohort study, cohort effect)

Cohort Effect   A change in rates that can be explained by the common experience or characteristic of a group of individuals. A cohort effect implies that current rates should not be directly extrapolated into the future.

Cohort Study   A study that begins by identifying individuals with and without a factor being investigated. These factors are identified without knowledge of which individuals have or will develop the outcome. Cohort studies may be concurrent or retrospective.

Concurrent Cohort Study   A cohort study in which an individual's group assignment is determined at the time that the study begins, and the study group and control group participants are followed forward in time to determine if the disease occur. (*Synonym:* prospective cohort study)

Confidence Interval (95%)   In statistical terms, the interval of numerical values within which one can be 95% confident that the value being estimated lies. (*Synonym:* interval estimate)

Confidence Limits   The upper and lower extremes of the confidence interval.

Confounding Variable   A variable that is distributed differently in the study group and control group and that affects the outcome being assessed. A confounding variable may be due to chance or bias. When it is due to bias in the assignment process, the resulting error is also called a selection bias. (*Synonym:* confounder)

Consensus Conference   As used here, a process for determining the presence or absence of a consensus by using face-to-face structured communication among a representative group of experts.

Continuous Data   A type of data with an unlimited number of equally spaced potential values (e.g., diastolic blood pressure, cholesterol).

Contributory Cause   Contributory cause is definitively established when all three of the following have been established: (a) the existence of an association between the cause and the effect at the level of the individual; (b) the cause precedes the effect in time; and (c) altering the cause alters the probability of occurrence of the effect.

Control Group   A group of subjects used for comparison with a study group. Ideally, the control group is identical to the study group except that it does not possess the characteristic or has not been exposed to the treatment under study.

Controlled Clinical Trial   *See:* randomized clinical trial

Convenience Sample   A subset from a population that is assembled because of the ease of collecting data without regard for the degree to which the sample is random or representative of the population of interest.

Conventional Care   The current level of intervention accepted as routine or standard care.

Correlation   A statistic used for studying the strength of an association between two variables, each of which has been sampled using a representative or naturalistic method from a population of interest.

Correlation Analysis   A class of statistical procedures that is used to estimate the strength of the relationship between a continuous dependent variable and a continuous independent variable when both the dependent variable and the independent variable are selected by naturalistic sampling.

Correlation Coefficient   An estimate of the strength of the association between a dependent variable and an independent variable when both are obtained using naturalistic sampling. (e.g., Peason's and Spearman's correlation coefficients.)

Cost-and-Effectiveness Studies   As used here, the type of decision analysis study that compares the cost of achieving a common unit of effectiveness, such as a life saved or a diagnosis made.

Cost-Benefit Analysis   The type of decision-making investigation that converts effectiveness as well as cost into monetary terms. Benefit in a cost-benefit analysis refers to net effectiveness, that is, the favorable minus the unfavorable outcomes.

Cost-Consequence Analysis   A type of cost-effectiveness analysis in which harms, benefits, and costs are measured or described but not directly combined or compared.

Cost-Effective   An alternative is considered cost-effective if the increase in effectiveness is considered worth the increase in cost; if the decreased effectiveness is considered worth the substantial reduction in costs; or if there is reduced cost plus increased effectiveness.

Cost-Effectiveness Analysis   A general term for the type of decision-making investigation in which costs are considered as well as harms and benefits.

Cost-Effectiveness Ratios   The average cost per QALY obtained. The comparison alternative in a cost-effectiveness ratio is not usually specified but should generally be considered to be the do-nothing or zero cost–zero effectiveness alternative.

Cost-QALY Graph   A graph that includes cost on the y-axis and QALY on the x-axis, and includes four quadrants with different interpretations related to cost-effectiveness. The intersection of the x- and y-axes represents the do-nothing or zero cost–zero effectiveness alternative.

Cost Savings   A reduction in cost that may be accompanied by a reduction or an increase in effectiveness.

Cost-Utility Analysis   The type of cost-effectiveness analysis that measures and combines benefits, harms, and costs, taking into account the probabilities and the utilities. Cost-utility investigations often use QALYs as the measure of effectiveness and thus may be called cost-effectiveness analysis using QALYs. (*Synonym:* QALY cost-effectiveness study)

Covariance   The statistic that is calculated to estimate how closely a dependent and an independent variable change together.

Cox Regression   See proportional hazards regression.

Credibility Intervals   A term used in decision-making investigations to present the results in a form that parallels confidence intervals. The Monte Carlo method may be used to generate credibility intervals by performing large numbers of simulation's using the investigation's own decision-making model.

Cross-Over Study   A type of paired design in which the same individual receives a study and a control therapy, and an outcome is assessed for each therapy.

Cross-Sectional Study   A study that identifies individuals with and without the condition or disease under study and the characteristic or exposure of interest at the same point in time. The independent and the dependent variables are measured at the same point in time, and thus data can be collect from a one-time survey. A cross-sectional study may be regarded as a special type of case-control study.

Cumulative Survival   The estimate of survival derived for a life-table analysis calculated by combining the probabilities from each time interval.

Database Research   Investigations done based on previously collected data. May be used as a synonym for retrospective cohort study when a study group and a control group are identified based on prior characteristics contained in a database.

Decision Analysis   As used in decision-making investigations, refers to the type of investigations in which benefits and harms are included but not costs. Often used generically to refer to all quantitative decision-making.

Decision-Making Model   A diagram or written description of the steps involved in each of the alternatives being considered in a decision-making investigation. A decision tree is a common method of presenting the decision-making model.

Decision Node   A square in a decision tree that indicates that a choice needs to be made. (*Synonym:* choice node)

Decision Tree   A graphic display of the decision alternatives, including the choices that need to be made and the chance events that occur.

Declining Exponential Approximation of Life Expectancy (DEALE)   A specialized life-expectancy measure which combines survival derived for a longitudinal life table and life expectancy based on age and other demographic factors derived from a cross-sectional life table.

Delphi Method   A formal method for reaching group agreement in which the participants do not communicate directly with each other.

Diagnostic Ability   A term used here to indicate that the measurement of a test's performance includes a weighting of false positives compared to false negatives in addition to the discriminant ability.

Diagnostic Test   A test conducted in the presence of symptoms with the intention of identifying the presence of disease.

Discriminant Ability   A measure of test performance that assumes that a false positive and a false negative are of equal importance. May be measured by the area under a ROC curve. (*Synonym:* area under ROC curve)

Dependent Variable   Generally, the outcome variable of interest in any type of research study. The outcome or endpoint that one intends to explain or estimate.

Describe a Population   In statistical terminology, indicates the distribution of the data in the larger population from which the samples are obtained.

Descriptive Study   An investigation that provides data on one group of individuals and does not include a comparison group, at least within the investigation itself. (*Synonym:* description study, case series, time series)

Direct Cause   A contributory cause that is the most directly known cause of a disease (e.g., hepatitis B virus is the direct cause of hepatitis B infection, and contaminated needles are an indirect cause). The direct cause is dependent on the current state of knowledge and may change as more immediate mechanisms are discovered.

Disability Adjusted Life Years (DALY))   A disease- or condition-specific measure of the number of life years lost from death and disability per population unit (such as per 100,000 people) compared to a population with the best current health status.

Discordant Pairs   In a case-control study, the pairs of subjects in which the study and control differ in their exposure or nonexposure to the potential risk factor.

Discounted Present Value   The amount of money that needs to be invested today to pay a bill of a particular size at a particular time in the future. (*Synonym:* present value)

Glossary

Discounting   A method used in decision-making investigations to take into account the reduced importance of benefits, harms, and costs that occur at a later period of time compared to those that occur immediately. The discount rate is the annual rate used to perform discounting.

Discrete Data   Data with a limited number of categories or potential values. Discrete data may be further classified as either nominal or ordinal data.

Dispersion   Spread of data around a measure of central tendency, such as a mean.

Distribution   Frequencies or relative frequencies of all possible values of a characteristic. Population and sample distributions can be described graphically or mathematically. One purpose of statistics is to estimate parameters of population distributions.

Distributional Effects   A term used in decision-making investigations that indicates that the average results do not take into account the distributions of the adverse and favorable outcomes among subgroups with different demographic characteristics.

Dominance   An alternative is dominant when a recommendation can be made on the basis of probabilities alone. That is, one alternative is preferred regardless of the utilities that are attached to particular favorable and unfavorable outcomes. In cost effectiveness, dominance refers to the situation in which an option is more effective and also less costly. Extended dominance then usually refers to the situation where effectiveness is approximately equal but one option is less costly than the other.

Do-Nothing Approach   The comparison alternative in decision-making investigations in which there is presumed to be zero cost and zero effectiveness.

Dose-Response Relationship   A dose-response relationship is present if changes in levels of an exposure are associated with changes in the frequency of the outcome in a consistent direction. A dose-response relationship is an ancillary or supportive criterion for contributory cause.

Ecological Fallacy   The type of error that can occur when the existence of a group association is used to imply the existence of a relationship that does not exist at the individual level. (*Synonym:* population fallacy)

Economies of Scale   Generally refers to reductions in cost that accompany increases in the scale of production. Diseconomies of scale imply increases in cost that accompany changes in the scale of production.

Effect   An outcome that is brought about, at least in part, by an etiological factor known as the cause, i.e., altering the probability that the cause occurs alters the probability that the effect occurs.

Effect of Observation   A type of assessment bias that results when the process of observation alters the outcome of the study.

Effect Size   A summary measure of the magnitude of the difference or association found in the sample.

Effectiveness   The extent to which a treatment produces a beneficial effect when implemented under the usual conditions of clinical care for a particular group of patients. In the context of cost-effectiveness, effectiveness incorporates desirable outcomes and undesirable outcomes, and may be referred to as net effectiveness

Efficacy   The extent to which a treatment produces a beneficial effect when assessed under the ideal conditions of an investigation.

Eligibility Criteria The combined set of inclusion and exclusion criteria that define those who are eligible for participation in an investigation (*Synonym:* entry criteria)

Estimate A value calculated from sample observations that are used to approximate a corresponding population value or parameter. Obtaining an estimate is one of the primary goals of statistical methods. (*See:* point estimate)

Event An episode or diagnosis of the condition or disease that appears in the numerator of a rate or proportion.

Evidence-Based Guideline Structured set of recommendations for clinical or public health practice indicating specific conditions for utilizing or not utilizing interventions. Based on evidence from the research literature combined with decision-maker preferences and expert opinion. (*Synonym:* evidence-based recommendation).

Exclusion Criteria Conditions which preclude entrance of candidates into an investigation even if they meet the inclusion criteria.

Expected Utility The results of multiplying the probability times the utility of a particular outcome. (*Synonym:* quality-adjusted probability)

Expected-Utility Decision Analysis The type of decision analysis that considers probabilities and utilities but does not explicitly incorporate life expectancy.

Expected Value A measure that incorporates cost as well as benefit and harm into a decision tree. The outcome is then measured in monetary terms.

Experimentwise Error The probability of making a Type I error for at least one comparison in an analysis that involves more than one comparison.

Exploratory Meta-analysis A meta-analysis in which there is not a specific hypothesis, and all potentially relevant investigations are included.

Extended Dominance *See:* dominance

Extrapolation Conclusions drawn about the meaning of the study for a target population. The target population may be similar to those included in the investigation or may include types of individuals or a range of data not represented in the study sample.

F **distribution** A standard distribution that can be used to calculate *P* values and confidence intervals in ANOVA, ANCOVA, multiple regression, and multiple correlation analysis procedures.

Factor A term used in ANOVA procedures to separate a collection of characteristics that define mutually exclusive and topically related categories, such as race. Statistical significance tests on factors are called tests of main effects in a factorial ANOVA. Also, less formally used to represent characteristics under investigation to determine if they are risk factors.

Fail-Safe N The number of studies which must be omitted from a meta-analysis before the results would no longer be statistically significant. These additional studies are assumed to be of the same average size as the included studies and have, on average, an effect size of 0 for differences or 1 for ratios.

False Negative An individual whose result on a test is negative but who has the disease or condition as determined by the reference standard.

False Positive An individual whose result on a test is positive but who does not have the disease or condition as determined by the reference standard.

Final Outcome An outcome that occurs at the completion of a decision option. This outcome is displayed at the right end of a decision tree.

Fisher's Exact Procedure   A method for calculating P values for data with one nominal dependent variable and one nominal independent variable when any of the frequencies predicted by the null hypothesis are less than 5.

Fixed Costs   Costs which do not vary with modest increases or decreases in the volume of services provided. Space and personnel costs are considered examples of fixed costs, which partly explains why institutional decision-making does not always conform to the recommendations of cost-effectiveness analysis.

Fixed-Effect Model   A type of statistical significance test that assumes that sub-groups all come from the same large population. In meta-analysis, implies that there is homogeneity across the investigations.

Folding Back the Decision Tree   A process in which probabilities are multiplied together to obtain a probability of a particular outcome known as a path probability. Calculations of path probabilities assume that the probability of each of the outcomes that occur along the path is independent of the other probabilities along the same path.

Funnel Diagram   A graphical method for evaluating whether publication bias is likely to be present in a meta-analysis.

Gaussian Distribution   A distribution of data assumed in many statistical procedures. The Gaussian distribution is a symmetrical, continuous, bell-shaped curve with its mean value corresponding to the highest point on the curve. (*Synonym:* normal distribution)

Generalized Regression Model   A statistical method that combines logistic regression methods for nominal or dichotomous outcome with multiple regression methods for continuous outcomes.

Gold Standard   *See:* reference standard

Group Association   The situation in which a characteristic and a disease both occur more frequently in one group of individuals compared with another. Group association does not necessarily imply that individuals with the characteristic are the same ones who have the disease. (*Synonym:* ecological association, ecological correlation)

Group Matching   A matching procedure used during assignment in an investigation that selects study and control individuals in such a way that the groups have a nearly equal distribution of a particular variable or variables. (*Synonym:* frequency matching)

Guideline   In practice guidelines, the term indicates a recommendation for (or against) an intervention except under specified exceptions. At times, used to indicate the special type of recommendation in which indications and contraindications are included. Guidelines developed based on evidence are increasingly referred to as evidence-based guidelines or evidence-based recommendations.

Health Adjusted Life Expectancy (HALE)   A measurement of life expectancy that includes a measure of the quality of health that may be measured as utilities.

Healthy-Worker Effect   A tendency for workers in an occupation to be healthier than the general population of individuals of the same age.

Heuristic   A rule of thumb or method used in nonquantitative or subjective decision-making that generally uses only a portion of the potentially available data and thus simplifies the decision-making process.

Historical Control   A control group from an earlier period of time that is used to compare outcomes with a study group in an investigation.

Homogeneous   When used in the context of a meta-analysis, homogeneous refers to investigations which can be combined into a single meta-analysis because the study characteristics being examined do not substantially affect the outcome.

Homoscedasticity   An assumption of statistical methods for a continuous dependent variable implying equal variance of the dependent variable values in the population for each value of the independent variable. (*Synonym:* assumption of equal variance)

Human Capital   An approach to converting effectiveness to monetary terms that uses the recipient's ability to contribute to the economy.

Hypothesis-Driven Meta-analysis   A meta-analysis in which a specific hypothesis is used as the basis for inclusion or exclusion of investigations.

Incidence Rate   The rate at which new cases of disease occur per unit of time. The incidence rate is theoretically calculated as the number of individuals who develop the disease over a period of time divided by the total person-years of observation. (*Synonym:* hazard)

Inclusion Criteria   Conditions which must be met by all potential candidates for entrance into an investigation.

Incremental Cost-effectiveness Ratio   The cost of obtaining one additional QALY using an alternative compared with the use of the conventional alternative.

Independence   Two events or two tests are independent if the results of the first do not influence the results of the second. (*Synonym:* independence assumption)

Independent Variable   Variable being measured to estimate the corresponding measurement of the dependent variable in any type of research study. Independent variables define the conditions under which the dependent variable is to be measured.

Index Test   The test of interest that is being evaluation by comparison with the reference standard test.

Indicator Variable   A variable that is used to represent the value of a nominal variable in ANCOVA. An indicator variable tells us how much the estimate of the continuous dependent variable differs between levels of the indicator variable. (*Synonym:* dummy variable)

Indirect Cause   A contributory cause that acts through a biological mechanism that is more closely related to the disease than it is to the direct cause (e.g., contaminated needles are an indirect cause of hepatitis B; the hepatitis B virus is a direct cause). (*See:* direct cause)

Inference   In statistical terminology, inference is the logical process that occurs during statistical significance testing in which conclusions concerning a population are obtained based on data from a random sample of the population. (*See:* statistical significance test)

Influence Diagram   An alternative to decision trees that displays the factors that influence events. Influence diagrams may be combined with a decision tree.

Information Bias   A systematic error introduced by the process of obtaining the investigation's measurement of outcome.

Intention to Treat   A method for data analysis in a randomized clinical trial in which individual outcomes are analyzed according to the group to which they have been randomized even if they never received the treatment to which they were assigned. (*Synonym:* per protocol)

Interaction   Occurs when the probability of an outcome resulting from the presence of one variable is altered by the level of a second variable. Interaction between variables may produce results that are more than additive or less than additive. Biological interaction may be distinguished from statistical interaction. The presence or absence of statistical interaction depends on the scale of measurement used. (*Synonym:* effect modification, synergy)

Intercept   The intercept estimates the mean of the dependent variable when the independent variables are equal to zero.

Interobserver Variation   Variation in measurement by different individuals.

Interpolation   The process of implying or filling in data values between the points that are actually measured. As opposed to extrapolation, which implies extending the data beyond the points actually measured.

Interpretation   The drawing of conclusions about the meaning of any differences found between the study group and the control group for those included in the investigation.

Interval Estimate   *See:* confidence interval

Intraobserver Variation   Variation in measurements by the same person at different times.

Kaplan-Meier Life Table   *See:* life table (cohort or longitudinal)

Kendall's Coefficient of Concordance   An estimate of the degree of correlation. This estimate can be used when the dependent variable and all the independent variables are ordinal.

Koch's Postulates   A set of criteria developed for demonstrating cause-and-effect that was extensively applied to infectious disease. Koch's postulates include necessary cause. What has been called modern Koch's postulates include epidemiological association, isolation, and transmission pathogenesis.

Kruskal-Wallis Test   A statistical significance test that can be used when there is an ordinal dependent variable and two or more nominal independent variables. Dunn's test may be used as an alternative test.

Lead-Time Bias   Overestimation of survival time due to earlier diagnosis of disease. Actual time of death does not change when lead-time bias is present despite the earlier time of diagnosis.

Least-Squares Regression   A method of regression analysis that selects numerical values for the slope and intercept which minimize the sum of the squared differences between the data observed in the sample and those estimated by the regression equation.

Length Bias   The tendency of a screening test to more frequently detect individuals with a slowly progressive disease compared with individuals with a rapidly progressive disease.

Life Expectancy   The average number of years of remaining life from a particular age based on the probabilities of death in each age group in one particular year. Life expectancy assumes a stationary population and the same age specific probabilities of death in subsequent years, or it is not an accurate prediction of the average number of years of remaining life.

Life Table (Cohort or Longitudinal)   A method for organizing data that allows examination of the experience of one or more groups of individuals over time when some individuals are followed for longer periods of time than others. (*Synonym:* Kaplan-Meier life tables)

Life Table (Cross-Sectional or Current)   A technique that uses mortality data from one year's experience and applies the data to a stationary population to calculate life expectancies.

Likelihood Ratio of Negative Test   A ratio of the probability of a negative test if the disease is present to the probability of a negative test if the disease is absent.

Likelihood Ratio of Positive Test   A ratio of the probability of a positive test if the disease is present to the probability of a positive test if the disease is absent.

Linear Extrapolation   A form of extrapolation that assumes, often incorrectly, that levels of a variable beyond the range of the data will continue to operate in the same manner that they operate in the investigation. Linear extrapolation is often used to extrapolate beyond the data by extending the straight-line relationship obtained from an investigation.

Linear Regression   A form of regression analysis in which there is only one dependent and one independent variable, and a straight-line or linear relationship is assumed to exist between the dependent and independent variable.

Location   A measure of central tendency of a distribution. Means and medians are examples of measures of location.

Log-Rank Test   A statistical significance test that is used in life-table analysis (*Synonym:* Mantel-Haenszel test)

Logistic Regression   A multivariable method used when there is a nominal dependent variable and a nominal and continuous independent variable that are not affected by time.

Main Effect   A term used in factorial ANOVA to indicate statistical tests used to examine each factor separately. May also refer to the relationship between the independent variable and the dependent variable that reflect the relationship stated in the study hypothesis.

Mann-Whitney Test   A statistical significance test that is used for an ordinal dependent variable and a nominal independent variable.

Mantel-Haenszel Test   *See:* log rank test

Marginal Cost   The impact on costs of greatly increasing the scale of operation of an intervention so that economies of scale and diseconomies of scale may impact the costs. Often but not always distinguished from incremental cost, which relates to the cost of one additional unit.

Markov Analysis   A method of analysis used in decision-making investigations to take into account recurrent events such as recurrence of previous disease or development of a second episode of disease.

Masked   *See:* blind assessment; blind assignment

Matched Test   A type of statistical significance test that is used to analyze data in which the special type of matching called pairing is used.

Matching   An assignment procedure in which study and control groups are chosen to ensure that a particular variable is the same in both groups. Pairing is a special type of matching in which study group and control group subjects are analyzed together.

Maximum Likelihood Regression   A regression method that chooses estimates for the regression coefficients to maximize the likelihood that the data observed would have resulted from sampling a population with those coefficients.

McNemar's Test   A statistical significance test for paired data when there is one nominal dependent variable and one nominal independent variable.

Mean   Sum of the measurements divided by the number of measurements being added together. The "center of gravity" of a distribution of observations. A special type of average in which all values are given the same weight.

Median   The mid-point of a distribution. The median is chosen so that half the data values occur above and half occur below the median.

Meta-analysis   A series of methods for systematically combining data from more than one investigation to draw a conclusion which could not be drawn solely on the basis of the single investigations. A specific type of systematic review in which there is a quantitative method used for combining the data from two or more studies.

Monte Carlo Simulation   A method used in cost-effectiveness analysis and other applications that repeatedly samples the same population to derive a large number of samples whose distribution can be used to calculate point estimates and confidence or credibility ranges.

Mortality Rate   A measure of the incidence of death. This rate is calculated as the number of deaths over a period of time divided by the product of the number of individuals times their period of follow-up.

Multicollinearity   Sharing of information among independent variables. In a regression method, the existence of multicollinearity poses an issue of which independent variables to include in a regression equation.

Multiple Correlation Analysis   Statistical methods used with one continuous dependent variable plus nominal and continuous independent variables when all variables are obtained by naturalistic sampling.

Multiple Regression Analysis   Statistical methods used with one continuous dependent variable and more than one continuous independent variable.

Multivariable Analysis   A statistical analysis in which there is one dependent variable and more than one independent variable.

Multivariate Analysis   A statistical analysis in which there is more than one dependent variable. Commonly but incorrectly used as a synonym for multivariable analysis.

Mutually Exclusive   Categories are mutually exclusive if any one individual can be included in only one category.

Natural Experiment   A special type of cohort study in which the study and control groups' outcomes are compared with their own outcomes before and after a change is observed in the exposure of the study group.

Naturalistic Sample   A set of observations obtained from a population in such a way that the sample distribution of independent variable values as well as dependent variable values is representative of their distribution in the population. (*Synonym:* representative sample)

Necessary Cause   A characteristic is a necessary cause if its presence is required to cause the disease.

Nested case-control study   A case-control study conducted using data originally obtained as part of a cohort study or randomized clinical trial.

Nominal Data   A type of data with named categories. Nominal data may have more than two categories that cannot be ordered (e.g., race, eye color). Nominal data may have only two categories, i.e., dichotomous data, that can be ordered one above another (e.g., dead/alive). Nominal data are represented by more than one nominal variable if there are more than two potential categories.

Nonparametric Statistics   Statistical procedures that do not make assumptions about the distribution of parameters in the population being sampled. Nonparametric statistical methods are not free of assumptions such as the assumption of random sampling. They are most often used for ordinal data but may be used for continuous data converted to an ordinal scale. (*Synonym:* distribution-free)

Normal Approximation   A statistical method that can be used to calculate approximate probabilities for binomial and Poisson distributions using the standard normal distribution.

Normal Distribution   *See:* Gaussian distribution

Null Hypothesis   The assertion that no association or difference between the independent variable of interest and the dependent variables exists in the larger population from which the study samples are obtained.

Number Needed to Treat   The number of patients, similar to the study patients, who need to be treated to obtain one fewer bad outcome or one more good outcome compared to the control group treatment.

Observational Study   An investigation in which the assignment is conducted by observing the subjects who meet the inclusion and exclusion criteria. Case-control and cohort studies are observational studies.

Observed Assignment   Refers to the method of assignment of individuals to study and control groups in observational studies when the investigator does not intervene to perform the assignment.

Odds   A ratio in which the numerator contains the number of times an event occurs and the denominator contains the number of times the event does not occur.

Odds Form of Bayes' Theorem   The formula for Bayes' theorem that indicates that the posttest odds of disease is equal to the pretest odds times the likelihood ratio.

Odds Ratio   A ratio measuring the strength of an association applicable to all types of studies employing nominal data but is required for case-control and cross-sectional studies. The odds ratio for case-control and cross-sectional studies is measured as the odds of having the risk factor if the condition is present divided by the odds of having the risk factor if the condition is not present.

Omnibus Null Hypothesis   A null hypothesis that addresses the relationship between the dependent variable and the entire collection of independent variables as a unit.

One-Tailed Test   A statistical significance test in which deviations from the null hypothesis in only one direction are considered. Use of a one-tailed test implies that the investigator does not consider a true deviation in the opposite direction to be possible.

Open label   Refers to an investigation usually of a therapeutic or preventive agent, in which there is no attempt to blind either the participants or the investigators.

Option   One alternative intervention being compared in a decision-making investigation. May also be used in practice guidelines to indicate that the evidence does not support a clear recommendation or that inadequate data are available to make a recommendation.

Ordinal Data   A type of data with a limited number of categories and with an inherent ordering of the categories from lowest to highest. Ordinal data, however, say nothing about the spacing between categories (e.g., Stage 1, 2, 3, and 4 cancer).

Outcome   The phenomenon being measured in the assessment process of an investigation. In case-control studies, outcome is a prior characteristic; in concurrent cohort studies and randomized clinical trials, the outcome is a future event which occurs subsequent to the assignment. (*Synonym:* endpoint)

Outcome Studies   A generic term which refers to investigations of the results of therapeutic interventions regardless of the type of investigation used.

Outcomes Profile   The type of decision analysis that measures the benefits and harms but does not directly compare them. (*Synonym:* balance sheet)

Outliers   An investigation included in a meta-analysis or a subject in an investigation whose results are substantially different from the vast majority of studies or subjects, suggesting a need to examine the situation to determine why such an extreme result has occurred.

Overmatching   The error which occurs when investigators attempt to study a factor closely related to a characteristic by which the groups have been matched or paired.

***P* Value**   The probability of obtaining data at least as extreme as the data obtained in the investigation's sample if the null hypothesis is true. The *P* value is considered the "bottom line" in statistical significance testing.

Paired Design   A study design in which the data are analyzed using the difference between the measurements on the two members of a pair.

Pairing   A special form of matching in which each study individual is paired with a control group individual and their outcomes are compared. When pairing is used, special statistical methods called matching methods should be used. These methods may increase the statistical power of the study.

Parameter   A value that summarizes the distribution of a large population. One purpose of statistical analysis is to estimate a population's parameter(s) from the sample's observations.

Partial Test   A statistical significance test of a null hypothesis that addresses the relationship between the dependent variable and one of the independent variables. (*Synonym:* pairwise test)

Path Probability   The probability of a final outcome in a decision-making investigation. Path probabilities are calculated by multiplying the probabilities of each of the outcomes that follow chance nodes and that lead to a final outcome.

Pearson's Correlation Coefficient   The correlation coefficient that may be used when the dependent variable and the independent variable are both continuous and both have been obtained by naturalistic sampling.

Per Treatment   Analysis of data based on the actual treatment received. (*Synonym:* as treated)

Period Prevalence   The number of cases of a condition or disease during a period of time. Period prevalence incorporates incidence and well as point prevalence.

Person-Years   A person-year is equivalent to one person observed for a period of 1 year. Person-years are used as a measure of total observation time in the denominator of a rate.

Perspective   In decision-making investigations, the perspective of an investigation asks what factors should be consider when measuring the impact of the benefits, harms, and costs from a particular point of view. (*See:* social perspective, user perspective)

Plateau Effect   A flat portion of a life-table curve at the right end of the curve that may reflect the fact that very few individuals remain in the investigation rather than indicating cure.

Point Estimate   A single value calculated from sample observations that is used as the estimate of the population value, or parameter.

Poisson Distribution   A special case of a binomial distribution that can be used when the nominal event, such as disease or death, is rarely observed and the number of observations is great.

Population   A large group often, but not necessarily, comprising individuals. In statistics, one attempts to draw conclusions about a population by obtaining a representative sample made up of individuals from the larger population.

Population-Attributable Risk Percentage   The percentage of the risk in a community, including individuals with and without a risk factor, that is associated with exposure to a risk factor. Population attributable risk does not necessarily imply a cause-and-effect relationship. (*Synonym:* attributable fraction [population], attributable proportion [population], etiological fraction [population])

Population Based   An investigation is population based if the prevalence of the risk factor in the investigation reflects the prevalence of the risk factor in the larger population. A population-based case-control study is one in which the ratio of cases to controls is representative of the ratio in the larger population.

Positive-if-All-Positive   As used here, a screening strategy in which a second test is administered to all those who have a positive result on the initial test. The results may be labeled positive only if both tests are positive. Also called serial or consecutive testing; however, these terms may cause confusion.

Positive-if-One-Positive   As used here, a screening strategy in which two or more tests are initially administered to all individuals and the screening is labeled as positive if one or more tests produce positive results. Also called parallel or alternative testing; however, these terms can cause confusion.

Power   The ability of an investigation to demonstrate statistical significance when a true association or difference of a specified strength exists in the population being sampled. Power equals 1 minus the Type II error. (*Synonym:* statistical power, resolving power)

Practice Guideline   A set of recommendations defining conditions for using or not using available interventions in clinical or public health practice. Practice guidelines may be evidence-based and referred to as evidence-based guidelines or evidence-based recommendations.

Precise   Without random error, without variability from measurement to measurement of the same phenomenon. (*Synonym:* reproducibility, reliability)

Prediction   A special form of extrapolation in which the investigator extrapolates to a future point in time. May also refer to effort to develop a prognosis or to predict the outcome for one particular individual. Prediction should not be used as a synonym for estimation.

Predictive Value of a Negative Test   The proportion of individuals with a negative test who do not have the condition or disease as measured by the reference standard. This measure incorporates the prevalence of the condition or disease. Clinically, the predictive value of a negative test is the probability that an individual does not have the disease if the test is negative. (*Synonym:* posttest probability after a negative test)

Predictive Value of a Positive Test   The proportion of people with a positive test who actually have the condition or disease as measured by the reference standard. This measure incorporates the prevalence of the condition or disease. Clinically, the predictive value of a positive test is the probability that an individual has the disease if the test is positive. (*Synonym:* posttest probability after a positive test)

Pretest Probability   The probability of disease before the results of a test are known. Pretest probability may be derived from disease prevalence and the presence or absence of risk factors when screening for disease or may also include the clinical symptoms with which a patient presents. The pretest probability may also be the posttest results or predictive value based on the results from a previous test.

Prevalence   The proportion of persons with a particular disease or condition at a point in time. Prevalence can also be interpreted as the probability that an individual selected at random from the population of interest will be someone who has the disease or condition. (*Synonym:* point prevalence; also see period prevalence)

Primary Endpoint   The outcome measurement in a study which is used to calculate the sample's size. It should be a frequently occurring and biologically important endpoint. (*See:* secondary endpoint)

Probability   A proportion in which the numerator contains the number of times an event occurs and the denominator includes the number of times an event occurs plus the number of times it does not occur.

Proportion   A fraction in which the numerator contains a subset of the individuals contained in the denominator.

Proportional Hazards Regression   A statistical procedure for a nominal dependent variable and a mixture of nominal and continuous independent variables that can be used when the dependent variable is affected by time (*Synonym:* Cox regression)

Proportionate Mortality Ratio   A fraction in which the numerator contains the number of individuals who die of a particular disease over a period of time and the denominator contains the number of individuals dying from all diseases over the same period of time.

Prospective Study   *See:* concurrent cohort study

Protocol Deviant   An individual in a randomized clinical trial whose treatment differs from that which the person would have received if the treatment had followed the rules contained in the investigation's protocol.

Proximal Cause   A legal term that implies an examination of the time sequence of cause-and-effect to determine the element in the constellation of causal factors that was most closely related in time to the outcome.

Pruning the Decision Tree   The process of reducing the complexity of a decision tree by combining outcomes and removing potential outcomes which are considered extremely rare or inconsequential.

Publication Bias   The tendency to not publish small studies that do not demonstrate a statistically significant difference between groups.

Purposive Sample   A set of observations obtained from a population in such a way that the sample's distribution of independent variable values is determined by the researcher and not necessarily representative of their distribution in the population.

QALY Decision Analysis   The form of decision analysis that uses QALYs as the outcome measure.

Quality Adjusted Life Years (QALYs)   A measure which incorporates probabilities, utilities, and life expectancies.

Quality-Adjusted Number Needed to Treat   As used here, a summary measurement that can be derived from an expected utility decision analysis that takes into account the utilities as well as the probabilities of the outcome. Measures the number of individuals, on average, who need to receive the better alternative in order to obtain one additional QALY.

Random Effects Model   A type of statistical significance test that does not assume that subgroups all come from the same large population. In meta-analysis, implies that there is heterogeneity across the investigations.

Random Error   Error which is due to the workings of chance, which can either operate in the direction of the study hypothesis or in the opposite direction.

Random Sampling   A method of obtaining a sample that ensures that each individual in the larger population has a known, but not necessarily equal, probability of being selected for the sample.

Randomization   A method of assignment in which individuals have a known, but not necessarily equal, probability of being assigned to a particular study group or control group. As distinguished from random sampling, the individuals being randomized may or may not be representative of a large target population. (*Synonym:* random assignment)

Randomized Clinical Trial   An investigation in which the investigator assigns individuals to study and control groups using a process known as randomization. (*Synonym:* controlled clinical trial, experimental study)

Range   The difference between the highest and lowest data values in a population or sample.

Range of Normal   *See:* reference interval

Rate   Commonly used to indicate any measure of disease or outcome occurrence. From a statistical point of view, rates or true rates, are those measures of disease occurrence that include time in the denominator (e.g., incidence rate).

Rate Ratio   A ratio of rates. The rate ratio may be used as an estimate of the relative risk even when there is no data relating the population outcomes to individual characteristics.

Ratio   A fraction in which the numerator is not necessarily a subset of the denominator, as opposed to a proportion.

Real Differences or Changes   Differences or changes in the measurement of occurrence which reflect differences or changes in the phenomenon under study as opposed to artifactual changes.

Real Rate of Return   The rate of return that is used when discounting. It is designed to take into account the fact that money invested rather than spent is expected to increase in value, on average, at a rate that approximates the rate of return for invested capital in the overall economy—that is, a rate above and beyond inflation.

Recall Bias   An assessment bias that occurs when individuals in one study or control group are more likely to remember past events than individuals in the other group. Recall bias is especially likely when a case-control study involves serious disease and the characteristics under study are commonly occurring, subjectively remembered events.

Receiver-Operator Characteristics (ROC) Curve   A method used to quantitate the discriminant ability of a test based on the area under the curve. ROC curves can also assist in identifying a separating or cutoff line for a positive and a negative test.

Reference Case   In decision-making investigations, a reference case is the accepted method for presenting the data using the social perspective, best guess, or baseline estimates for variables, a 3% discount rate, and a series of other generally accepted assumptions.

Reference Interval   The interval of test results obtained from a reference sample group which reflects the variation among those who are free of the disease. (*Synonym:* range of normal)

Reference Sample Group   The sample used to represent the population of individuals who are believed to be free of the disease. The characteristics of the sample chosen may affect the reference interval derived from the reference sample group. (*Synonym:* disease-free source group)

Reference Standard   The criterion used to unequivocally define the presence and absence of the condition or disease under study. (*Synonym:* gold standard)

Regression Coefficient   In a regression analysis, an estimate of the amount that the dependent variable changes in value for each change in the corresponding independent variable.

Regression Techniques   A series of statistical methods useful for describing the association between one dependent variable and one or more independent variables. Regression techniques are often used to perform adjustment for confounding variables.

Regression to the Mean   A statistical principle based on the fact that unusual events are unlikely to recur. By chance alone, measurements subsequent to an unusual measurement are likely to be closer to the mean.

Relative Risk   A ratio of the probability of developing the outcome in a specified period of time if the risk factor is present divided by the probability of developing the outcome in that same period of time if the risk factor is not present. The relative risk is a measure of the strength of association applicable to cohort and randomized clinical trials. In case-control studies, the odds ratio often can be used to approximate the relative risk.

Reportable Diseases   Diseases or conditions that are expected to be reported by clinicians and laboratories to a governmental organization, often the local health department.

Reporting Bias   An assessment bias that occurs when individuals in one study or control group are more likely to report past events than individuals in the other group. Reporting bias is especially likely to occur when one group is under disproportionate pressure to report confidential information.

Reproducibility   *See:* precision

Residuals   The difference between the observed numerical values of the dependent variable and those estimated by the regression equation. Residuals indicate how well the regression equation estimates the dependent variable.

Results   The comparison of the outcome of the study and control groups. Includes issues of estimation, inference, and adjustment.

Retrospective Cohort Study   A cohort study in which an individual's group assignment is determined before the investigator is aware of the outcome even though the outcome has already occurred. A retrospective cohort study uses a previously collected database. (*Synonym:* nonconcurrent cohort study, database research)

Retrospective Study   *See:* case-control study

Reverse Causality   The situation in which the apparent "effect" is actually the "cause."

Risk   The probability of an event occurring during a specified period of time. For the risk of disease, the numerator of risk contains the number of individuals who develop the disease during the time period; the denominator contains the number of disease-free persons at the beginning of the time period. (*Synonym:* absolute risk, cumulative probability)

Risk Factor   A characteristic or factor that has been shown to be associated with an increased probability of developing a condition or disease. A risk factor does not necessarily imply a cause-and-effect relationship. In this book, a risk factor implies that at least an association has been established on an individual level. A risk factor that implies only an association may be called a risk marker, while a risk factor that precedes the outcome may also be called a determinant.

Risk-Neutral   Decision-making investigations are risk-neutral if the choice of alternatives is governed by expected utility and is not influenced by the tendency to either choose a risk-seeking or a risk-avoiding alternative.

Robust   A statistical procedure is robust if its assumptions can be violated without substantial effects on its conclusions.

Rule of Three   The number of individuals who must be observed to be 95% confident of observing at least one case of an adverse effect is three times the denominator of the true probability of occurrence of the adverse effect.

Run-In Period   Prerandomization observation of patients usually designed to ensure that they are appropriate candidates for entrance into a randomized clinical trial, especially with regard to their adherence to therapy.

Sample   A subset of a larger population obtained for investigation to draw conclusions or make estimates about the larger population.

Sampling Error   An error introduced by chance differences between the estimate obtained in a sample and the true value in the larger population from which the sample was drawn. Sampling error is inherent in the use of sampling methods and its magnitude is measured by the standard error.

Satisficing   A decision-making approach in which the goal is not to maximize expected utility but to maximize the chances of achieving a satisfactory solution.

Screening Test   Test conducted on an individual who is asymptomatic for a particular disease as part of a testing strategy to diagnose that particular disease.

Secondary Endpoint   An endpoint which is of interest and importance, such as death, but which occurs too infrequently to use to calculate the sample's size.

Secular Trend   Long-term real changes in rates (*Synonym:* temporal trend)

Selection Bias   A bias in assignment that occurs when the study and control groups are chosen so that they differ from each other by one or more factors that affect the outcome of the study. A special type of confounding variable that results from study design rather than chance. (*See:* confounding variable)

Self-Selection Bias   A bias related to the assignment process in screening that may occur when volunteers are used in an investigation. The bias results from differences between volunteers and the larger population of interest, i.e., the target population.

Sensitivity   The proportion of those with the disease or condition, as measured by the reference standard, who are positive by the test being studied. (*Synonym:* positive-in-disease)

Sensitivity Analysis   A method used in decision-making investigations that alters one or more factors from their best guess or baseline estimates and examines the impact on the results. One-way, multiple-way, best-case/worst-case sensitivity analyses, and threshold analyses are special types of sensitivity analyses.

Sentinel Sites   A sentinel site is a location such as an emergency department in which the first cases of a condition are likely to be identified.

Sequential Analyses   Methods of analysis that seek to determine whether an investigation should continue. Sequential analysis methods may permit an investigation to be terminated at an earlier time.

Simple Random Sample   A random sample in which the sample is drawn to represent the overall larger population without stratification to ensure greater representation of particular groups within the population.

Slope   The regression coefficient in linear regression analysis. The slope of a linear equation in linear regression estimates the amount that the mean of the dependent variable changes for each unit change in the numerical value of the independent variable.

Social Perspective   The perspective that takes into account all health-related impacts of the benefits, harms, and costs regardless of who experiences these outcomes or who pays these costs. The social perspective is considered the appropriate perspective for decision-making investigations.

Spearman's Correlation Coefficient   A correlation coefficient that can be obtained in a bivariable analysis when the dependent variable and the independent variable are both ordinal and are obtained through naturalistic sampling.

Specificity   The proportion of those without the disease or condition, as measured by the reference standard, who are negative by the test being studied. (*Synonym:* negative-in-health)

Spectrum Bias   A bias in testing in which the participants do not reflect the spectrum of disease in the target population, such as not including those with other diseases of the same organ system that may produce false negative or false positive results.

Standard Deviation   A commonly used measure of the spread or dispersion of data. The standard deviation squared is known as the variance.

Standard Distribution   Distribution for which statistical tables have been developed. Use of standard distributions, when chosen appropriately, simplify the calculation of *P* values and confidence intervals.

Standard Error   The spread or dispersion of point estimates, such as the mean obtained from all possible samples of a specified size. The standard error is equal to the standard deviation divided by the square root of the sample size. (*See:* sampling error)

Standardization (of a rate)   An effort to take into account or adjust for the effects of a factor such as age or sex on the obtained rates. (*See:* adjustment)

Standardized Mortality Ratio   A ratio in which the numerator contains the observed number of deaths and the denominator contains the number of deaths that would be expected based on a comparison population. A standardized mortality ratio implies that indirect standardization has been used to control for confounding variables. Note that the terms "standardized mortality ratio" and "proportionate mortality ratio" are not synonymous.

Stationary Population   A population often defined as 100,000 birth that experiences no entry or exit from the population except for birth or death. Often used as the population for cross-sectional life table and life expectancy calculations.

Statistic   A value calculated from sample data that is used to estimate a value or parameter in the larger population from which the sample was obtained.

Statistical Significance Test   A statistical technique for determining the probability that the data observed in a sample, or more extreme data, could occur by chance if there is no true difference or association in the larger population (i.e., if the null hypothesis is true). (*Synonym:* inference, hypothesis testing)

Stratification   In general, stratification means to divide into groups. Stratification often refers to a process to control for differences in confounding variables by making separate estimates for groups of individuals who have the same values for the confounding variable.

Stratified Analysis   Statistical procedures that can be used when there is a nominal dependent variable and more than one nominal independent variable. Stratified analysis produces stratum-specific point estimates.

Stratified Random Sampling   A purposive sampling method that is designed to over-sample rare categories of an independent variable.

Stratum   When data are stratified or divided into groups using a characteristic such as age, each group is known as a stratum.

Student-Newman-Keuls Test   A partial statistical significance test for a continuous dependent variable and more than one independent variable.

Student's *t* Distribution   A standard distribution that is used to obtain *P* values and confidence intervals for a continuous dependent variable. The Student's *t* distribution is used to obtain the Student's *t* test of statistical significance.

Study Group   In a cohort study or randomized clinical trial, a group of individuals who possess the characteristics or who are exposed to the factors under study. In case-control or cross-sectional study, a group of individuals who have developed the disease or condition being investigated.

Study Hypothesis   An assertion that an association or difference exists between two or more variables in the population sampled. A study hypothesis can be one-tailed (considering associations or differences in one direction only) or two-tailed (not specifying the direction of the association or difference).

Study Population   The population of individuals from which samples are obtained for inclusion in an investigation. (*Synonym:* study's population)

Subgroup Analysis   Examination of the relationship between variables in subgroups, such as gender or age groups, obtained from the original study and control groups.

Subjective Probabilities   Probabilities that are obtained based on perceived probabilities.

Sufficient Cause   A characteristic is a sufficient cause if its presence in and of itself will cause the disease.

Supportive Criteria   When contributory cause cannot be established, additional criteria can be used to develop a judgment regarding the existence of a contributory cause. These include strength of association, dose-response relationship, consistency of the relationship, and biological plausibility. (*Synonym:* adjunct, ancillary criteria)

Surrogate Endpoint   The use of measurements such as test results instead of clinically important outcome measures to assess the outcomes of an investigation. In order to be an appropriate measure of outcome, surrogate endpoints requires a strong association between the surrogate endpoint and a relevant clinical outcome.

Survival Plot   A graphic display of the results of a cohort or longitudinal life table.

Systematic Review   An evaluation of research that addresses a focused question using methods designed to reduce the possibility of bias. Systematic reviews may use qualitative as well as quantitative methods.

Target Population   The group of individuals to whom one wishes to apply the results of an investigation. The target population may be, and often is, different from the study population from which the sample used in an investigation is obtained.

Test-Based Confidence Interval   Confidence interval derived using the same data and same basic process as that used to perform a statistical significance test on a particular set of data.

Testwise Error   The probability of making a Type I error for any one particular comparison.

Threshold Analysis   A special type of sensitivity analysis in which the threshold levels are determined—that is, the levels for particular factors that alter the conclusion of a decision-making investigation.

Time Frame   The point in the course of the disease when the alternatives are being applied. When considering disease that is already fully developed, prevention may not be an available alternative because it is not within the time frame of the investigation.

Time Horizon   The follow-up period of time used to determine which potential outcomes that occur in the future will be included in a model for a decision-making investigation. (*Synonym:* analysis horizon)

Transformation   Methods used to mathematically express the data, usually from a continuous dependent variable, in a different way that fulfills the assumptions of a statistical method, especially the assumptions of Gaussian distribution and homoscedasticity.

True Negative   An individual who does not have the disease or condition, as measured by the reference standard, and has a negative test result.

True Positive   An individual who has the disease or condition, as measured by the reference standard, and has a positive test result.

Two-Tailed Test   A statistical significance test in which deviations from the null hypothesis in either direction are considered. Use of a two-tailed test implies that the investigator was willing to consider deviations in either direction before data were collected.

Type I Error   An error that occurs when data demonstrate a statistically significant result when no true association or difference exists in the population. The alpha level is the size of the Type I error which will be tolerated (usually 5%).

Type II Error   An error that occurs when the sample's observations fail to demonstrate statistical significance when a true association or difference actually exists in the population. The beta level is the size of the Type II error that will be tolerated. (*See:* power)

Unbiased   Lack of systematic error. *See:* bias

Univariable Analysis   Statistical analysis in which there is one dependent variable and no independent variable.

User Perspective   Perspective that takes into account the impacts of benefits, harms, and cost as they affect a particular user of the decision-making investigation. User perspectives include payer, provider, and patient perspectives.

Utility   A measure of the value of a particular health state measured on a scale of 0 to 1. Utilities are measured on the same scale as probabilities in order to multiply utilities and probabilities in decision-making investigations. A variety of methods exist for measuring utilities, including the rating scale, time trade-off, and reference gamble methods.

Valid   A measurement is valid if it is appropriate for the question being addressed and is accurate, precise, and complete. Validity implies that the measurement measures what it intends to measure. Discipline-specific definitions of validity exist that often define the methods used to establish validity. At times, validity may be used as a synonym for accuracy.

Variable   Generally refers to a characteristic for which measurements are made in a study. In strict statistical terminology, a variable is the representation of those measurements in an analysis. Continuous or ordinal scale data are expressed using one variable, as are nominal data with only two categories. However, nominal data with more than two categories must be expressed using more than one variable.

Variance   Variance is the mean square deviation of data from the mean. (*See:* standard deviation)

Verification Bias   A bias in testing that may occur when participants are chosen because they have previously undergone the index test and agree to subsequently undergo the reference standard test.

Weighting   A method used in adjustment to take into account the relative importance of a specific stratum. Each stratum is given a weight prior to combining its data.

Wilcoxon Signed-Rank Test   A statistical significance test that can be used for univariable analysis of an ordinal dependent variable.

Willingness to Pay   An approach to converting effectiveness to monetary terms that uses past choices made in specific situations to estimate how much society is willing to pay to obtain a specific outcome.

Subject Index